About Your
Medicines®

By authority of the
United States Pharmacopeial Convention, Inc.

Contents

When purchasing a medicine, whether over-the-counter (nonprescription) or with a doctor's prescription, you may have questions about its usefulness to you, the best way to take it, possible side effects, and advisable precautions. For instance, some medicines should be taken with meals, others between meals. Some may make you drowsy while others may tend to keep you awake. Alcoholic or other beverages, other medicines, certain foods, or smoking may affect the way your medicine works. As for side effects, some are merely bothersome and may go away while others may require medical attention.

About Your Medicines contains information which may provide general answers to some of your questions as well as suggestions for the correct use of your medicine. *It is important to remember, however, that the human body is very complex and medicines may act differently on different people—and even in the same person at different times. If you feel that you need additional information about your medicine or its possible side effects, ask your doctor, nurse, or pharmacist. They are there to help you.*

Organization of Information

About Your Medicines contains a section of general information about the correct use of any medicine (see Appendix I), as well as individual discussions of a wide variety of commonly and not so commonly used medicines. *You should read both the general information and the information specific to the medicine you are taking.*

Each medicine appears under its generic rather than brand name. If you already know the generic name of your medicine, you can find it listed in alphabetic order beginning on page 1. If not, look in the index. Common brand names are given in the index also. It is a good idea for you to learn both the generic and the brand names of the medicines you are using and even to write them down and keep them for future use.

Because of space constraints, monographs for only the more commonly used medicines have been included in this volume. In the case of some combination products, the reader is referred to the monographs of the individual ingredients which make up the combination. In these cases, however, please keep in mind that, because of the unique properties of certain combinations, some of the information provided in the individual listings may not be relevant to the combination product, or the combination product itself may have additional or different properties from those listed for the individual ingredients.

Information for each medicine is divided according to the area of the body which is affected. The common divisions used are:

- *SYSTEMIC*—For general effects throughout the body; applies to most medicines when taken by mouth or given by injection.
- *TOPICAL*—For local effects when applied directly to the skin.
- *NASAL*—For local effects when used in the nose.
- *INHALATION*—For local, and in some cases systemic, effects when inhaled into the lungs.
- *OPHTHALMIC*—For local effects when applied directly to the eyes.

As a general rule, information for one type of use will not be the same as for other types of use. Thus, if you take tetracycline capsules by mouth for their systemic effect in treating an infection, the information will not be the same as for tetracycline ointment which is applied directly to the skin for its topical effects.

Notice

The information about the drugs contained herein is general in nature and is not intended to replace specific instructions, directions, or warnings given to you by your physician or other prescriber or accompanying a particular product. The information is selective and it is not claimed that it includes all known precautions, contraindications, effects, or interactions possibly related to the use of a drug. The information may differ from that contained in the product labeling required by law. The information is not sufficient to make an evaluation as to the risks and benefits of taking a particular drug in a particular case or to provide medical advice for individual problems and should not alone be relied upon for these purposes. Since the inclusion or exclusion of particular information about a drug is judgmental in nature and since opinion as to drug usage may differ, you may wish to consult additional sources. Should you desire additional information or if you have any questions as to how this information may relate to you in particular, ask your doctor, nurse, pharmacist, or other health care provider.

There are many brands of drugs on the market. The listing of selected brand names is intended only for ease of reference. The inclusion of a brand name does not mean the USPC has any particular knowledge that the brand listed has properties different from other brands of the same drug, nor should it be interpreted as an endorsement by the USPC. Similarly, the fact that a particular brand name has not been included does not indicate that brand has been judged to be unsatisfactory or unacceptable.

If any of the information in this book causes you special concern, do not decide against taking any medicine prescribed for you without first checking with your doctor.

About USP

The information in this volume is prepared by the United States Pharmacopeial Convention, Inc. (USPC), the organization which sets the official standards of strength, quality, purity, packaging, and labeling for medical products used in the United States.

The United States Pharmacopeial Convention is an independent, nonprofit corporation composed of representatives from accredited colleges of medicine and pharmacy in the U.S.; state medical and pharmaceutical associations; many national associations concerned with medicines, such as the American Medical Association, the American Nurses Association, the American Dental Association, and the American Pharmaceutical Association; and various departments of the federal government, including the Food and Drug Administration. It was established more than 160 years ago, and is the only national body that represents the professions of both pharmacy and medicine. See Appendix II for a listing of current members.

The first convention came into being on January 1, 1820, and within the year published the first national drug formulary of the United States. The U.S. Pharmacopeia of 1820 contained 217 drug names, divided into two groups according to the level of general acceptance and usage.

When Congress passed the first major drug safety law in 1906, the standards recognized by that statute were those set forth in the United States Pharmacopeia and in the National Formulary. Today, the USP and NF continue to be the official U.S. compendia for standards for drugs and for the inactive ingredients in drug dosage forms. The United States Pharmacopeia is now the world's oldest regularly revised pharmacopeia and is generally accepted as being the most influential.

The work of the USPC is carried out by the Committee of Revision. This committee of experts is elected by the Convention and currently consists of 95 outstanding physicians, pharmacists, dentists, nurses, chemists, and other individuals particularly qualified to judge the merits of drugs and the standards and information that should apply to them. Committee members serve without pay and are assisted by numerous advisory panels, other outside reviewers, and USPC staff.

About USP DI

About Your Medicines contains information extracted from *Advice for the Patient* (Volume II of *USP DI*). Volume I contains drug use information in technical language for the doctor, pharmacist, nurse, or other health care provider, and Volume II is its lay-language counterpart for use by consumers. Together they form the foundation of a coordinated approach to drug-use education.

USP DI was first published in 1980. It is a continuously reviewed and revised base of drug information for use by prescribers, dispensers, and consumers of medications. The information is developed by the consensus of the USP Committee of Revision and its Advisory Panels and anyone, including users of medicines, may contribute through review of and comment on drafts of the monographs published in *USP DI Review.*

To receive further information about *USP DI* or to comment on how the information published in this volume might better meet your information needs, please contact:

USP Drug Information Division
12601 Twinbrook Parkway
Rockville, MD 20852
(301) 881-0666

United States Pharmacopeial Convention 1985-1990

MURRAY S. COOPER, PH.D.
Islamarada, FL

LLOYD E. DAVIS, D.V.M., PH.D.
Urbana, IL

CLYDE R. ERSKINE, B.S., M.B.A.
Philadelphia, PA

JAMES D. FINKELSTEIN, M.D.
Washington, DC

HARRY W. FISCHER, M.D.
Rochester, NY

EDWARD A. FITZGERALD, PH.D.
Bethesda, MD

DOUGLAS R. FLANAGAN, PH.D.
Iowa City, IA

JOHN P. FLETCHER, M.S.
South Charleston, WV

KLAUS G. FLOREY, PH.D.
New Brunswick, NJ

WILLIAM O. FOYE, PH.D.
Boston, MA

EDWARD D. FROHLICH, M.D.
New Orleans, LA

SALVATORE A. FUSARI, PH.D.
St. Clair Shores, MI

JOSEPH F. GALLELLI, PH.D.
Bethesda, MD

BURTON J. GOLDSTEIN, M.D.
Miami, FL

ALAN GRAY, PH.D.
West Point, PA

MARVIN F. GROSTIC, PH.D.
Kalamazoo, MI

MICHAEL J. GROVES, PH.D.
Chicago, IL

J. KEITH GUILLORY, PH.D.
Iowa City, IA

JOHN J. HALKI, M.D., PH.D.
Dayton, OH

SAMIR A. HANNA, PH.D.
Syracuse, NY

STANLEY L. HEM, PH.D.
West Lafayette, IN

DAVID W. HUGHES, PH.D.
Ottawa, Ontario, Canada

RAYMOND N. JOHNSON, PH.D.
Rouses Point, NY

RODNEY D. ICE, PH.D.
Edmond, OK

HERBERT E. KAUFMAN, M.D.
New Orleans, LA

DONALD KAYE, M.D.
Philadelphia, PA

WILLIAM J. KELLER, PH.D.
Monroe, LA

B.J. KENNEDY, M.D.
Minneapolis, MN

JAY S. KEYSTONE, M.D.
Toronto, Ontario, Canada

BOEN T. KHO, PH.D.
Plattsburgh, NY

LEWIS J. LEESON, PH.D.
Summit, NJ

ROBERT D. LINDEMAN, M.D.
Washington, DC

CHARLES H. LOCHMULLER, PH.D.
Durham, NC

DEAN H. LOCKWOOD, M.D.
Rochester, NY

JENNIFER M. H. LOGGIE, M.D.
Cincinnati, OH

EDWARD G. LOVERING, PH.D.
Ottawa, Ontario, Canada

JOHN R. MARKUS, B.S.
Rockville, MD

ROBERT A. MATHEWS, PH.D.
Washington, DC

WARREN A. MCALLISTER, PH.D.
Greenville, NC

THOMAS MEDWICK, PH.D.
Piscataway, NJ

ROBERT F. MORRISSEY, PH.D.
Somerville, NJ

TERRY E. MUNSON
Rockville, MD

HAROLD R. NACE, PH.D.
Barrington, RI

WENDEL L. NELSON, PH.D.
Seattle, WA

STANLEY P. OWEN, PH.D.
Kalamazoo, MI

JAMES W. PATE, M.D.
Memphis, TN

GARNET E. PECK, PH.D.
West Lafayette, IN

ROBERT V. PETERSEN, PH.D.
Salt Lake City, UT

JAMES R. RANKIN, B.S.
Taos, NM

CHRISTOPHER T. RHODES, PH.D.
Kingston, RI

JAY ROBERTS, PH.D.
Philadelphia, PA

JOSEPH R. ROBINSON, PH.D.
Madison, WI

THEODORE J. ROSEMAN, PH.D.
Morton Grove, IL

VIRGINIA C. ROSS
Silver Spring, MD

LEONARD RYBAK, M.D., PH.D.
Springfield, IL

ANDREW J. SCHMITZ, JR., M.S.
New York, NY

STEPHEN G. SCHULMAN, PH.D.
Gainesville, FL

RALPH F. SHANGRAW, PH.D.
Baltimore, MD

ALBERT L. SHEFFER, M.D.
Boston, MA

ELI SHEFTER, PH.D
Wilmington, DE

ERIC B. SHEININ, PH.D.
Washington, DC

JANE C. SHERIDAN, PH.D.
Nutley, NJ

EDWARD B. SILBERSTEIN, M.D.
Cincinnati, OH

JOSEPH E. SINSHEIMER, PH.D.
Ann Arbor, MI

Headquarters Staff

Drug Information Division Advisory Panels
1980-1985

Members of the Subcommittee who served as Chairmen or Co-chairmen are listed first.

The information presented in this text represents an ongoing review of the drugs contained herein and represents a consensus of various viewpoints expressed. The individuals listed below have been or are currently on the USP Advisory Panels and have contributed to the development of the 1986 USP DI data base. Such listing does not imply that these individuals have reviewed all of the material in this text or that they individually agree with all statements contained herein.

Panel on Allergy, Immunology, and Connective Tissue Disease— ALBERT L. SHEFFER, M.D., Boston, MA; RONALD ANDERSON, M.D., Boston, MA; EDWARD K. DUNHAM, M.D., Seal Harbor, ME; ELLIOT F. ELLIS, M.D., Buffalo, NY; STEPHEN R. KAPLAN, M.D., Providence, RI; DANIEL J. STECHSCHULTE, M.D., Kansas City, KS; MARTIN D. VALENTINE, M.D., Baltimore, MD.

Panel on Analgesics, Sedatives, and Anti-Inflammatory Agents— LOUIS HARRIS, PH.D., Richmond, VA; WILLIAM H. BARR, PHARM.D., PH.D., Richmond, VA; JOHN BAUM, M.D., Rochester, NY; THOMAS G. KANTOR, M.D., New York, NY; WILLIAM R. MARTIN, M.D., Lexington, KY; EDWARD B. NELSON, M.D., PH.D., Houston, TX; A. S. RIDOLFO, M.D., PH.D., Indianapolis, IN; ADA G. ROGERS, R.N., New York, NY; ERNEST W. SMALL, D.D.S., M.S., Blacksburg, VA; MURRAY WEINER, M.D., Cincinnati, OH; MICHAEL L. WEINTRAUB, M.D., Rochester, NY.

Panel on Anesthesiology—WALTER L. WAY, M.D., San Francisco, CA; ROY CRONNELLY, M.D., PH.D., San Francisco, CA; BRADLEY SMITH, M.D., Nashville, TN; PAUL WHITE, M.D., PH.D., Palo Alto, CA.

Panel on Cardiovascular Drugs—EDWARD D. FROHLICH, M.D., New Orleans, LA; JAMES E. DOHERTY, M.D., Little Rock, AR; THOMAS M. GLENN, PH.D., Summit, NJ; JOHN L. JUERGENS, M.D., Rochester, MN; BENEDICT R. LUCCHESI, M.D., PH.D., Ann Arbor, MI; PATRICK A. McKEE, M.D., Durham, NC; BERNARD L. MIRKIN, M.D., PH.D., Minneapolis, MN; EMANUEL M. PAPPER, M.D., Miami, FL; SHAHBUDIN H. RAHIMTOOLA, M.D., Los Angeles, CA; ARNOLD SCHWARTZ, PH.D., Cincinnati, OH.

Panel on Consumer Interest—JAMES R. RANKIN, Taos, NM; ESTELLE COHEN, Baltimore, MD; BOBBY F. DURAN, Taos, NM; JOAN HAMBURG, New York, NY; EDWARD JAMES, Pendleton, OR; ANNE KASPER, Bethesda, MD; RAYMOND F. LOPEZ, Albuquerque, NM; ESTHER PETERSON, Washington, DC; EDWARD SIMPSON, Squantum, MA; REV. AUGUSTUS R. TAYLOR, JR., PH.D., Los Angeles, CA.

Panel on Dentistry—SEBASTIAN G. CIANCIO, D.D.S., Buffalo, NY; PRISCILLA C. BOURGAULT, PH.D., Maywood, IL; ALFRED E. CIARLONE, D.D.S., PH.D., Augusta, GA; RICHARD E. CORPRON, D.D.S., Ann Arbor, MI; FREDERICK A. CURRO, D.M.D., PH.D., Hackensack, NJ; TOMMY W. GAGE, D.D.S., Dallas, TX; JOSEPH MARGARONE, D.D.S., Buffalo, NY; H. DEAN MILLARD, D.D.S., M.S., Ann Arbor, MI; RICHARD WYNN, PH.D., Baltimore, MD.

Panel on Dermatology—D. MARTIN CARTER, M.D., New York, NY; WILLIAM EAGLSTEIN, M.D., Pittsburgh, PA; WILLIAM EPSTEIN, M.D., San Francisco, CA; THOMAS FRANZ, M.D., Seattle, WA; HENRY JOLLY, M.D., New Orleans, LA; MILTON ORKIN, M.D., Minneapolis, MN; DAVID RAMSAY, M.D., New York, NY; EDGAR

BENTON SMITH, M.D., Galveston, TX; ROBERT STERN, M.D., Boston, MA; JOHN STRAUSS, M.D., Iowa City, IA; DENNIS WEST, M.S., Chicago, IL.

Panel on Diagnostic Agents (Non-Radioactive) and Radiological Contrast Media—HARRY W. FISCHER, M.D., Rochester, NY.

Panel on Electrolytes, Large-volume Parenterals and Renal Drugs—ROBERT D. LINDEMAN, M.D., Washington, DC; WILLIAM M. BENNETT, M.D., Portland, OR; WILLIAM O. BERNDT, PH.D., Omaha, NE; RALPH E. CUTLER, M.D., Loma Linda, CA; STANLEY J. DUDRICK, M.D., Houston, TX; LAURENCE FINBERG, M.D., Brooklyn, NY; JOHN F. MAHER, M.D., Bethesda, MD; VICTOR E. POLLAK, M.D., Cincinnati, OH; WILLIAM J. STONE, M.D., Nashville, TN; CARLOS A. VAAMONDE, M.D., Miami, FL; RONALD L. WILLIAMS, PH.D., Covington, LA.

Panel on Endocrinology—EDWIN D. BRANSOME, JR., M.D., Augusta, GA; LOUIS V. AVIOLI, M.D., St. Louis, MO; SALVADOR CASTELLS, M.D., Brooklyn, NY; KARL ENGELMAN, M.D., Philadelphia, PA; ARTHUR L. HERBST, M.D., Chicago, IL; P. REED LARSEN, M.D., Boston, MA; MARVIN E. LEVIN, M.D., St. Louis, MO; JAMES M. MOSS, M.D., Alexandria, VA; JOHN A. OWEN, JR., M.D., Charlottesville, VA; E. BRADBRIDGE THOMPSON, M.D., Galveston, TX.

Panel on Family Practice—JOHN S. DERRYBERRY, M.D., Shelbyville, TN; ROBERT H. BARR, M.D., Houston, TX; PAUL C. BRUCKER, M.D., Philadelphia, PA; PENNY W. BUDOFF, M.D., Woodbury, NY; W. RAY BURNS, PHARM.D., Spartanburg, SC; ROBERT E. DAVIS, PHARM.D., Lexington, SC; DENNIS K. HELLING, PHARM.D., Iowa City, IA; JULIAN F. KEITH, JR., M.D., Winston-Salem, NC; CHARLES M. PLOTZ, M.D., Brooklyn, NY; R. STEPHEN PORTER, PHARM.D., Philadelphia, PA; JACK M. ROSENBERG, PHARM.D., PH.D., Brooklyn, NY; ROBERT SMITH, M.D., Cincinnati, OH; KENNETH W. WITTE, PHARM.D., Chicago, IL.

Panel on Gastroenterology and Nutrition—MURRAY DAVIDSON, M.D., Jamaica, NY; PAUL BASS, PH.D., Madison, WI; LLOYD J. FILER, JR., M.D., Iowa City, IA; DONALD J. GLOTZER, M.D., Boston, MA; YOUNG S. KIM, M.D., San Francisco, CA; WALTER RUBIN, M.D., Philadelphia, PA; DAVID B. SACHAR, M.D., New York, NY; HAROLD H. SANDSTEAD, M.D., Boston, MA; JOHN T. SESSIONS, JR., M.D., Chapel Hill, NC; M. MICHAEL THALER, M.D., San Francisco, CA.

Panel on Geriatrics—JAY ROBERTS, PH.D., Philadelphia, PA; REUBIN ANDRES, M.D., Baltimore, MD; EVELYN BENSON, R.N., Havertown, PA; DAVID J. GREENBLATT, M.D., Boston, MA; DANIEL A. HUSSAR, PH.D., Philadelphia, PA; LINDA JARRETT, R.N., New Paltz, NY; PETER P. LAMY, PH.D., Baltimore, MD; RICHARD W. LINDSAY, M.D., Charlottesville, VA; MARCUS M. REIDENBERG, M.D., New York, NY; JOHN W. ROWE, xii

For the 1985–1990 Revision Cycle

At the March 22–24, 1985, meeting of the United States Pharmacopeial Convention, a new Committee of Revision was elected to serve for the 1985–1990 revision period. The following individuals have been elected and will establish advisory panels to serve from 1985 to 1990.

ACETAMINOPHEN (Systemic)

This information applies to the following medicines:

Acetaminophen (a-seat-a-MEE-noe-fen)
Acetaminophen and Caffeine
Buffered Acetaminophen

Some commonly used brand names or other names are:

For Acetaminophen†

A'Cenol	Mejoral without
A'Cenol D.S.	Aspirin
Aceta	Neopap
Ace-Tabs*	Oraphen-PD
Acephen	Pain Relief without
Actamin	Aspirin
Anacin-3	Panadol
Anuphen	Panex
APAP	Paracetamol
Apo-Acetaminophen*	Paraphen*
Atasol*	Pedric
Banesin	Peedee Dose
Bayapap	Aspirin
Campain*	Alternative
C2A*	Phenaphen
Conacetol	Robigesic*
Dapa	Rounox*
Datril	St. Joseph Aspirin-
Dolanex	Free
Dorcol	Sudoprin
Exdol*	Suppap
Genapap	Tapanol
Genebs	Tapar
Genetabs	Tempra
Halenol	Tenol
Liquiprin	Tylenol
Meda Cap	Ty-Tab
Meda Tab	Valadol
Mejoralito	Valorin

For Acetaminophen and Caffeine
Aspirin-Free Excedrin   Summit

For Buffered Acetaminophen
Bromo-Seltzer

*Not available in the United States.
†Generic name product may also be available.

Acetaminophen is a medicine used to relieve pain and reduce fever. Unlike aspirin, it does not relieve the redness, stiffness, or swelling caused by rheumatoid arthritis. However, it may relieve the pain caused by mild forms of arthritis. Acetaminophen can be taken by mouth or used rectally in the form of suppositories.

Buffered acetaminophen is used only to relieve pain, especially when an antacid is also needed to relieve an upset stomach.

This medicine is available without a prescription; however, your physician or dentist may have special instructions on the proper dose of acetaminophen for your medical condition.

Before Using This Medicine

Before you use acetaminophen, check with your doctor, nurse, or pharmacist:

—if you have ever had any unusual or allergic reaction to acetaminophen.

—if you are on a low-salt, low-sugar, or any other special diet, or if you are allergic to any substance, such as sulfites or other preservatives or dyes. Most medicines contain more than their active ingredient, and many liquid medicines contain alcohol. Your doctor or pharmacist can help you avoid products that may cause a problem.

—if you are pregnant or if you intend to become pregnant while taking this medicine. Although acetaminophen has not been shown to cause birth defects or other problems in humans, the chance always exists. Studies on birth defects have not been done in humans.

—if you are breast-feeding an infant. Although acetaminophen has not been shown to cause problems in humans, the chance always exists. Acetaminophen passes into the breast milk in small amounts.

—if you are now taking any of the following medicines or types of medicine:

    Anticoagulants (blood thinners)
    Anticonvulsants (seizure medicine)
    Antineoplastics (medicine for cancer)
    Aspirin, ibuprofen, or other medicine for pain and inflammation
    Barbiturates
    Chloroquine
    Contraceptives, oral (birth control pills)
    Dantrolene
    Estrogens
    Diflunisal
    Hydroxychloroquine
    Ketoconazole
    Methimazole
    Propylthiouracil
    Rifampin
    Sulfonamides (sulfa medicines)

—if you are taking buffered acetaminophen effervescent granules and are also taking any of the following medicines or types of medicine:

    Adrenocorticoids (cortisone-like medicines)
    Tetracycline

—if you are taking any of the products containing caffeine and are also taking any of the following medicines or types of medicine:

    Amantadine
    Aminophylline
    Amphetamines
    Appetite suppressants (diet pills)
    Chlophedianol
    Dyphylline
    Epinephrine
    Lithium
    Medicine for asthma or breathing problems (including oral inhalations)
    Medicine for hay fever or other allergies (including nose drops or sprays)
    Methylphenidate
    Oxtriphylline
    Pemoline
    Theophylline

—if you have any of the following medical problems:

    Kidney disease (severe)
    Liver disease
    Virus infection of the liver

Proper Use of This Medicine

Unless otherwise directed by your physician or dentist:

• **Do not take more of this medicine than is recommended on the package label. If too much is taken, liver damage may occur.**

• Children up to 12 years of age should not take this medicine more than 5 times a day or for more than 5 days in a row.

• Adults should not take this medicine for more than 10 days in a row.

If you have been directed to take this medicine for a longer period of time, especially in large doses, it is important that your doctor check your progress at regular visits.

This medicine will not relieve the redness, stiffness, or swelling that may occur with rheumatoid arthritis. If you plan to take this medicine for arthritic or rheumatic conditions, check with your doctor first.

For patients taking buffered acetaminophen effervescent granules:

• Pour the amount of granules directed on the package into a glass.

• Add ½ glass (4 ounces) of cool water.

• Drink all of the liquid in order to be sure you get the full dose of medicine.

• You may drink the liquid while it is still fizzing or after the fizzing stops.

For patients using the suppository dosage form of acetaminophen:

• How to insert suppository: First remove the foil wrapper and moisten the suppository with water. Lie down on one side and push the suppository well up into the rectum with a finger.

How to store this medicine:

• Store away from heat and direct light.

• **Keep out of the reach of children.**

• Do not store in the bathroom medicine cabinet because the heat or moisture may cause the medicine to break down.

• Keep the liquid and suppository forms of this medicine from freezing.

• Do not keep outdated medicine or medicine no longer needed. Flush the contents of the container down the toilet, unless otherwise directed.

Precautions While Using This Medicine

Check with your physician or dentist:

—if your symptoms do not improve or if they get worse.

—if you are taking this medicine to bring down a fever, and the fever lasts for more than 3 days or returns.

Check the labels of all over-the-counter (OTC), nonprescription, and prescription medicines you now take. If any contain acetaminophen be especially careful, since taking them while taking this medicine may lead to overdose. If you have any questions about this, check with your physician, dentist, or pharmacist.

There may be a greater risk of liver damage if you drink large amounts of alcoholic beverages regularly while taking this medicine, especially if you take more acetaminophen than is recommended on the package label or if you take it regularly for a long period of time.

Too much use of acetaminophen together with certain other medicines may increase the chance of kidney problems. Therefore, do not regularly take acetaminophen with any of the following, unless directed to do so by your physician or dentist:

> Aspirin, diflunisal, or other salicylates
> Fenoprofen
> Ibuprofen

> Indomethacin
> Meclofenamate
> Mefenamic acid
> Naproxen
> Oxyphenbutazone
> Phenylbutazone
> Piroxicam
> Sulindac
> Tolmetin

If you think that you or anyone else may have taken an overdose of acetaminophen, get emergency help at once, even if there are no signs of poisoning. Signs of severe poisoning may not appear for 2 to 4 days after the overdose is taken, but treatment to prevent liver damage or death must be started within 24 hours or less after the overdose is taken.

For patients taking buffered acetaminophen effervescent granules:

• If you are also taking a tetracycline antibiotic, do not take the two medicines within 1 hour of each other. Taking them together may prevent the tetracycline from being absorbed by your body. If you have any questions about this, check with your doctor or pharmacist.

• **If you have heart or blood vessel disease or if you are on a sodium-restricted (low salt) diet, do not take the buffered acetaminophen effervescent granules without first checking with your doctor.** This medicine contains a large amount of sodium.

Side Effects of This Medicine

Along with its needed effects, a medicine may cause some unwanted effects. Although not all of these side effects appear very often, when they do occur they may require medical attention. **Check with your doctor immediately** if any of the following side effects occur:

Rare

> Yellowing of eyes or skin

Signs of overdose
  Diarrhea
  Loss of appetite
  Nausea or vomiting
  Stomach cramps or pain
  Swelling or tenderness in the upper
    abdomen or stomach area
  Unusual increase in sweating

Also check with your doctor as soon as possible if any of the following side effects occur:
  Rare
  Bloody or cloudy urine
  Difficult or painful urination
  Skin rash, hives, or itching
  Sudden decrease in amount of urine
  Unexplained sore throat and fever
  Unusual bleeding or bruising
  Unusual tiredness or weakness

Other side effects not listed above may also occur in some patients. If you notice any other effects, check with your doctor.

ACETAMINOPHEN AND SALICYLATES (Systemic)

This information applies to the following medicines:

Acetaminophen and Aspirin (a-seat-a-MEE-noe-fen and AS-pir-in)
Acetaminophen, Aspirin, and Salicylamide (sal-i-SILL-a-mide)
Acetaminophen and Salicylamide
Acetaminophen and Sodium Salicylate (SOE-dee-um sa-LI-si-late)

Some commonly used brand names are:	Generic names:
Double-A Gemnisyn	Acetaminophen and Aspirin

APAP Fortified Duradyne Dynosal Excedrin Goody's Extra Strength Tablets Goody's Headache Powders Salatin Trigesic	Acetaminophen, Aspirin, and Caffeine
Buffets II Supac Vanquish	Buffered Acetaminophen, Aspirin, and Caffeine
Saleto Salocol	Acetaminophen, Aspirin, Salicylamide, and Caffeine
Presalin	Buffered Acetaminophen, Aspirin, Salicylamide, and Caffeine
Arthralgen Banesin Dinol Duoprin Duoprin-S Salimeph Forte	Acetaminophen and Salicylamide
Accurate Forte* 445 Anti-Pain Compound* Rid-A-Pain Compound S-A-C	Acetaminophen, Salicylamide, and Caffeine
Tisma	Acetaminophen, Sodium Salicylate, and Caffeine
Gaysal-S	Buffered Acetaminophen and Sodium Salicylate

*Not available in the United States.

Acetaminophen and salicylate combination medicines are taken by mouth to relieve pain and to reduce fever. They may be used to relieve occasional pain caused by mild inflammation or arthritis (rheumatism). However, neither acetaminophen nor salicylamide is as effective as aspirin or sodium salicylate for treating chronic or severe pain, or other symptoms, caused by inflammation or arthritis. Some of these combination medicines do not contain any aspirin or sodium salicylate. Even those that do contain aspirin or sodium salicylate may not contain enough to be effective in treating these conditions.

A few reports have suggested that acetaminophen and salicylates may work together to cause kidney damage or cancer of the kidney or urinary bladder. This may occur if large amounts of both medicines are taken together for a very long period of time. However, taking usual amounts of these combination medicines for short periods of time has not been shown to cause these unwanted effects. Also, these effects have not been reported with either acetaminophen or a salicylate used alone, even if large amounts have been taken for a long time. Therefore, for long-term use, it may be best to use either acetaminophen or a salicylate, but not both, unless you are under a doctor's care.

Before giving any of these combination medicines to a child, check the package label very carefully. Some of these medicines are too strong for use in children. If you are not certain whether a specific product can be given to a child, or if you have any questions about the amount to give, check with your doctor, nurse, or pharmacist.

There have been a few reports suggesting that use of aspirin in children with fever due to a viral infection (especially flu or chicken pox) may cause a serious illness called Reye's syndrome. Do not give a medicine containing aspirin or other salicylates to a child with flu or chicken pox without first discussing this with your child's doctor.

These medicines are available without a prescription. However, your doctor may have special instructions on the proper dose of these medicines for your medical condition.

For information about the precautions and side effects of the medicines in this combination, see:

Acetaminophen (Systemic)
Salicylates (Systemic)

Combination products are designed for specific uses. These uses may not be the same as the uses of the individual ingredients. Therefore, some of the information provided in the individual listings may not be relevant to the combination listings product. If questions arise, check with your doctor, nurse, or pharmacist.

ADRENOCORTICOIDS (Inhalation)

This information applies to the following medicines:

Beclomethasone (be-kloe-METH-a-sone)
Dexamethasone (dex-a-METH-a-sone)
Flunisolide (floo-NISS-oh-lide)
Triamcinolone (trye-am-SIN-oh-lone)

Some commonly used brand names are:	Generic names
Beclovent Vanceril	Beclomethasone
Decadron Respihaler	Dexamethasone
AeroBid	Flunisolide
Azmacort	Triamcinolone

Inhalation adrenocorticoids (a-dree-noe-KOR-ti-koids) are cortisone-like medicines. They belong to the general family of medicines called steroids. These medicines are inhaled (breathed in) through the mouth to help prevent asthma attacks. However, they will not relieve an asthma attack that has already started.

Adrenocorticoids may slow or stop growth in children when used for long periods of time. Before this medicine is given to a child, you and your child's doctor should talk about the good this medicine will do as well as the risks of using it. Follow the doctor's directions very carefully in order to lessen the chance that these unwanted effects will occur.

Inhalation adrenocorticoids are available only with your doctor's prescription.

Before Using This Medicine

In order to decide on the best treatment for your medical problem, your doctor should be told:

—if you have ever had any unusual or allergic reaction to adrenocorticoids or aerosol spray inhalation medicines.

—if you are allergic to any substance, such as certain preservatives or dyes. Most medicines contain more than their active ingredient. Your doctor or pharmacist can help you avoid products that may cause a problem.

—if you are pregnant or if you intend to become pregnant while using this medicine. In one study, use of beclomethasone inhalation by pregnant women did not cause birth defects or other problems. Studies on birth defects with dexamethasone, flunisolide, or triamcinolone inhalations have not been done in humans. However, too much use of an adrenocorticoid during pregnancy may cause the baby to have problems after birth, such as slower growth. Also, studies in animals have shown that adrenocorticoids cause birth defects affecting the mouth, tongue, or bones, or other unwanted effects.

—if you are breast-feeding an infant. Many adrenocorticoids pass into the breast milk and cause problems with growth or other unwanted effects in breast-fed infants.

It is not known whether beclomethasone, flunisolide, or triamcinolone passes into the breast milk. Although they have not been shown to cause problems in breast-fed infants, the chance always exists.

Dexamethasone passes into the breast milk and may cause problems in breast-fed infants. It may be necessary for you to take another medicine or to stop breast-feeding during treatment. Be sure you have discussed the risks and benefits of this medicine with your doctor.

—if you are using any inhalation adrenocorticoid and have an infection of the mouth, throat, or lungs, or if you have ever had tuberculosis (TB).

—if you are using dexamethasone or triamcinolone inhalation aerosol and have any of the following medical problems:
Bone disease
Colitis
Diabetes mellitus (sugar diabetes)
Diverticulitis
Fungal infection
Glaucoma
Heart disease
Herpes simplex (virus) infection of the
    eye
High blood pressure
High cholesterol levels
Kidney disease or kidney stones
Liver disease
Myasthenia gravis
Stomach ulcer or other stomach problems
Underactive thyroid

—if you are using any inhalation adrenocorticoid and are also using another aerosol spray inhalation for asthma.

—if you are using dexamethasone or triamcinolone inhalation aerosol and are now taking or receiving any of the following medicines or types of medicine:
Acetazolamide
Amphotericin B
Anticoagulants (blood thinners)
Antidiabetics, oral (diabetes medicine
    you take by mouth)
Aspirin or other salicylates
Dichlorphenamide
Digitalis glycosides (heart medicine)
Diuretics (water pills or high blood
    pressure medicine)
Heparin

Inflammation medicine (for example, arthritis medicine)
Insulin
Methazolamide
Potassium supplements
Somatropin (growth hormone)
Streptozocin

Proper Use of This Medicine

In order for this medicine to help prevent asthma attacks, it must be taken every day in regularly spaced doses as ordered by your doctor. Up to four weeks may pass before you feel its full effects. However, this may take less time if you have been taking certain other medicines for your asthma.

Do not use this medicine to treat an asthma attack that has already started, because it will not work. However, continue to take this medicine at the usual time, even if you use another medicine to relieve the asthma attack.

Do not use more of this medicine, and do not use it more often, than your doctor ordered. To do so may increase the chance of absorption into the body and the chance of unwanted effects.

Inhalation adrenocorticoids are used with a special inhaler and usually come with patient directions. Read the directions carefully before using. If you do not understand the directions, or if you are not sure how to use the inhaler, check with your doctor, nurse, or pharmacist.

The inhaler should be cleaned every day as directed. If you do not receive instructions with the inhaler, or if you are not certain how to clean it, check with your pharmacist.

Gargling and rinsing your mouth after each dose may help prevent hoarseness, throat irritation, and infection in the mouth.

If you miss a dose of this medicine, use it as soon as possible. However, if it is almost time for your next dose, skip the missed dose and go back to your regular dosing schedule. Do not double doses.

Check with your pharmacist to see if you should save the inhaler piece that comes with this medicine. Refill units may be available at lower cost. However, remember that the inhaler is meant to be used only for the medicine that comes with it. Do not use the inhaler for any other inhalation aerosol medicine, even if the cartridge fits.

How to store this medicine:

• Store away from heat and direct light.

• **Keep out of the reach of children.**

• Do not store in the bathroom medicine cabinet because the heat or moisture may cause the medicine to break down.

• Keep the medicine from freezing.

• Do not puncture, break, or burn the aerosol container, even after it is empty.

• Do not keep outdated medicine or medicine no longer needed.

Precautions While Using This Medicine

Check with your doctor:

—if you go through a period of unusual stress.

—if you have an asthma attack that does not improve after you take a bronchodilator medicine.

—if signs of mouth, throat, or lung infection occur.

—if your symptoms do not improve.

—if your condition gets worse.

Also, check with your doctor immediately if any of the following side effects occur while you are using this medicine:

Abdominal or back pain
Dizziness or fainting
Fever

Muscle or joint pain
Nausea or vomiting
Prolonged loss of appetite
Shortness of breath
Unusual tiredness or weakness
Unusual weight loss

Your doctor may want you to carry a medical identification card stating that you are using this medicine and may need additional medicine during times of emergency, a severe asthma attack or other illness, or unusual stress.

Before you have any kind of surgery (including dental surgery) or emergency treatment, tell the physician or dentist in charge that you are using this medicine.

For patients who are also using a bronchodilator inhalation aerosol:

• Unless otherwise directed by your doctor, **use the bronchodilator aerosol first, then wait about 15 minutes before using this medicine.** In order to lessen the chance of unwanted effects, it is best not to use the two kinds of aerosols too close together.

For patients who are also regularly taking an adrenocorticoid in tablet or liquid form:

• **Do not stop taking the other adrenocorticoid without your doctor's advice, even if your asthma seems better.** Your doctor may want you to reduce gradually the amount you are taking before stopping completely, in order to lessen the chance of unwanted effects.

• When your doctor tells you to reduce the dose, or to stop taking the other adrenocorticoid, follow the directions carefully. Your body may need time to adjust to the change. The length of time this takes may depend on the amount of medicine you were taking and how long you took it. **It is especially important that your doctor check your progress at regular visits during this period of time.**

Also, ask your doctor if there are special directions you should follow if you have a severe asthma attack, if you need any other medical or surgical treatment, or if certain side effects occur. Be certain that you understand these directions, and follow them carefully.

Side Effects of This Medicine

Along with its needed effects, a medicine may cause some unwanted effects. Although not all of these side effects appear very often, when they do occur they may require medical attention. **Check with your doctor immediately** if any of the following side effects occur just after you use this medicine:

Rare

Shortness of breath, troubled breathing, tightness in chest, or wheezing

Also, check with your doctor as soon as possible if any of the following side effects occur:

More common

Any sign of possible infection, such as chest pain, chills, fever, cough, congestion, ear pain, eye pain, red or teary eyes, runny nose, sneezing, or sore throat
Creamy white, curd-like patches inside the mouth
Nausea or vomiting
Skin rash or itching
Unusually fast or pounding heartbeat

Less common

Decreased or blurred vision
Frequent urination
Hives
Increased thirst
Mental depression or other mood or mental changes

Rare

Difficulty in swallowing
Increased blood pressure
Swelling of feet or lower legs
Unusual weight gain

Additional side effects may occur after you have been using this medicine for a long period of time. Check with your doctor as soon as possible if any of the following side effects occur:

Acne or other skin problems
Back or rib pain
Bloody or black tarry stools
Filling or rounding out of the face (moon face)
Irregular heartbeats
Menstrual problems
Muscle weakness, cramps, or pains
Stomach pain or burning (severe and continuing)
Unusual tiredness or weakness
Wounds that will not heal

Other side effects may occur which usually do not require medical attention. These side effects may go away during treatment as your body adjusts to the medicine. However, check with your doctor if any of the following side effects continue or are bothersome:

More common

Abdominal or stomach pain (mild)
Bloated feeling or gas
Constipation
Diarrhea
Dizziness or lightheadedness
Headache
Heartburn or indigestion
Loss of smell or taste sense
Nervousness or restlessness
Unpleasant taste

Less common or rare

Cough without other signs of infection
Dry or irritated nose, mouth, tongue, or throat
False sense of well-being
General feeling of discomfort, illness, shakiness, or faintness
Hoarseness or other voice changes without other signs of infection
Increase or decrease in appetite
Trouble in sleeping
Unexplained nosebleeds
Unusual increase in sweating

Some of the above side effects have been reported for dexamethasone or flunisolide, but not for beclomethasone or triamcinolone. However, all of the inhalation adrenocorticoids are similar.

Therefore, the chance always exists that these side effects may occur with beclomethasone or triamcinolone also, especially if large amounts are used for a long time.

Other side effects not listed above may also occur in some patients. If you notice any other effects, check with your doctor.

ADRENOCORTICOIDS (Systemic)
Combined Glucocorticoid and Mineralocorticoid Effects

This information applies to the following medicines:

Betamethasone (bay-ta-METH-a-sone)
Corticotropin (kor-ti-koe-TROE-pin)
Cortisone (KOR-ti-sone)
Dexamethasone (dex-a-METH-a-sone)
Hydrocortisone (hye-droe-KOR-ti-sone)
Methylprednisolone (meth-ill-pred-NISS-oh-lone)
Paramethasone (par-a-METH-a-sone)
Prednisolone (pred-NISS-oh-lone)
Prednisone (PRED-ni-sone)
Triamcinolone (trye-am-SIN-oh-lone)

The following information does *not* apply to desoxycorticosterone or fludrocortisone.

Some commonly used brand names or other names are:

For Betamethasone†

Betameth	Cel-U-Jec
Betnelan*	Prelestone
Celestone	Selestoject

For Corticotropin

ACTH	Cortrophin Gel
Acthar	Cortrophin Zinc
Cortigel	Cotropic Gel
	H P Acthar Gel

For Cortisone†
Cortone

For Dexamethasone†

Ak-Dex	Dexacen
Baycadron	Dexasone
BayDex	Dexo-LA
Dalalone	Dexon
Decadrol	Dexone
Decadron	Dezone
Decaject	Hexadrol
Decameth	Savacort-D
Deronil*	SK-Dexamethasone
	Solurex

For Hydrocortisone†

A-hydroCort	Cortisol
Biosone	Hydrocortone
Cortef	Lifocort
Cortenema	S-Cortilean*
Cortifoam	Solu-Cortef

For Methylprednisolone†

A-methaPred	Med-Depo
BayMep	Medralone
depMedalone	Medrol
Depoject	Medrone
Depo-Medrol	Mepred
Depo-Pred	Methylone
D-Med	M-Prednisol
Duralone	Pre-Dep
Durameth	Rep-Pred
	Solu-Medrol

For Paramethasone
    Haldrone

For Prednisolone†

Articulose	Nor-Pred T.B.A.
Cortalone	Predaject
Delta-Cortef	Predcor
Duapred	Prednisol TBA
Hydeltrasol	PSP-IV
Hydeltra-T.B.A.	Savacort
Key-Pred	Solu-Predalone
Metalone T.B.A.	Sterane
Niscort	TBA-Pred

For Prednisone†

Apo-Prednisone*	Orasone
Colisone*	Panasol
Cortan	Paracort*
Deltasone	Prednicen-M
Liquid Pred	SK-Prednisone
Meticorten	Winpred*

For Triamcinolone†

Acetospan	Kenalone
Amcort	Tramacort
Aristocort	Triacilon
Aristospan	Triacin
Articulose-L.A.	Triacort
BayTac	Triam
Cenocort	Triamolone
Cino-40	Triamonide
Kenacort	Tri-Kort
Kenaject	Trilog
Kenalog	Trilone
	Tristoject

*Not available in the United States.
†Generic name product may also be available.

Adrenocorticoids (a-dree-noe-KOR-ti-koids) (cortisone-like medicines) belong to the general family of medicines called steroids. Your body naturally produces certain cortisone-like hormones which are necessary to maintain good health. If your body does not produce enough, your doctor may have prescribed this medicine to help make up the difference.

Cortisone-like medicines are used also to provide relief for inflamed areas of the body. They lessen swelling, redness, itching, and allergic reactions. They are often used as part of the treatment for a number of different diseases, such as severe allergies or skin problems, asthma, or arthritis. They may also be used for other conditions as determined by your doctor.

Corticotropin is not an adrenocorticoid. It is a hormone which occurs naturally in the body. Corticotropin is known as an adrenocorticotropic hormone, which means it causes the adrenal glands to produce cortisone-like hormones. Corticotropin is used as a test to determine whether your adrenal glands are producing enough hormones. Also, it may be used instead of adrenocorticoids to treat many of the same medical problems.

Adrenocorticoids are very strong medicines. In addition to their helpful effects in treating your medical problem, they have side effects that can be very serious. If your adrenal glands are not producing enough cortisone-like hormones, taking this medicine is not likely to cause problems unless you take too much of it. If you are taking this medicine to treat another medical problem, be sure that you discuss the risks and benefits of this medicine with your doctor.

Adrenocorticoids may slow or stop growth in children, especially when they are used for a long time. Before this medicine is given to children you should discuss the use of it with your doctor and then carefully follow your doctor's instructions.

Adrenocorticoids are taken by mouth, given by injection, or used rectally. Corticotropin is given by injection because it is destroyed by digestion when taken by mouth.

These medicines are available only with your doctor's prescription.

Before Using This Medicine

In order to decide on the best treatment for your medical problem, your doctor should be told:

—if you have ever had any unusual or allergic reaction to adrenocorticoids or to corticotropin.

—if you are receiving corticotropin and have ever had any unusual or allergic reaction to pork products (corticotropin is often obtained from pigs).

—if you are on a low-salt, low-sugar, or any other special diet, or if you are allergic to any substance, such as sulfites or other preservatives or dyes. Most medicines contain more than their active ingredient, and many liquid medicines contain alcohol. Your doctor or pharmacist can help you avoid products that may cause a problem.

—if you are pregnant or if you intend to become pregnant while taking this medicine. Studies on birth defects with adrenocorticoids or with corticotropin have not been done in humans. However, too much use of adrenocorticoids during pregnancy may cause the baby to have problems after birth, such as slower growth. Also, studies in animals have shown that adrenocorticoids cause birth defects and that corticotropin may cause other unwanted effects in the fetus.

—if you are breast-feeding an infant. Adrenocorticoids pass into breast milk and may cause problems with growth or other unwanted effects in infants of mothers taking this medicine. Depending on the amount of medicine you are taking every day, it may be necessary for you to take another medicine or to stop breast-feeding during treatment. Be sure you have discussed the risks and benefits of the medicine with your doctor.

Although corticotropin has not been shown to cause problems in humans, the chance always exists.

—if you have an infection at the place of treatment.

—if you have recently had surgery or a serious injury.

—if you have any of the following medical problems:

> Bone disease
> Colitis
> Diabetes mellitus (sugar diabetes)
> Diverticulitis
> Fungus infection or any other infection
> Glaucoma
> Heart disease
> Herpes simplex infection of the eye
> High blood pressure
> High cholesterol levels
> Kidney disease or kidney stones
> Liver disease
> Myasthenia gravis
> Overactive thyroid
> Stomach ulcer or other stomach or intestine problems
> Tuberculosis (active TB, nonactive TB, or past history of)
> Underactive thyroid

—if you regularly take large amounts of antacids.

—if you regularly use any medicine that contains a large amount of sodium (salt).

—if you are now taking or receiving any of the following medicines or types of medicine:

Acetazolamide
Amphotericin B
Anabolic steroids
Androgens (male hormones)
Anticoagulants, oral (blood thinners you take by mouth)
Anticonvulsants (seizure medicine)
Antidepressants, tricyclic (medicine for depression)
Antidiabetics, oral (diabetes medicine you take by mouth)
Aspirin or other salicylates
Barbiturates
Dichlorphenamide
Digitalis glycosides (heart medicine)
Diuretics (water pills—also used for high blood pressure)
Ephedrine
Estrogens (female hormones)
Folic acid
Heparin
Inflammation medicine (for example, arthritis medicine)
Insulin
Isoniazid (medicine for TB)
Methazolamide
Oral contraceptives (birth control pills)
Potassium supplements
Rifampin
Somatropin (growth hormone)
Thyroid hormones
Troleandomycin

Proper Use of This Medicine

Use this medicine only as directed by your doctor. Do not use more or less of it, do not use it more often, and do not use it for a longer period of time than your doctor ordered. To do so may increase the chance of side effects.

For patients taking this medicine by mouth:
• **Take this medicine with food** to help prevent stomach upset. If stomach upset, burning, or pain continues, check with your doctor.

• Stomach problems may be more likely to occur if you drink alcoholic beverages while being treated with this medicine. You should not drink alcoholic beverages while taking this medicine, unless you have first checked with your doctor.

For patients using this medicine rectally:
• This medicine usually comes with patient directions. Read them carefully before using this medicine.

• For patients using hydrocortisone enema:

—For best results, use this medicine right after a bowel movement (BM). Lie on your left side and stay there for at least 30 minutes after the enema is given so the medicine can work. If you can, keep the enema inside all night.

—Gently insert the rectal tip of the enema applicator to prevent damage to the rectal wall.

—Each bottle contains a single dose. Use it all, unless otherwise directed by your doctor.

• For patients using hydrocortisone acetate rectal aerosol foam:

—This medicine is used with a special applicator. Do not insert any part of the aerosol container into the rectum.

• For patients using methylprednisolone acetate for enema:

—Gently insert the rectal tip of the enema applicator to prevent damage to the rectal wall.

—Shake the bottle every half-hour while you are giving the enema.

—Each bottle contains a single dose. Use it all, unless otherwise directed by your doctor.

—Save your applicator. Refill units of this medicine may be available at lower cost.

If you miss a dose of this medicine and your dosing schedule is one dose to be taken:

Every other day—Take the missed dose as soon as possible if you remember it the same morning, then go back to your regular dosing schedule. If you do not remember the missed dose until later, wait and take it the following morning. Then skip a day and start your regular dosing schedule again.

Once a day—Take the missed dose as soon as possible, then go back to your regular dosing schedule. If you do not remember until the next day, skip the missed dose and do not double the next one.

Several times a day—Take the missed dose as soon as possible, then go back to your regular dosing schedule. If you do not remember until your next dose is due, double the next dose.

If you have any questions about this, check with your doctor, nurse, or pharmacist.

How to store tablet, liquid, or enema forms of this medicine:

• Store away from heat and direct light.

• **Keep out of the reach of children.**

• Do not store in the bathroom medicine cabinet because the heat or moisture may cause the medicine to break down.

• Keep the liquid dosage forms of this medicine, including enemas, from freezing.

• Do not keep outdated medicine or medicine no longer needed. Flush the contents of the container down the toilet, unless otherwise directed.

How to store hydrocortisone rectal aerosol foam:

• Store away from heat and direct light.

• **Keep out of the reach of children.**

• Do not store in the bathroom medicine cabinet because the heat or moisture may cause the medicine to break down.

• Keep the medicine from freezing.

• Do not puncture, break, or burn the aerosol container, even after it is empty.

• Do not keep outdated medicine or medicine no longer needed.

Precautions While Using This Medicine

Your doctor should check your progress at regular visits. Your progress may have to be checked also after you have stopped using this medicine, since some of the effects may continue.

Do not stop using this medicine without first checking with your doctor. Your doctor may want you to reduce gradually the amount you are using before stopping completely.

Check with your doctor if your condition reappears or worsens after the dose has been reduced or treatment with this medicine is stopped.

If you will be using adrenocorticoids or corticotropin for a long time:

• **Your doctor may want you to follow a low-salt diet and/or a potassium-rich diet.**

• Your doctor may want you to watch your calories to prevent weight gain.

• Your doctor may want you to add extra protein to your diet.

• Your doctor may want you to have your eyes examined by an ophthalmologist before and also sometime later during treatment.

• Your doctor may want you to carry a medical identification card stating that you are using this medicine.

Tell the doctor in charge that you are using this medicine:

—**before having a vaccination, other immunizations, or skin tests.**

—**before having any kind of surgery (including dental surgery) or emergency treatment.**

—**if you get a serious infection or injury.**

Diabetics—This medicine may cause your blood sugar levels to rise. If you notice a change in the results of your urine or blood sugar test or if you have any questions, check with your doctor, nurse, or pharmacist.

For patients having this medicine injected into their joints:

• If this medicine is injected into one of your joints, you should be careful not to put too much stress or strain on it for a while, even if it begins to feel better. Make sure your doctor has told you how much you are allowed to move this joint while it is healing.

• If redness or swelling occurs at the place of injection, and continues or gets worse, check with your doctor.

For patients using this medicine rectally:

• Check with your doctor if you notice rectal bleeding, pain, burning, itching, blistering, or other sign of irritation not present before you started using this medicine, or if signs of infection occur.

Side Effects of This Medicine

Adrenocorticoids or corticotropin may lower your resistance to infections. Also, any infection you get may be harder to treat. Always check with your doctor as soon as possible if you notice any signs of a possible infection, such as sore throat, fever, sneezing, or coughing.

Along with its needed effects, a medicine may cause some unwanted effects. Although not all of these side effects appear very often, when they do occur they may require medical attention. When this medicine is used for short periods of time, side effects usually are rare. However, check with your doctor as soon as possible if any of the following side effects occur:

Less common

Decreased or blurred vision
Decreased or slow growth (in children)
Frequent urination
Increased thirst
Rectal bleeding, blistering, burning, itching, or pain not present before treatment (when used rectally)

Rare

Burning, numbness, pain, or tingling at or near place of injection
Hallucinations (seeing, hearing, or feeling things that are not there)
Mental depression or other mood or mental changes
Redness, swelling, or other sign of infection at place of injection
Skin rash or hives

Additional side effects may occur if you take this medicine for a long period of time. Check with your doctor if any of the following side effects occur:

Abdominal or stomach pain or burning (continuing)
Acne or other skin problems
Bloody or black tarry stools
Filling or rounding out of the face
Hip pain
Increase in blood pressure
Irregular heartbeats
Menstrual problems
Muscle cramps or pain
Muscle weakness
Nausea or vomiting
Pain in back, ribs, arms, or legs
Pitting or depression of skin at place of injection
Reddish purple lines on arms, face, legs, trunk, or groin
Swelling of feet or lower legs

Thin, shiny skin
Unusual bruising
Unusual tiredness or weakness
Unusual weight gain
Wounds that will not heal

Other side effects may occur which usually do not require medical attention. These side effects may go away during treatment as your body adjusts to the medicine. However, check with your doctor if any of the following side effects continue or are bothersome:

More common

False sense of well-being
Indigestion
Increase in appetite
Loss of appetite (for triamcinolone only)
Nervousness or restlessness
Trouble in sleeping

Less common or rare

Darkening or lightening of skin color
Dizziness or lightheadedness
Headache
Increase in joint pain (after injection into a joint)
Unusual increase in hair growth on body or face

After you stop using this medicine, your body may need time to adjust. The length of time this takes depends on the amount of medicine you were using and how long you used it. If you have taken large doses of this medicine for a long period of time, your body may need one year to adjust. During this period of time, **check with your doctor immediately if any of the following side effects occur:**

Abdominal or stomach or back pain
Dizziness or fainting
Fever
Loss of appetite (continuing)
Muscle or joint pain
Nausea or vomiting
Shortness of breath
Unexplained headaches (frequent or continuing)
Unusual tiredness or weakness
Unusual weight loss

Some of the above side effects, especially bone problems, may be more likely to occur in children and in the elderly, who are usually more sensitive to some of the effects of these medicines.

Other side effects not listed above may also occur in some patients. If you notice any other effects, check with your doctor.

ADRENOCORTICOIDS (Topical)

This information applies to the following medicines:

Amcinonide (am-SIN-oh-nide)
Betamethasone (bay-ta-METH-a-sone)
Clocortolone (kloe-KOR-toe-lone)
Desonide (DESS-oh-nide)
Desoximetasone (des-ox-i-MET-a-sone)
Dexamethasone (dex-a-METH-a-sone)
Diflorasone (dye-FLOR-a-sone)
Flumethasone (floo-METH-a-sone)
Fluocinolone (floo-oh-SIN-oh-lone)
Fluocinonide (floo-oh-SIN-oh-nide)
Fluorometholone (flure-oh-METH-oh-lone)
Flurandrenolide (flure-an-DREN-oh-lide)
Halcinonide (hal-SIN-oh-nide)
Hydrocortisone (hye-droe-KOR-ti-sone)
Methylprednisolone (meth-ill-pred-NISS-oh-lone)
Prednisolone (pred-NISS-oh-lone)
Triamcinolone (trye-am-SIN-oh-lone)

Some commonly used brand names or other names are:

For Amcinonide
    Cyclocort

For Betamethasone†

Alphatrex	Diprolene
Beben*	Diprosone
Benisone	Ectosone*
Betacort Scalp Lotion*	Metaderm*
Betaderm*	Novobetamet*
Betatrex	Uticort*
Beta-Val	Valisone
Betnovate*	Valnac
Celestoderm-V*	

For Clocortolone
  Cloderm

For Desonide
  DesOwen   Tridesilon

For Desoximetasone
  Topicort

For Dexamethasone†
  Aeroseb-Dex   Decadron
  Decaderm   Decaspray

For Diflorasone
  Florone   Flutone*
                           Maxiflor

For Flumethasone*
  Locacorten*

For Fluocinolone†
  Dermophyl   Fluonide*
  Fluocet   Flurosyn
  Fluoderm*   Psoranide
  Fluolar*   Synalar
  Fluolean*   Synamol*
  Fluonid   Synemol

For Fluocinonide
  Lidemol*   Lidex-E
  Lidex   Lyderm*
                           Topsyn*

For Fluorometholone*

For Flurandrenolide
  Cordran   Cordran SP
                           Drenison*

For Halcinonide
  Halog   Halog-E

For Hydrocortisone†
  Acticort   Cortef
  Aeroseb-HC   Corticreme*
  Bactine Hydrocortisone   Cortisol
  CaldeCort   Cortizone
  Cetacort   Cortoderm
  Clinicort   Delacort
  Cortaid   Dermacort
  Cortate*   DermiCort
  Cort-Dome

Dermolate Anti-Itch   Microcort*
Dermolate Scalp Itch   MyCort
Dermtex HC   Novohydrocort*
Eldecort   nutracort
Emo-Cort*   Penecort
Epifoam   Pharma-Cort
Gynecort   Pro-Cort
HC-Jel   Pro-Cort M
Hi-Cor   Racet-SE
H_2 Cort   Resicort
Hyderm*   Rhulicort
Hydro-Cortilean*   Synacort
Hydro-tex   Texacort Scalp
Hytone   Lotion
Lanacort   Unicort*
Locoid   Westcort

For Methylprednisolone
  Medrol

For Prednisolone*

For Triamcinolone
  Aristocort   Kenalog-H
  Aristocort-A   Triacet
  Cremocort*   Triaderm*
  Flutex   Trialean*
  Kenac   Triamalone
  Kenalog   Triderm
  Kenalog-E*   Trymex

*Not available in the United States.
†Generic name product may also be available.

This medicine is an adrenocorticoid (a-dree-noe-KOR-ti-koid) (cortisone-like medicine). It belongs to the general family of medicines called steroids. Topical cortisone-like medicines are applied to the skin to help relieve redness, swelling, itching, and discomfort of many skin problems.

Topical adrenocorticoids are absorbed through the skin and may rarely affect growth in children. Before using this medicine in children, you should discuss the use of it with your doctor.

Most adrenocorticoids are available only with your doctor's prescription. Some strengths of hydrocortisone are available without a prescription; however, your doctor may have special instructions on its proper use for your medical condition.

Before Using This Medicine

In order to decide on the best treatment for your medical problem, your doctor should be told:

—if you have ever had any unusual or allergic reaction to adrenocorticoids.

—if you are allergic to any substance, such as certain preservatives or dyes. Most medicines contain more than their active ingredient. Your doctor or pharmacist can help you avoid products that may cause a problem.

—if you are pregnant or if you intend to become pregnant while using this medicine. Studies on birth defects have not been done in humans. However, studies in animals have shown that topical adrenocorticoids, when used in large amounts or for a long period of time, cause birth defects.

—if you are breast-feeding an infant. Although topical adrenocorticoids have not been shown to cause problems in humans, the chance always exists. Other adrenocorticoids pass into breast milk and may interfere with the infant's growth.

—if you have any of the following medical problems:

    Diabetes mellitus (sugar diabetes)
    Infection or ulceration at the place of treatment
    Tuberculosis

Proper Use of This Medicine

Do not use this medicine more often or for a longer period of time than your doctor ordered or than recommended on the package label. To do so may increase the chance of absorption through the skin and the chance of side effects. In addition, too much use, especially on thin skin areas (for example, face, armpits, groin), may result in thinning of the skin and stretch marks.

If this medicine has been prescribed for you, it is meant to treat a specific skin problem. **Do not use it for other skin problems, and do not use nonprescription hydrocortisone for skin problems that are not listed on the package label, without first checking with your doctor.** Topical adrenocorticoids should not be used on many kinds of bacterial, viral, or fungal skin infections.

Be very careful not to get this medicine in your eyes. If you are using this medicine on your face, it may be best to apply it with a cotton-tipped applicator or a gauze pad.

Do not bandage or otherwise wrap the area of the skin being treated unless directed to do so by your doctor.

If your doctor has ordered an occlusive dressing (for example, kitchen plastic wrap) to be applied over this medicine, make sure you know how to apply it. Since occlusive dressings increase the amount of medicine absorbed through your skin and the possibility of side effects, use them only as directed. If you have any questions about this, check with your doctor.

For patients using the topical aerosol form of this medicine:

    • This medicine usually comes with patient directions. Read them carefully before using this medicine.

    • It is important to avoid breathing in the vapors from the spray.

    • Do not use near heat, near an open flame, or while smoking.

For patients using flurandrenolide tape:

    • This medicine usually comes with patient directions. Read them carefully before using this medicine.

If your doctor has ordered you to use this medicine on a regular schedule and you miss a dose, apply it as soon as possible. But if it is almost time for your next dose, just skip the missed dose and apply it at the next regularly scheduled time.

How to store aerosol forms of this medicine:
- Store away from heat and direct light.
- **Keep out of the reach of children.**
- Do not store in the bathroom medicine cabinet because the heat or moisture may cause the medicine to break down.
- Keep the medicine from freezing.
- Do not puncture, break, or burn the aerosol container.
- Do not keep outdated medicine or medicine no longer needed.

How to store other forms of this medicine:
- Store away from heat and direct light.
- **Keep out of the reach of children.**
- Do not store in the bathroom medicine cabinet because the heat or moisture may cause the medicine to break down.
- Keep the medicine from freezing.
- Do not keep outdated medicine or medicine no longer needed. Flush the contents of the container down the toilet, unless otherwise directed.

Precautions While Using This Medicine

Children who must use this medicine should be followed closely by their doctor since this medicine may be absorbed through the skin and can affect growth or cause other unwanted effects.

If this medicine is to be used on the diaper area, avoid using tight-fitting diapers or plastic pants on the child. Wearing these may increase the chance of absorption of the medicine through the skin and the chance of side effects.

Side Effects of This Medicine

Along with its needed effects, a medicine may cause some unwanted effects. Although not all of these side effects appear very often, when they do occur they may require medical attention. Check with your doctor as soon as possible if any of the following side effects occur:

Signs of infection such as pain, redness, or pus-containing blisters
Signs of irritation such as burning, itching, blistering, or peeling not present before using this medicine

Additional side effects may occur if you use this medicine for a long period of time. Check with your doctor if any of the following side effects occur:

Acne or oily skin
Filling or rounding out of the face
Reddish purple lines on arms, face, legs, trunk, or groin
Thinning of skin with easy bruising
Unusual increase in hair growth, especially on the face
Unusual loss of hair, especially on the scalp

When the gel, solution, lotion, or aerosol form of this medicine is applied, a mild, temporary stinging may be expected.

Other side effects not listed above may also occur in some patients. If you notice any other effects, check with your doctor.

ALBUTEROL (Systemic)

Some commonly used brand names or other names are Proventil, Salbutamol, and Ventolin.

Albuterol (al-BYOO-ter-ole) is taken by oral inhalation or by mouth to treat lung diseases such as bronchial asthma, chronic bronchitis, and emphysema. It relieves wheezing, shortness of breath, and troubled breathing.

Albuterol is also taken by oral inhalation to prevent bronchospasm (wheezing or difficulty in breathing) caused by exercise.

This medicine is available only with your doctor's prescription.

Before Using This Medicine

In order to decide on the best treatment for your medical problem, your doctor should be told:

—if you have ever had any unusual or allergic reaction to albuterol or other aerosol inhalation medicines.

—if you are on a low-salt, low-sugar, or any other special diet, or if you are allergic to any substance, such as sulfites or other preservatives or dyes. Most medicines contain more than their active ingredient, and many liquid medicines contain alcohol. Your doctor or pharmacist can help you avoid products that may cause a problem.

—if you are pregnant or if you intend to become pregnant while using this medicine. Studies on birth defects in humans have not been done. However, in some animal studies, albuterol has been shown to cause birth defects when given in doses up to many times the usual human dose. Although albuterol has been reported to delay preterm labor when taken by mouth, it has not been shown to stop preterm labor or prevent labor at term.

—if you are breast-feeding an infant. Although it is not known whether albuterol passes into the breast milk and this medicine has not been shown to cause problems in humans, the chance always exists.

—if you have any of the following medical problems:
  Diabetes mellitus (sugar diabetes)
  Enlarged prostate
  Heart or blood vessel disease
  High blood pressure
  Overactive thyroid

—if you are now taking any of the following medicines or types of medicine:
  Acebutolol
  Amantadine
  Aminophylline
  Amphetamines
  Antihypertensives (high blood pressure medicine)
  Appetite suppressants (diet pills)
  Atenolol
  Caffeine
  Chlophedianol
  Digitalis glycosides (heart medicine)
  Dyphylline
  Epinephrine
  Labetalol
  Levodopa
  Medicine for hay fever or other allergies (including nose drops or sprays)
  Methylphenidate
  Metoprolol
  Nadolol
  Nitrates (medicine for angina)
  Other medicine (including oral inhalations) for asthma or breathing problems
  Oxtriphylline
  Pemoline
  Pindolol
  Propranolol
  Theophylline
  Thyroid hormones
  Timolol

—if you are now taking tricyclic antidepressants (medicine for depression), such as:
  Amitriptyline
  Amoxapine
  Clomipramine
  Desipramine
  Doxepin
  Imipramine
  Nortriptyline
  Protriptyline
  Trimipramine

—if you are now taking monoamine oxidase (MAO) inhibitors, such as:
  Furazolidone
  Isocarboxazid
  Pargyline
  Phenelzine
  Procarbazine
  Tranylcypromine

Proper Use of This Medicine

It is very important that you use this medicine only as directed. Do not use more of it and do not use it more often than your doctor ordered. To do so may increase the chance of serious side effects. Inhalation aerosol medicines similar to albuterol have been reported to cause death when too much of the medicine was used.

If you are using this medicine regularly and you miss a dose, use it as soon as possible. However, if it is almost time for your next dose, skip the missed dose and go back to your regular dosing schedule. Do not double doses.

For patients using the inhalation aerosol form of this medicine:

• This medicine usually comes with patient directions. Read them carefully before using this medicine.

• Keep spray away from the eyes.

How to store this medicine:

• Store away from heat.

• Store the syrup or tablet form of this medicine away from direct light and the inhalation aerosol form of this medicine away from direct sunlight.

• **Keep out of the reach of children.**

• Do not store in the bathroom medicine cabinet because the heat or moisture may cause the medicine to break down.

• Keep the inhalation aerosol form of this medicine from freezing.

• Do not puncture, break, or burn the inhalation aerosol container, even if it is empty.

• Do not keep outdated medicine or medicine no longer needed. Flush the syrup or tablet form of this medicine down the toilet, unless otherwise directed.

Precautions While Using This Medicine

Check with your doctor at once:

—if you still have trouble breathing 1 hour after using this medicine.

—if your symptoms return within ⌐ hours after using this medicine.

—if your condition gets worse.

Dryness of the mouth and throat may occu after using this medicine. Rinsing th mouth with water after each dose ma help prevent the dryness.

For patients using the inhalation aeros form of albuterol:

• If you use all of the medicine in on canister (container) in less than 2 weeks, check with your doctor. You may be using too much of the medicine.

• If you are also using the inhalation aerosol form of an adrenocorticoid (cortisone-like medicine, such as beclomethasone, dexamethasone, flunisolide, or triamcinolone), **allow 15 minutes between using the albuterol and an adrenocorticoid,** unless otherwise directed by your doctor. This will help to reduce the possibility of side effects.

Side Effects of This Medicine

In some animal studies, albuterol was shown to cause benign (not cancerous) tumors. The doses given were many times the dose of albuterol given to humans. It is not known if albuterol causes tumors in humans.

Along with its needed effects, a medicine may cause some unwanted effects. Although not all of these side effects appear very often, when they do occur they may require medical attention. Check with your doctor as soon as possible if any of the following side effects occur:

Signs of overdose
    Chest pain
    Dizziness (severe)
    Headache (severe or continuing)

Increase in blood pressure (severe)
Nausea or vomiting (continuing)
Unusually fast or pounding heartbeat
(continuing)
Unusual nervousness or restlessness

Other side effects may occur which usually do not require medical attention. These side effects may go away during treatment as your body adjusts to the medicine. However, check with your doctor if any of the following side effects continue or are bothersome:

More common
Nausea
Nervousness
Trembling
Unusually fast or pounding heartbeat

Less common
Difficult urination
Dizziness or lightheadedness
Dryness or irritation of mouth and throat
Headache
Heartburn
Increase or decrease in blood pressure
Restlessness
Trouble in sleeping
Unusual taste in mouth
Vomiting

Other side effects not listed above may also occur in some patients. If you notice any other effects, check with your doctor.

ALLOPURINOL (Systemic)

Some commonly used brand names are:

Alloprin*	Purinol*
Apo-Allopurinol*	Roucol*
Lopurin	Zyloprim
Novopurol*	

Generic name product may also be available.

---

*Not available in the United States.

Allopurinol (al-oh-PURE-i-nole) is taken by mouth to treat chronic gout or gouty arthritis. These conditions are caused by too much uric acid in the blood. It works by causing less uric acid to be produced by the body. Allopurinol will not relieve a gout attack that has already started. Also, it does not cure gout, but it will help prevent gout attacks. However, it works only after you have been taking it regularly for a few months. Also, allopurinol will help prevent gout attacks only as long as you continue to take it.

Allopurinol is also used to prevent or treat other medical problems that may occur if too much uric acid is present in the body. These include certain kinds of kidney stones or other kidney problems.

Allopurinol is available only with your doctor's prescription.

Before Using This Medicine

In order to decide on the best treatment for your medical problem, your doctor should be told:

—if you have ever had any unusual or allergic reaction to allopurinol.

—if you are on a low-salt, low-sugar, or any other special diet, or if you are allergic to any substance, such as sulfites or other preservatives or dyes. Most medicines contain more than their active ingredient. Your doctor or pharmacist can help you avoid products that may cause a problem.

—if you are pregnant or if you intend to become pregnant while taking this medicine. Although studies on birth defects have not been done in humans, allopurinol has not been reported to cause problems in humans. In one study in mice, large amounts of allopurinol caused birth defects and other unwanted effects. However, allopurinol did not cause birth defects or other problems in rats or rabbits given doses up to 20 times the amount usually given to humans.

—if you are breast-feeding an infant. Although allopurinol has not been shown to cause problems in humans, the chance always exists. Allopurinol passes into the breast milk.

—if you have kidney disease.

—if you are now taking any of the following medicines or types of medicine:

Aminophylline
Ampicillin
Anticoagulants (blood thinners)
Antineoplastics (medicine for cancer)
Azathioprine
Bacampicillin
Chlorpropamide (diabetes medicine you take by mouth)
Dacarbazine
Diazoxide
Diuretics (water pills)
Hetacillin
Mecamylamine
Medicine to make the urine more acid
Other gout medicine
Oxtriphylline
Pyrazinamide
Theophylline
Vidarabine

Proper Use of This Medicine

In order for this medicine to help you, it must be taken regularly as ordered by your doctor.

If this medicine upsets your stomach, it may be taken after meals. If stomach upset (nausea, vomiting, diarrhea, or stomach pain) continues, check with your doctor.

To help prevent kidney stones while taking allopurinol, adults should drink at least 10 to 12 full glasses (8 ounces each) of fluids each day unless otherwise directed by their doctor. Check with the doctor about the amount of fluids that children should drink each day while receiving this medicine. Also, your doctor may want you to take another medicine to make your urine less acid. It is important that you follow your doctor's instructions very carefully.

For patients taking allopurinol for gout:

• After you begin to take allopurinol, gout attacks may continue to occur for a while. However, if you take this medicine regularly as directed by your doctor, the attacks will gradually become less frequent and less painful. After you have been taking allopurinol for several months, they may stop completely.

• Allopurinol is used to help prevent gout attacks. It will not relieve an attack that has already started. **Even if you take another medicine for gout attacks, continue to take this medicine also.**

If you miss a dose of allopurinol and your dosing schedule is one dose to be taken:

Once a day—
Take the missed dose as soon as possible. However, if you do not remember the missed dose until the next day, skip the missed dose and go back to your regular dosing schedule. Do not double the next day's dose.

More than once a day—
Take the missed dose as soon as possible. However, if it is almost time for your next dose, and each regular dose is one 100-mg tablet, double the next dose. If each regular dose is two 100-mg tablets, take three tablets for the next dose. Then go back to your regular dosing schedule.

How to store this medicine:

• Store away from heat and direct light.

• **Keep out of the reach of children.**

• Do not store in the bathroom medicine cabinet because the heat or moisture may cause the medicine to break down.

• Do not keep outdated medicine or medicine no longer needed. Flush the contents of the container down the toilet, unless otherwise directed.

Precautions While Using This Medicine

Your doctor should check your progress at regular visits. A blood test may be needed in order to make sure that this medicine is working properly and is not causing unwanted effects.

Drinking too much alcohol may increase the amount of uric acid in the blood and lessen the effects of allopurinol. Therefore, **do not drink alcoholic beverages while taking this medicine,** unless you have first checked with your doctor.

Taking too much vitamin C may make the urine more acidic and increase the possibility of kidney stones forming while you are taking allopurinol. Therefore, do not take vitamin C while taking this medicine, unless you have first checked with your doctor.

Check with your doctor immediately:

• **if you notice a skin rash, hives, or itching while taking allopurinol.**

• **if chills, fever, muscle aches or pains, or nausea or vomiting occur together with or shortly after a skin rash.**

Very rarely, these effects may be the first signs of a serious allergic reaction to the medicine, especially during the first few months of treatment.

Allopurinol may cause some people to become drowsy or less alert than they are normally. **Make sure you know how you react to this medicine before you drive, use machines, or do other jobs that require you to be alert.**

Side Effects of This Medicine

Along with its needed effects, a medicine may cause some unwanted effects. Although not all of these side effects appear very often, when they do occur they may require medical attention. **Check with your doctor immediately** if any of the following side effects occur:

More common

Skin rash, hives, or itching

Rare

Chills, fever, muscle aches and pains, nausea, or vomiting occurring with or shortly after a skin rash
Red, thickened, or scaly skin
Sore throat and fever
Sudden decrease in amount of urine
Unusual bleeding or bruising
Unusual tiredness or weakness
Yellowing of eyes or skin

Also, check with your doctor as soon as possible if any of the following side effects occur:

Rare

Blood in urine
Difficult or painful urination
Numbness, tingling, pain, or weakness in hands or feet
Pain in lower back

Other side effects may occur which usually do not require medical attention. These side effects may go away during treatment as your body adjusts to the medicine. However, check with your doctor if any of the following side effects continue or are bothersome:

Less common

Diarrhea
Drowsiness
Nausea or vomiting occurring without a skin rash
Stomach pain

Other side effects not listed above may also occur in some patients. If you notice any other effects, check with your doctor.

AMANTADINE (Systemic)
A commonly used brand name is Symmetrel.

Amantadine (a-MAN-ta-deen) belongs to the general family of medicines called antivirals. It is used to prevent or treat certain flu infections (type A). It is given alone by mouth or may be given along with flu shots. Amantadine will not work for colds, other types of flu, or other virus infections.

Amantadine also belongs to the general family of medicines called antidyskinetics. It is used to treat Parkinson's disease, sometimes called paralysis agitans or shaking palsy. It may be given alone or with other medicines for Parkinson's disease. By improving muscle control and reducing stiffness, this medicine allows more normal movements of the body as the disease symptoms are reduced.

Amantadine is available only with your doctor's prescription.

Before Using This Medicine

In order to decide on the best treatment for your medical problem, your doctor should be told:

—if you have ever had any unusual or allergic reaction to amantadine.

—if you are on a low-salt, low-sugar, or any other special diet, or if you are allergic to any substance, such as sulfites or other preservatives or dyes. Most medicines contain more than their active ingredient, and many liquid medicines contain alcohol. Your doctor or pharmacist can help you avoid products that may cause a problem.

—if you are pregnant or if you intend to become pregnant while taking this medicine. Studies have not been done in humans. However, studies in some animals have shown that amantadine taken in high doses causes birth defects and harms the fetus. Lower doses have not been shown to cause problems.

—if you are breast-feeding an infant. Use is not recommended in nursing mothers since amantadine passes into the breast milk and may cause vomiting, difficult urination, and skin rash in the infant.

—if you have any of the following medical problems:
Blood vessel disease of brain
Eczema (recurring)
Epilepsy or other seizures
Heart disease or other circulation problems
Kidney disease
Mental or emotional illness
Stomach or intestinal ulcers
Swelling of feet and ankles

—if you are now taking any of the following medicines or types of medicine:
Amphetamines
Antihistamines
Appetite suppressants (diet pills)
Caffeine
Carbidopa and levodopa
Chlophedianol
Diarrhea medicine
Doxapram
Levodopa
Medicine for abdominal or stomach spasms or cramps
Medicine for asthma or other breathing problems
Medicine for hay fever or other allergies (including nose drops or sprays)
Methylphenidate
Other medicine for Parkinson's disease
Pemoline
Phenothiazines (tranquilizers)

—if you are now taking tricyclic antidepressants (medicine for depression) such as:
Amitriptyline
Amoxapine
Desipramine
Doxepin
Imipramine
Nortriptyline
Protriptyline
Trimipramine

Proper Use of This Medicine

For patients taking amantadine to prevent or treat flu infections:

• This medicine is best taken before exposure, or as soon as possible after exposure, to people who have the flu.

• To help keep you from getting the flu, **keep taking this medicine for the full time of treatment.** Or if you already have the flu, you should still continue taking this medicine for the full time of treatment even if you begin to feel better after a few days. This will help to clear up your infection completely. If you stop taking this medicine too soon, your symptoms may return.

• If using the oral liquid form of amantadine, use a specially marked measuring spoon or other device to measure each dose accurately since the average household teaspoon may not hold the right amount of liquid.

• This medicine works best when there is a constant amount in the blood. **To help keep this amount constant, do not miss any doses. Also, it is best to take each dose at evenly spaced times day and night.** For example, if you are to take 2 doses a day, each dose should be spaced about 12 hours apart. If this interferes with your sleep or other daily activities, or if you need help in planning the best times to take your medicine, check with your doctor, nurse, or pharmacist.

• If you do miss a dose of this medicine, take it as soon as possible. This will help to keep a constant amount of medicine in the blood. However, if it is almost time for your next dose, skip the missed dose and go back to your regular dosing schedule. Do not double doses.

For patients taking amantadine for Parkinson's disease:

• **Take this medicine exactly as directed by your doctor.** Do not miss any doses and do not take more medicine than your doctor ordered.

• If you do miss a dose of this medicine, take it as soon as possible. If your next scheduled dose is within 4 hours, do not take the missed dose at all and do not double the next one. Instead, go back to your regular dosing schedule.

• Improvement in the symptoms of Parkinson's disease usually occurs in about 2 days. However, in some patients this medicine must be taken for up to 2 weeks before full benefit is seen.

How to store this medicine:

• Store away from heat and direct light.

• **Keep out of the reach of children.**

• Do not store in the bathroom medicine cabinet because the heat or moisture may cause the medicine to break down.

• Keep the liquid form of this medicine from freezing.

• Do not keep outdated medicine or medicine no longer needed. Flush the contents of the container down the toilet, unless otherwise directed.

Precautions While Using This Medicine

Drinking alcoholic beverages while taking this medicine may cause increased side effects such as circulation problems, dizziness, lightheadedness, fainting, or confusion. Therefore, **you should not drink alcoholic beverages while you are taking this medicine.**

This medicine may cause some people to become dizzy, confused, or lightheaded, or to have blurred vision or trouble concentrating. **Make sure you know how you react to this medicine before you drive, use machines, or do other jobs that require you to be alert or to see clearly.**

Getting up suddenly from a lying or sitting position may also be a problem because of the dizziness, lightheadedness, or fainting that may be caused by this medicine. Getting up slowly may help. If this problem continues or gets worse, check with your doctor.

Your mouth, nose, and throat may feel very dry while you are taking this medicine. To help relieve mouth dryness, chew sugarless gum or dissolve bits of ice in your mouth.

This medicine may cause purplish red, net-like, blotchy spots on the skin. This problem occurs more often in females and usually occurs on the legs and/or feet after taking this medicine regularly for a month or more. Although the blotchy spots may remain as long as you are taking this medicine, they usually go away gradually within 2 to 12 weeks after you stop taking this medicine. If you have any questions about this, check with your doctor.

For patients taking amantadine to prevent or treat flu infections:
• If your symptoms do not improve within a few days, or if they become worse, check with your doctor.

For patients taking amantadine for Parkinson's disease:
• **Patients with Parkinson's disease must be careful not to overdo physical activities as their condition improves and body movements become easier,** since injuries resulting from falls may occur. Such activities must be gradually increased to give your body time to adjust to changing balance, circulation, and coordination.

• Some patients may notice that this medicine gradually loses its effect while they are taking it regularly for a few months. If you notice this, check with your doctor. Your doctor may want to adjust the dose or stop the medicine for a while and then restart it to restore its effect.

• **Do not suddenly stop taking this medicine without first checking with your doctor** since your Parkinson's disease may get worse very quickly. Your doctor may want you to reduce your dose gradually before stopping completely.

Side Effects of This Medicine

Along with its needed effects, a medicine may cause some unwanted effects. Although not all of these side effects appear very often, when they do occur they may require medical attention. Check with your doctor as soon as possible if any of the following side effects occur:

More common
    Confusion, especially in elderly patients
    Hallucinations (seeing, hearing, or feeling things that are not there)
    Mood or other mental changes

Less common
    Difficult urination, especially in elderly patients
    Fainting

Rare
    Slurred speech
    Sore throat and fever
    Uncontrolled rolling of eyes

Usually only with long-term therapy
    Swelling of feet or lower legs
    Unexplained shortness of breath
    Weight gain (rapid)

Signs of overdose
    Confusion (severe)
    Convulsions (seizures)
    Mood or other mental changes (severe)
    Trouble in sleeping or nightmares (severe)

Other side effects may occur which usually do not require medical attention. These side effects may go away during treatment as your body adjusts to the medicine. However, check with your doctor if any of the following side effects continue or are bothersome:

More common
    Difficulty concentrating
    Dizziness or lightheadedness
    Irritability
    Loss of appetite

Nausea
Nervousness
Purplish red, net-like, blotchy spots on skin
Trouble in sleeping or nightmares

Less common or rare
Blurred vision
Constipation
Dry mouth, nose, and throat
Headache
Skin rash
Unusual tiredness or weakness
Vomiting

Other side effects not listed above may also occur in some patients. If you notice any other effects, check with your doctor.

ANESTHETICS (Topical)

This information applies to the following medicines:

Benzocaine (BEN-zoe-kane)
Butamben (byoo-TAM-ben)
Cyclomethycaine (sye-kloe-METH-i-kane)
Dibucaine (DYE-byoo-kane)
Lidocaine (LYE-doe-kane)
Pramoxine (pra-MOX-een)
Tetracaine (TET-ra-kane)

Some commonly used brand names and other names are:	Generic names:
aeroCAINE‡	
aeroTHERM‡	
Americaine	
Anbesol‡	
Benzocal	
BiCozene‡	
Burntame‡	
Chiggerex‡	
Chiggertox‡	Benzocaine†
Dermacoat‡	
Derma-Medicone‡	
Dermoplast‡	
Ethyl aminobenzoate	
Foille‡	
Ivy-Dry Cream‡	
Lanacane‡	
Medicone Dressing‡	
Soft-N-Soothe‡	
Solarcaine‡	
Tega Caine‡	Benzocaine†
Unguentine Spray	
Velvacaine A&O‡	
Butesin Picrate	
Butyl aminobenzoate	Butamben
Surfacaine	Cyclomethycaine
Nupercainal	Dibucaine
Bactine‡	
Clinicaine‡	
Lida-Mantle	
Lignocaine	
Mercurochrome II‡	Lidocaine†
Unguentine Plus‡	
Xylocaine	
Proxine	
Tronothane	Pramoxine
Pontocaine Cream	
Pontocaine Ointment‡	Tetracaine

†Generic name product may also be available (benzocaine cream and lidocaine ointment only).

‡Contains other active ingredients in addition to the topical local anesthetic.

This medicine belongs to a group of medicines known as topical local anesthetics (an-ess-THET-iks). Topical anesthetics are used to relieve the pain, itching, and redness of minor skin disorders. These include sunburn or other minor burns, insect bites or stings, poison ivy, poison oak, and minor cuts and scratches.

Topical anesthetics deaden the nerve endings in the skin. They do not cause drowsiness or unconsciousness as general anesthetics used for surgery do.

Benzocaine (present in many of these topical medicines) may be absorbed through the skin of young children and cause unwanted effects. Before benzocaine is used for children under 2 years of age, you should discuss the use of it with your doctor.

Many of the products containing topical anesthetics also contain other ingredients. The following information applies mostly to the local anesthetics contained in these products. However, if you have any questions about the other ingredients, check with your doctor, nurse, or pharmacist.

Most topical anesthetics are available without a prescription; however, your doctor may have special instructions on the proper use and dose for your medical problem.

Before Using This Medicine

Before you use a topical anesthetic, check with your doctor, nurse, or pharmacist:

—if you have ever had any unusual or allergic reaction to this medicine or to a local anesthetic, especially when applied to the skin or other areas of the body.

—if you have ever had any unusual or allergic reaction to para-aminobenzoic acid or PABA (present in some sun screens), to parabens (preservatives in many foods and medicines), or to para-phenylenediamine (a hair dye).

—if you are allergic to any substance, such as other preservatives or dyes. Most medicines contain more than their active ingredient. Your doctor or pharmacist can help you avoid products that may cause a problem.

—if you are pregnant or if you intend to become pregnant while using this medicine. Although topical anesthetics have not been shown to cause problems in humans, the chance always exists. Studies on birth defects have not been done in humans.

—if you are breast-feeding an infant. Although topical anesthetics have not been shown to cause problems, the chance always exists.

—if you have any of the following medical problems:
>   Infection at or near place of application
>   Large sores, broken skin, or severe injury at area of application

—if you are planning to use one of the products containing benzocaine, butamben, cyclomethycaine, or tetracaine and are now taking any of the following medicines or types of medicine:
>   Antimyasthenics (medicine for myasthenia gravis)
>   Long-acting eye drops or ointment for glaucoma, including demecarium, echothiophate, or isoflurophate
>   Sulfonamides (sulfa medicine).

–if you are planning to use one of the products containing lidocaine and are also taking any of the following medicines:
>   Acebutolol
>   Atenolol
>   Cimetidine
>   Labetalol
>   Metoprolol
>   Nadolol
>   Oxprenolol
>   Pindolol
>   Propranolol
>   Timolol

Proper Use of This Medicine

For safe and effective use of this medicine:
- Follow your doctor's instructions if this medicine was prescribed.

- Follow the manufacturer's package directions if you are treating yourself.

- Unless otherwise directed by your doctor, **do not use this medicine on large areas, especially if the skin is broken or scraped. Also, do not use it more often than directed on the package label, or for more than a few days at a time.** To do so may increase the chance of absorption through the skin and the chance of unwanted effects.

This medicine should be used only for problems being treated by your doctor or those listed in the package directions. **Check with your doctor before using it for other problems, especially if you think that an infection may be present.** This medicine should not be used to treat certain kinds of skin infections or for treating serious problems, such as severe burns.

Read the package label very carefully to see if the product contains any alcohol. Alcohol is flammable and can catch on fire. **Do not use any product containing alcohol near a fire or open flame, or while smoking. Also, do not smoke after applying one of these products until after it has completely dried.**

If you are using this medicine on your face, **be very careful not to get it in your eyes.** If you are using an aerosol or spray form of this medicine, spray it on your hand or an applicator (for example, a sterile gauze pad or a cotton swab) before applying it to your face.

For patients using butamben:
- Butamben may stain clothing. To avoid this, do not touch your clothing while applying the medicine. Also, cover the area with a loose bandage after applying butamben in order to protect your clothes.

If your doctor has ordered you to use this medicine according to a regular schedule and you miss a dose, use it as soon as possible. However, if it is almost time for your next dose, skip the missed dose and use your next dose at the regularly scheduled time.

How to store aerosol spray forms of this medicine:
- Store away from heat and direct light.
- **Keep out of the reach of children.**

- Do not store in the bathroom medicine cabinet because the heat or moisture may cause the medicine to break down.
- Keep the medicine from freezing.
- Do not puncture, break, or burn the aerosol container.
- Do not keep outdated medicine or medicine no longer needed.

How to store other forms of this medicine:
- Store away from heat and direct light.
- **Keep out of the reach of children.**
- Do not store in the bathroom medicine cabinet because the heat or moisture may cause the medicine to break down.
- Keep the medicine from freezing.
- Do not keep outdated medicine or medicine no longer needed. Flush the contents of the container down the toilet, unless otherwise directed.

Precautions While Using This Medicine

Stop using this medicine and check with your doctor:

—**if your condition does not improve within a few days, or if it gets worse.**

—**if the area you are treating becomes infected.**

—**if you notice a skin rash, burning, stinging, swelling, or any other sign of new irritation that was not present when you began using this medicine.**

—**if you swallow any of the medicine.**

Side Effects of This Medicine

Along with its needed effects, a medicine may cause some unwanted effects. Although not all of these side effects appear very often, when they do occur they may require medical attention. **Check with your doctor immediately** if any of the following side effects occur:

Less common
　　Swelling of skin, mouth, or throat

Signs of too much medicine being absorbed by the body—very rare

Blurred or double vision
Convulsions (seizures)
Dizziness
Drowsiness
Ringing or buzzing in the ears
Shivering or trembling
Unusual anxiety, excitement, nervousness, or restlessness
Unusual increase in sweating
Unusually slow or irregular heartbeat
Unusual paleness

Also, check with your doctor as soon as possible if any of the following side effects occur:

Burning, stinging, or tenderness not present before treatment
Skin rash, redness, itching, or hives

Other side effects not listed above may also occur in some patients. If you notice any other effects, check with your doctor.

ANTACIDS (Oral)

Note: For quick reference the following antacids are numbered to match the corresponding brand names.

This information applies to the following medicines:

1. Alumina (a-LOO-mi-na) and Magnesia (mag-NEE-zha)
2. Alumina, Magnesia, and Calcium Carbonate (KAL-see-um KAR-boe-nate)
3. Alumina, Magnesia, and Simethicone (si-METH-i-kone)
4. Alumina and Magnesium Carbonate (mag-NEE-zhum KAR-boe-nate)
5. Alumina, Magnesium Carbonate, and Calcium Carbonate
6. Alumina, Magnesium Carbonate, and Magnesium Oxide (OX-ide)
7. Alumina and Magnesium Trisilicate (mag-NEE-zhum trye-SILL-i-kate)
8. Alumina, Magnesium Trisilicate, and Sodium Bicarbonate (SOE-dee-um bye-KAR-boe-nate)
9. Aluminum Carbonate (a-LOO-mi-num KAR-boe-nate), Basic
10. Aluminum Hydroxide (hye-DROX-ide)†
11. Calcium Carbonate†
12. Calcium Carbonate and Magnesia
13. Calcium and Magnesium Carbonates
14. Calcium and Magnesium Carbonates and Magnesium Oxide
15. Dihydroxyaluminum Aminoacetate (dye-hye-DROX-ee-a-LOO-mi-num a-mee-noe-ASS-e-tate)
16. Dihydroxyaluminum Aminoacetate, Magnesia, and Alumina
17. Dihydroxyaluminum Sodium (SOE-dee-um) Carbonate
18. Magaldrate (MAG-al-drate)
19. Magaldrate and Simethicone
20. Magnesia, Milk of†
21. Magnesium Carbonate (mag-NEE-zhum KAR-boe-nate) and Sodium Bicarbonate
22. Magnesium Oxide (mag-NEE-zhum OX-ide)
23. Magnesium Trisilicate
24. Magnesium Trisilicate, Alumina, and Magnesia
25. Magnesium Trisilicate, Alumina, and Magnesium Carbonate
26. Simethicone, Alumina, Magnesium Carbonate, and Magnesia

Some commonly used brand names:

Alagel[10]	Calglycine[11]
Algenic Alka[1]	Camalox[2]
Alka-Mints[11]	Chooz[11]
Alkets[14]	Creamalin[1]
Almacone[3]	Delcid[1]
Almacone II[3]	Dialume[10]
Alma-Mag Improved[3]	Dicarbosil[11]
Alma-Mag #4 Improved[3]	Di-Gel[3] [26]
ALternaGEL[10]	Diovol[*3]
Alu-Cap[10]	Diovol Ex[*1]
Aludrox[1]	Duracid[5]
Alumid[1]	Equilet[11]
Alumid Plus[3]	Escot[25]
Alu-Tab[10]	Estomul-M[4] [6]
Amitone[11]	Gaviscon[4] [7]
Amphojel[10]	Gaviscon-2[7]
Amphojel 500[*1]	Gelamal[1]
Amphojel Plus[*3]	Gelusil[3]
AntaGel[3]	Gelusil[*1]
AntaGel-II[3]	Gelusil-400[*1]
Basaljel[9]	Gelusil-II[3]
Bisodol[12] [21]	Gelusil Extra
Calcilac[11]	Strength[*1]
	Gelusil-M[3]

Gustalac[11]
Kolantyl[1]
Kudrox[1]
Lo-Sal[12]
Lowsium[18]
Lowsium Plus[19]
Maalox[1]
Maalox No. 1[1]
Maalox No. 2[1]
Maalox Plus[3]
Maalox TC[1]
Magmalin[1]
Magnagel[4]
Magnatril[24]
Mag-Ox 400[22]
Maox[22]
Marblen[13]
Mi-Acid[3]
Mintox[1]
M.O.M.[20]
Mygel[3]
Mygel II[3]
Mylanta[3]
Mylanta-2*[3]
Mylanta-2 Extra
  Strength*[3]
Mylanta-II[3]
Nephrox[10]
Neutralca-S*[1]

Noralac[25]
Pama No. 1[11]
Par-Mag[22]
Phillips' Milk of
  Magnesia[20]
Riopan[18]
Riopan Plus[19]
Robalate*[15]
Rolaids[17]
Rolox[1]
Rulox[1]
Rulox No. 1[1]
Rulox No. 2[1]
Silain-Gel[3]
Simaal Gel[3]
Simaal 2 Gel[3]
Simeco[3]
Spastosed[13]
Tempo[26]
Titracid[11]
Titralac[11]
Tralmag[16]
Triconsil[6]
Tums[11]
Tums E-X[11]
Univol*[1]
Uro-Mag[22]
WinGel[1]

---

*Not available in the United States.
†Generic name product may also be available.

Antacids are taken by mouth to relieve heartburn, sour stomach, or acid indigestion. They work by neutralizing the excess stomach acid. Some antacid combinations also contain simethicone. Simethicone may relieve the painful symptoms of too much gas in the stomach and intestines. Antacids alone or in combination with simethicone may be used to treat the symptoms of stomach or duodenal ulcers.

With larger doses than those used for the antacid effect, magnesium oxide and milk of magnesia antacids produce a laxative effect. The information that follows applies only to their use as an antacid.

Some antacids, like aluminum carbonate and aluminum hydroxide, may be prescribed with a low-phosphate diet to treat hyperphosphatemia (too much phosphate in the blood). Aluminum carbonate and aluminum hydroxide may also be used with a low-phosphate diet to prevent the formation of some kinds of kidney stones. Aluminum hydroxide may also be used for other conditions as determined by your doctor.

Calcium carbonate may also be used to prevent or treat hypocalcemia (not enough calcium in the blood). In addition it may be used as a dietary supplement for patients who are unable to get enough calcium in their regular diet or have a need for more calcium, when recommended by their doctor. The information about calcium carbonate that follows applies only when used as an antacid.

Antacids should not be given to young children (up to 6 years of age) unless prescribed by their doctor. Since children cannot usually describe their symptoms very well, a doctor should check the child before giving this medicine. This is to prevent an unknown condition from getting worse and to avoid causing unwanted effects in the child. In addition, magnesium-containing medicines may cause serious side effects when given to very young children, especially those with kidney disease or who are dehydrated.

These medicines are available without a prescription; however, your doctor may have special instructions on the proper use and dose for your medical problem.

Before Using This Medicine

Before you use this medicine, check with your doctor, nurse, or pharmacist:

—if you have ever had any unusual or allergic reaction to aluminum-, calcium-, magnesium-, sodium bicarbonate-, or simethicone-containing medicines.

—if you are on a low-salt, low-sugar, or any other special diet, or if you are allergic to any substance, such as sulfites or other preservatives or dyes. Most medicines contain more than their active ingredient. Your doctor or pharmacist can help you avoid products that may cause a problem.

—if you are pregnant or if you intend to become pregnant while taking this medicine. Studies have not been done in either animals or humans; however, there are reports of antacids causing side effects in babies whose mothers took antacids for a long period of time, especially in high doses.

Also, sodium-containing medicines should be avoided if you tend to retain (keep) body water.

—if you are breast-feeding an infant, although these medicines have not been shown to cause problems in humans.

—if you have any of the following medical problems:

Appendicitis (or signs of)
Bone fractures
Colitis
Colostomy
Constipation (severe and continuing)
Diarrhea (chronic)
Edema (swelling of feet or lower legs)
Heart disease
High blood pressure
Ileostomy
Inflamed bowel
Intestinal blockage
Intestinal or rectal bleeding (of unknown cause)
Kidney disease
Liver disease
Sarcoidosis
Toxemia of pregnancy
Underactive parathyroid glands

—if you are now taking *any* other medicines by mouth, especially:

Adrenocorticoids
Cellulose sodium phosphate
Ketoconazole
Mecamylamine
Methenamine
Sodium polystyrene sulfonate resin (SPSR)
Tetracyclines

Proper Use of This Medicine

For safe and effective use of this medicine:

• Follow your doctor's instructions if this medicine was prescribed.

• Follow the manufacturer's package directions if you are treating yourself.

If you are taking the chewable tablet form of this medicine, chew the tablets well before swallowing. This is to allow the medicine to work faster and be more effective.

When taking this medicine for a stomach or duodenal ulcer:
—take it exactly as directed and for the full time of treatment as ordered by your doctor to obtain maximum relief of your symptoms.

—take it 1 to 3 hours after meals and at bedtime for best results, unless otherwise directed by your doctor.

If this medicine has been ordered by your doctor to be taken on a regular schedule and you miss a dose, take it as soon as possible. However, if it is almost time for your next dose, skip the missed dose and go back to your regular dosing schedule. Do not double doses.

How to store this medicine:

• Store away from heat and direct light.

• **Keep out of the reach of children.**

• Do not store in the bathroom medicine cabinet because the heat or moisture may cause the medicine to break down.

• Keep the liquid dosage form of this medicine from freezing.

• Do not keep outdated medicine or medicine no longer needed. Flush the contents of the container down the toilet, unless otherwise directed.

Precautions While Using This Medicine

Before you have any test in which a radiopharmaceutical will be used, tell the doctor in charge that you are taking this medicine. The results of the test may be affected by aluminum-containing antacids.

If this medicine has been ordered by your doctor and if you will be taking it in large doses, or for a long period of time, your doctor should check your progress at regular visits. This is to make sure the medicine does not cause unwanted effects.

Patients on a sodium-restricted diet—This medicine may contain a large amount of sodium. If you have any questions about this, check with your doctor or pharmacist.

Do not take this medicine:

—**if you have any signs of appendicitis or inflamed bowel** (such as stomach or lower abdominal pain, cramping, bloating, soreness, nausea, or vomiting). Instead, check with your doctor as soon as possible.

—**within 1 to 2 hours of taking other medicine by mouth.** To do so may keep the other medicine from working as well.

—**for more than 2 weeks** or if the problem comes back often. Instead, check with your doctor. Antacids should be used only for occasional relief, unless otherwise directed by your doctor.

For patients taking calcium-containing antacids:

• **Do not take with large amounts of milk or milk products.** To do so may increase the chance of side effects.

Side Effects of This Medicine

Along with its needed effects, a medicine may cause some unwanted effects. Although the following side effects occur very rarely when this medicine is taken as recommended, they may be more likely to occur if:

—too much medicine is taken.
—it is taken in large doses.
—it is taken for a long period of time.
—it is taken by patients with kidney disease.

Check with your doctor as soon as possible if any of the following side effects or signs of overdose occur:

For aluminum-containing antacids (including magaldrate)
  Bone pain
  Constipation (severe and continuing)
  Feeling of discomfort (continuing)
  Loss of appetite (continuing)
  Mood or mental changes
  Muscle weakness
  Swelling of wrists or ankles
  Unusual loss of weight

For calcium-containing antacids
  Constipation (severe and continuing)
  Cramping
  Difficult or painful urination
  Frequent urge to urinate
  Headache (continuing)
  Loss of appetite (continuing)
  Mood or mental changes
  Muscle pain or twitching
  Nausea or vomiting
  Nervousness or restlessness
  Stomach or lower abdominal pain (severe)
  Unpleasant taste in mouth
  Unusually slow breathing
  Unusual tiredness or weakness

For magnesium-containing antacids (including magaldrate)
  Difficult or painful urination (with magnesium trisilicate)
  Dizziness or lightheadedness

Irregular heartbeat
Mood or mental changes
Unusual tiredness or weakness

For sodium bicarbonate–containing antacids

Frequent urge to urinate
Headache (continuing)
Loss of appetite (continuing)
Mood or mental changes
Muscle pain or twitching
Nausea or vomiting
Nervousness or restlessness
Swelling of feet or lower legs
Unpleasant taste in mouth
Unusually slow breathing
Unusual tiredness or weakness

Other side effects may occur which usually do not require medical attention. These side effects may go away during treatment as your body adjusts to the medicine. However, check with your doctor if any of the following side effects continue or are bothersome:

More common
Belching
Chalky taste
Swelling of stomach or gas

Less common
Constipation (mild)
Diarrhea or laxative effect
Speckling or whitish discoloration of stools
Stomach cramps

Other side effects not listed above may also occur in some patients. If you notice any other effects, check with your doctor.

ANTICOAGULANTS (Systemic)

This information applies to the following medicines:

Anisindione (an-iss-in-DYE-one)
Dicumarol (dye-KOO-ma-role)
Phenindione (fen-in-DYE-one)

Phenprocoumon (fen-proe-KOO-mon)
Warfarin (WAR-far-in)

This information does *not* apply to heparin.

Some commonly used brand names are:	Generic names:
Miradon	Anisindione
	Dicumarol†
	Phenindione*
Liquamar	Phenprocoumon
Coumadin Panwarfin Warfilone* Warnerin*	Warfarin†

*Not available in the United States.
†Available by generic name.

Anticoagulants decrease the clotting ability of the blood and therefore help to prevent harmful clots from forming in the blood vessels. They are given by mouth; warfarin is also given by injection. These medicines are sometimes called blood thinners, although they do not actually thin the blood. They also will not dissolve clots which already have formed, but they may prevent the clots from becoming larger and causing more serious problems. They are often used as treatment for certain blood vessel, heart, and lung conditions.

In order for an anticoagulant to help you without causing serious bleeding, it must be used properly and all of the precautions concerning its use must be followed exactly. Be sure that you have discussed the use of this medicine with your doctor. It is very important that you understand all of your doctor's orders and that you are willing and able to follow them exactly.

Anticoagulants are available only with your doctor's prescription.

Before Using This Medicine

In order to decide on the best treatment for your medical problem, your doctor should be told:

—if you have ever had any unusual or allergic reaction to anticoagulants.

—if you are on a low-salt, low-sugar, or any other special diet, or if you are allergic to any substance, such as sulfites or other preservatives. Most medicines contain more than their active ingredient. Your doctor or pharmacist can help you avoid products that may cause a problem.

—if you are pregnant or if you intend to become pregnant while taking this medicine. Anticoagulants may cause birth defects. They may also cause other problems affecting the physical or mental growth of the fetus. In addition, use of this medicine during the last 6 months of pregnancy may increase the chance of severe, possibly fatal, bleeding in the fetus. If taken during the last few weeks of pregnancy, anticoagulants may cause severe bleeding in both the fetus and mother before or during delivery and in the newborn infant.

Do not begin taking this medicine during pregnancy, and do not become pregnant while taking this medicine, unless you have first discussed the possible effects of this medicine with your doctor. Also, if you suspect that you may be pregnant and you are already taking an anticoagulant, check with your doctor at once. Your doctor may suggest that you take a different anticoagulant, which is less likely to harm the fetus or the newborn infant, during all or part of your pregnancy. Anticoagulants may also cause severe bleeding in the mother if taken soon after the baby is born.

—if you are breast-feeding an infant. Most anticoagulants pass into the breast milk and may cause bleeding problems in nursing infants.

—if you have any other medical problems, or if you are now being treated by any other physician or dentist, since many medical problems and treatments affect the way your body responds to this medicine.

—if you have recently had any of the following conditions or medical procedures:

Childbirth
Falls or blows to the body or head
Fever lasting more than a couple of days
Heavy or unusual menstrual bleeding
Insertion of intrauterine device (IUD)
Medical or dental surgery
Severe or continuing diarrhea
Spinal anesthesia
X-ray treatment

—if you are taking **any** medicine, including over-the-counter (OTC) or nonprescription medicines such as aspirin, laxatives, or antacids.

Proper Use of This Medicine

Take this medicine only as directed by your doctor. Do not take more or less of it, do not take it more often, and do not take it for a longer period of time than your doctor ordered.

Your doctor should check your progress at regular visits. A blood test must be taken regularly to see how fast your blood is clotting. This will help your doctor decide on the proper amount of anticoagulant you should be taking each day.

If you miss a dose of this medicine, take it as soon as possible. Then go back to your regular dosing schedule. If you do not remember until the next day, do not take the missed dose at all and do not double the next one. **Doubling the dose may cause bleeding.** Instead, go back to your regular dosing schedule. It is recommended that you keep a record of each dose as you take it in order to avoid mistakes. Also, be sure to give your doctor a record of any doses you miss. If you have any questions about this, check with your doctor.

How to store this medicine:

• Store away from heat and direct light.

• **Keep out of the reach of children.**

• Do not store in the bathroom medicine cabinet because the heat or moisture may cause the medicine to break down.

• Do not keep outdated medicine or medicine no longer needed. Flush the contents of the container down the toilet, unless otherwise directed.

Precautions While Using This Medicine

Tell all physicians and dentists you go to that you are taking this medicine.

Check with your doctor, nurse, or pharmacist before you start or stop taking any other medicine. This includes any over-the-counter (OTC) or nonprescription medicine, even aspirin or acetaminophen. Many medicines change the way this medicine affects your body. You may not be able to take the other medicine, or the dose of your anticoagulant may need to be changed.

It is recommended that you carry identification stating that you are using this medicine. If you have any questions about what kind of identification to carry, check with your doctor, nurse, or pharmacist.

While you are taking this medicine, it is very important that you avoid sports and activities which may cause you to be injured. Report to your doctor any falls, blows to the body or head, or other injuries, since serious internal bleeding may occur without your knowing about it.

Be careful to avoid cutting yourself. This includes taking special care in brushing your teeth and in shaving. Use a soft toothbrush and floss gently. Also, it is best to use an electric shaver rather than a blade.

Drinking too much alcohol may change the way this anticoagulant affects your body. You should not drink regularly on a daily basis or take more than 1 or 2 drinks at any time. If you have any questions about this, check with your doctor.

The foods that you eat may also affect the way that this medicine affects your body. Eat a normal, balanced diet while you are taking this medicine. Do not go on a reducing diet, make other changes in your eating habits, start taking vitamins, or begin using other nutrition supplements unless you have first checked with your doctor, nurse, or pharmacist. Also, check with your doctor if you are unable to eat for several days or if you have continuing stomach upset, diarrhea, or fever.

After you stop taking this medicine, your body will need time to recover before your blood clotting abilities return to normal. Your pharmacist or doctor can tell you how long this will take depending on which anticoagulant you were taking. Use the same caution during this period of time as you did while you were taking the anticoagulant.

Side Effects of This Medicine

Along with its needed effects, a medicine may cause some unwanted effects. Although not all of these side effects appear very often, when they do occur they may require medical attention. **Check**

with your doctor immediately if any of the following side effects occur:

Less common or rare
Blue or purple color of toes and pain in toes
Cloudy or dark urine
Difficult or painful urination
Sores, ulcers, or white spots in mouth or throat
Sore throat and fever or chills
Sudden decrease in amount of urine
Swelling of feet or lower legs
Unusual tiredness or weakness
Unusual weight gain
Yellowing of eyes or skin

Since many things can affect the way your body reacts to this medicine, you should always watch for signs of unusual bleeding. Unusual bleeding may mean that your body is getting more medicine than it needs. **Check with your doctor immediately if any of the following signs of overdose occur:**
Bleeding from gums when brushing teeth
Unexplained bruising or purplish areas on skin
Unexplained nosebleeds
Unusually heavy bleeding or oozing from cuts or wounds
Unusually heavy or unexpected menstrual bleeding

Signs of bleeding inside the body
Abdominal or stomach pain or swelling
Back pain or backaches
Blood in urine
Bloody or black tarry stools
Constipation
Coughing up blood
Dizziness
Headache (severe or continuing)
Joint pain, stiffness, or swelling
Vomiting blood or material that looks like coffee grounds

Also, check with your doctor as soon as possible if any of the following side effects occur:

Less common or rare
Diarrhea (more common for dicumarol)
Nausea or vomiting
Skin rash, hives, or itching
Stomach cramps or pain

If you are taking anisindione tablets or phenindione tablets:
• Depending on your diet, this medicine may cause the urine to turn orange. Since it may be hard to tell the difference between blood in the urine and this normal color change, check with your doctor if you notice any color change in your urine.

Other side effects may occur which usually do not require medical attention. These side effects may go away during treatment as your body adjusts to the medicine. However, check with your doctor if any of the following side effects continue or are bothersome:

More common
Bloated stomach or gas (for dicumarol)
Less common
Blurred vision or other vision problems (for anisindione or phenindione)
Loss of appetite
Unusual hair loss

Other side effects not listed above may also occur in some patients. If you notice any other effects, check with your doctor.

ANTICONVULSANTS, HYDANTOIN (Systemic)

This information applies to the following medicines:

Ethotoin (ETH-oh-toyn)
Mephenytoin (me-FEN-i-toyn)
Phenytoin (FEN-i-toyn)

Some commonly used brand names and other names are:	Generic names:
Peganone	Ethotoin
Mesantoin	Mephenytoin

Dilantin
Dilantin Infatabs
Dilantin Kapseals
Dilantin-30 Pediatric   Phenytoin†
Dilantin-125
Diphenylan
Diphenylhydantoin
Novophenytoin*

---

*Not available in the United States.
†Generic name product may also be available.

Hydantoin anticonvulsants (hye-DAN-toyn an-tye-kon-VUL-sants) are used most often to control certain convulsions or seizures in the treatment of epilepsy. Phenytoin may also be used for other conditions as determined by your doctor.

These medicines act on the central nervous system (CNS) to reduce the number and severity of seizures. Hydantoin anticonvulsants may also produce some unwanted effects. These depend on the patient's individual condition, the amount of medicine taken, and the length of time it has been taken. It is important that you know what the side effects are and when to call your doctor.

Hydantoin anticonvulsants are available only with your doctor's prescription.

Before Using This Medicine

In order to decide on the best treatment for your medical problem, your doctor should be told:

—if you have had any unusual or allergic reaction to any hydantoin anticonvulsant medicine.

—if you are on a low-salt, low-sugar, or any other special diet, or if you are allergic to any substance, such as sulfites or other preservatives or dyes. Most medicines contain more than their active ingredient, and many liquid medicines contain alcohol. Your doctor or pharmacist can help you avoid products that may cause a problem.

—if you are pregnant or if you intend to become pregnant while using this medicine. Although most mothers who take medicine for seizure control deliver normal babies, there have been reports of increased birth defects when these medicines were used during pregnancy. It is not definitely known if any of these medicines are the cause of such problems.

Also, pregnancy may cause a change in the way hydantoin anticonvulsants are absorbed in your body. You may have more seizures, even though you are taking your medicine regularly. Your doctor may need to increase the anticonvulsant dose during your pregnancy.

In addition, when taken during pregnancy, there may be bleeding problems in the mother during delivery and in the newborn. This may be prevented by administration of vitamin K to the mother 1 month before and during delivery, and to the baby immediately after birth.

—if you are breast-feeding an infant. Phenytoin passes into the breast milk in small amounts. Although it has not been shown to cause unwanted effects in the breast-fed infant, the chance always exists. It may be necessary for you to take another medicine or to stop breast-feeding during treatment. It is not known whether ethotoin or mephenytoin pass into breast milk.

—if you have any of the following medical problems:
   Alcoholism
   Blood disease
   Diabetes mellitus (sugar diabetes)
   Heart disease

Kidney disease
Liver disease
Thyroid disease

—if you are now taking any of the following medicines or types of medicine:

Acetaminophen
Adrenocorticoids (cortisone-like medicines)
Anticoagulants (blood thinners)
Antidiabetics, oral (diabetes medicine you take by mouth)
Birth-control pills
Calcifediol
Chloramphenicol
Cimetidine
Disulfiram (medicine for alcoholism)
Doxycycline
Folic acid (contained in some vitamin formulas)
Insulin
Isoniazid (INH)
Levodopa
Medicine for heart disease
Medicine for mental illness
Medicine for asthma
Methadone
Methylphenidate
Miconazole
Nomifensine
Other anticonvulsants (medicine for seizures)
Oxyphenbutazone
Phenylbutazone
Pimozide
Sulfonamides (sulfa drugs)
Thyroid medicine
Vitamin D

—if you are now taking antidepressants (medicine for depression) such as:

Amitriptyline
Amoxapine
Clomipramine
Desipramine
Doxepin
Imipramine
Maprotiline
Nomifensine
Nortriptyline
Protriptylne
Trazodone
Trimipramine

—if you are now taking or have taken within the past 2 weeks monoamine oxidase (MAO) inhibitors such as:

Furazolidone
Isocarboxazid
Pargyline
Phenelzine
Procarbazine
Tranylcypromine

Proper Use of This Medicine

Take this medicine every day exactly as ordered by your doctor in order to control your medical problem. To help you remember, try to get into the habit of taking your medicine at the same times each day.

If this medicine upsets your stomach, take it with food or milk, unless otherwise directed by your doctor.

For patients taking the liquid form of this medicine:
• Shake the bottle well before using.
• Use a specially marked measuring spoon or other device to measure each dose accurately since the average household teaspoon may not hold the right amount of liquid.

For patients taking the chewable tablet form of this medicine:
• Chew or crush the tablet before swallowing it.

If you miss a dose of this medicine and your dosing schedule is one dose to be taken: Once a day—
Take the missed dose as soon as possible. However, if you do not remember the missed dose until the next day, skip it and go back to your regular dosing schedule. Do not double doses.

Several times a day—
Take the missed dose as soon as possible. However, if it is within 4 hours of your next dose, skip the missed dose and go back to your regular dosing schedule. Do not double doses.

If you miss doses for 2 or more days, check with your doctor.

How to store this medicine:

• Store away from heat and direct light.

• **Keep out of the reach of children.**

• Do not store in the bathroom medicine cabinet because the heat or moisture may cause the medicine to break down.

• Keep the liquid from freezing.

• Do not keep outdated medicine or medicine no longer needed. Flush the contents of the container down the toilet, unless otherwise directed.

Precautions While Using This Medicine

Your doctor should check your progress at regular visits, especially during the first few months you take this medicine. During this time the amount of medicine you are taking may have to be changed often to meet your individual needs.

Do not stop or start taking any other medicine without your doctor's advice. Other medicines may affect the way this medicine works.

Drinking alcohol may change the way this medicine works. Check with your doctor before drinking alcoholic beverages while you are taking this medicine.

Do not change brands or dosage forms of phenytoin without first checking with your doctor. Different products may not work the same way. If you refill your medicine and it looks different, check with your pharmacist.

If you have been taking this medicine regularly for several weeks or more, do not suddenly stop taking it. Your doctor may want you to reduce gradually the amount you are taking before stopping completely.

Your doctor may want you to carry a medical identification card or bracelet stating that you are taking this medicine.

Diabetic patients—This medicine may affect blood sugar levels. If you notice a change in the results of your urine sugar tests or if you have any questions, check with your doctor.

Before having any kind of surgery (including dental surgery), or emergency treatment, tell the physician or dentist in charge that you are taking this medicine.

This medicine may cause some people to become dizzy, lightheaded, drowsy, or less alert than they are normally. After you have taken this medicine for a while, this effect may not be so bothersome. **Make sure you know how you react to this medicine before you drive, use machines, or do other jobs that require you to be alert.**

For patients taking phenytoin or mephenytoin:

• In some patients (usually younger patients), tenderness, swelling, or bleeding of the gums may appear soon after starting treatment with phenytoin. Brushing and flossing your teeth carefully and regularly and massaging your gums may help prevent this. **See your dentist regularly to have your teeth cleaned. Check with your doctor or dentist if you have any questions about how to take care of your teeth and gums, or if you notice any tenderness, swelling, or bleeding of your gums.**

Side Effects of This Medicine

Along with its needed effects, a medicine may cause some unwanted effects. Although not all of these side effects appear very often, when they do occur they may require medical attention. Check with your doctor as soon as possible if any of the following side effects or signs of overdose occur:

More common

Behavior changes
Bleeding, tender, or enlarged gums
Clumsiness or unsteadiness (rare with ethotoin)
Confusion
Continuous, uncontrolled back-and-forth or rolling eye movements
Increase in convulsions (seizures)
Mood or mental changes
Muscle weakness
Slurring of speech
Trembling of hands
Unusual excitement, nervousness, or irritability

Less common

Enlarged glands in neck or underarms
Fever
Skin rash

Rare

Bone malformations
Darkening of urine
Frequent breaking of bones
Light gray–colored stools
Loss of appetite
Slowed growth
Sore throat and fever
Stomach pain (severe)
Unusual bleeding or bruising
Yellowing of eyes or skin

Signs of overdose

Blurred or double vision
Clumsiness or unsteadiness
Confusion
Dizziness or drowsiness (severe)
Hallucinations (seeing, feeling, or hearing things that are not there)
Nausea
Slurred speech
Staggering walk
Uncontrolled eye movements

Other side effects may occur which usually do not require medical attention. These side effects may go away during treatment as your body adjusts to the medicine. However, check with your doctor if any of the following side effects continue or are bothersome:

More common

Constipation
Dizziness (mild)
Drowsiness (mild)
Unusual and excessive hair growth on body and face (more common with phenytoin)
Nausea and vomiting

Less common or rare

Diarrhea (with ethotoin)
Enlargement of jaw
Headache
Muscle twitching
Thickening of lips
Trouble in sleeping
Widening of nose tip

The above side effects, especially the signs of overdose, are more likely to occur in elderly patients and patients with liver disease, who are usually more sensitive to the effects of hydantoin anticonvulsants.

Other side effects not listed above may also occur in some patients. If you notice any other effects, check with your doctor.

ANTIDEPRESSANTS, MONOAMINE OXIDASE (MAO) INHIBITOR (Systemic)

This information applies to the following medicines:

Isocarboxazid (eye-soe-kar-BOX-a-zid)
Phenelzine (FEN-el-zeen)
Tranylcypromine (tran-ill-SIP-roe-meen)

This information does *not* apply to furazolidone, pargyline, or procarbazine.

Some commonly used brand names are:	Generic names:
Marplan	Isocarboxazid
Nardil	Phenelzine
Parnate	Tranylcypromine

These medicines are also known as MAO inhibitors or MAOIs. They are taken by mouth to relieve certain types of mental depression. They do this by inhibiting an enzyme in the nervous system known as monoamine oxidase (MAO).

It is important to avoid certain foods, beverages, and medicines while you are being treated with an MAOI. Your pharmacist or doctor will help you obtain a list of them that you can carry in your wallet or purse as a reminder.

MAO inhibitors are available only with your doctor's prescription.

Before Using This Medicine

In order to decide on the best treatment for your medical problem, your doctor should be told:

—if you have ever had any unusual or allergic reaction to monoamine oxidase inhibitors.

—if you are on a low-salt, low-sugar, or any other special diet, or if you are allergic to any substance, such as sulfites or other preservatives or dyes. Most medicines contain more than their active ingredient. Your doctor or pharmacist can help you avoid products that may cause a problem.

—if you are pregnant or if you intend to become pregnant while taking this medicine. Studies have not been done in humans. However, studies in animals have shown that MAO inhibitors caused a reduced growth rate and an increase in excitement in the newborn when very large doses were given to the mother.

—if you are breast feeding an infant. MAO inhibitors have not been shown to cause problems in humans; however, studies in animals have shown that this medicine passes into breast milk.

—if you have any of the following medical problems:

Alcoholism
Angina (chest pain)
Asthma or bronchitis
Diabetes mellitus (sugar diabetes)
Epilepsy
Headache (severe or frequent)
Heart or blood vessel disease
High blood pressure
Kidney disease
Liver disease
Mental illness (or history of)
Overactive thyroid
Parkinson's disease
Pheochromocytoma (PCC)

—if you have recently had a stroke or heart attack.

—if you are planning to have surgery of any kind.

—if you are now taking any of the following medicines or types of medicine:

Antidiabetics, oral (sugar diabetes medicine you take by mouth)
Antihypertensives (high blood pressure medicine)
Appetite suppressants (medicine for reducing appetite)
Asthma medicine
Caffeine-containing medicine
Diuretics (water pills)
Insulin
Levodopa
Nasal decongestants or other cold medicines
Nomifensine

—if you are now taking or have taken within the past 2 weeks any other monoamine oxidase (MAO) inhibitors including furazolidone, pargyline, or procarbazine.

—if you are now taking tricyclic anti-depressants (medicine for depression) such as:

Amitriptyline
Amoxapine
Clomipramine
Desipramine
Doxepin
Imipramine
Nortriptyline
Protriptyline
Trimipramine

—if you are now taking central nervous system (CNS) depressants such as:

Alcohol
Anticonvulsants (seizure medicine)
Antihistamines or medicine for hay fever, other allergies, or colds
Barbiturates
Muscle relaxants
Narcotics
Prescription pain medicine
Sedatives, tranquilizers, or sleeping medicine

—if you use cocaine. Cocaine use by persons taking MAO inhibitors, including furazolidone, pargyline, and procarbazine, may cause a severe increase in blood pressure.

Proper Use of This Medicine

Take this medicine only as directed by your doctor. Do not take more of it, do not take it more often, and do not take it for a longer period of time than your doctor ordered.

Sometimes this medicine must be taken for several weeks before you begin to feel better. **Your doctor should check your progress at regular visits.**

If you miss a dose of this medicine, take it as soon as possible. However, if it is within 2 hours of your next dose, skip the missed dose and go back to your regular dosing schedule. Do not double doses.

How to store this medicine:

• Store away from heat and direct light.

• **Keep out of the reach of children.**

• Do not store in the bathroom medicine cabinet because the heat or moisture may cause the medicine to break down.

• Do not keep outdated medicine or medicine no longer needed. Flush the contents of the container down the toilet, unless otherwise directed.

Precautions While Using This Medicine

Check with your doctor or hospital emergency room immediately if severe headache, stiff neck, chest pains, rapid heartbeat, or nausea and vomiting occur while you are taking this medicine. These may be symptoms of a serious side effect which should have a doctor's attention.

When taken with certain foods, drinks, or other medicines, MAO inhibitors can cause very dangerous reactions. To avoid such reactions, **obey the following rules of caution:**

• Do not eat foods that have a high tyramine content (most common in foods that are aged or fermented to increase their flavor), such as cheeses, yeast or meat extracts, fava or broad bean pods, smoked or pickled fish, beef or chicken liver, fermented sausage (bologna, pepperoni, salami, and summer sausage) or other unfresh meat, or any overripe fruit. If a list of these foods and beverages is not given to you, ask your doctor, nurse, or pharmacist to provide one.

• Do not drink alcoholic beverages, including beer and wines (especially chianti and other hearty red wines).

• Do not eat or drink any more than small amounts of caffeine-containing food or beverages such as chocolate, coffee, tea, or cola.

• Do not take any other medicine unless prescribed by your doctor. This especially includes over-the-counter (OTC) or nonprescription medicine such as that for colds (including nose drops), cough, asthma, hay fever, appetite control, or "keep awake" products.

Do not stop taking this medicine without first checking with your doctor. Your doctor may want you to reduce gradually the amount you are using before stopping completely.

After you stop using this medicine, you must continue to obey the rules of caution concerning food, drink, and other medicine for at least 2 weeks since they may continue to react with MAO inhibitors.

Before having any kind of surgery (including dental surgery) or emergency treatment, tell the physician or dentist in charge that you are using this medicine or have used it within the past 2 weeks.

Your doctor may want you to carry an identification card stating that you are using this medicine.

Patients with angina (chest pain)—This medicine may cause you to have an unusual feeling of health and energy. However, **do not suddenly increase the amount of exercise you get without discussing it with your doctor** since that could bring on an attack of angina.

Diabetic patients—This medicine may affect blood sugar levels. While you are using this medicine, be especially careful in testing for sugar in your urine. If you have any questions about this, check with your doctor.

Dizziness, lightheadedness, or fainting may occur, especially when you get up from a lying or sitting position. **Getting up slowly may help.** When you get up from lying down, sit on the edge of the bed with your feet dangling for 1 or 2 minutes. Then stand up slowly. If the problem continues or gets worse, check with your doctor.

This medicine may cause some people to become drowsy or less alert than they are normally. **Make sure you know how you react to this medicine before you drive, use machines, or do other jobs that require you to be alert.**

Side Effects of This Medicine

Along with its needed effects, a medicine may cause some unwanted effects. Although not all of these side effects appear very often, when they do occur they may require medical attention. **Stop taking this medicine and get emergency help immediately if any of the following side effects occur:**

Signs of unusually high blood pressure

Chest pain (severe)
Enlarged pupils
Headache (severe)
Increased sensitivity of eyes to light
Nausea and vomiting
Stiff or sore neck
Unusually rapid or slow heartbeat
Unusual sweating (possibly with fever or cold, clammy skin)

Check with your doctor as soon as possible if any of the following side effects occur:

More common

Dizziness or lightheadedness (severe), especially when getting up from a lying or sitting position

Less common

Diarrhea
Swelling of feet or lower legs
Unusual excitement or nervousness
Unusually rapid or pounding heartbeat

Rare

Dark urine
Skin rash
Yellowing of eyes and skin

Signs of overdose
  Anxiety
  Confusion
  Convulsions (seizures)
  Cool, clammy skin
  Dizziness (severe)
  Drowsiness (severe)
  Fever
  Hallucinations (seeing, hearing, or
    feeling things that are not there)
  High or low blood pressure
  Rapid and irregular pulse
  Sweating
  Trouble in sleeping (severe)
  Troubled breathing
  Unusual irritability

Other side effects may occur which usually do not require medical attention. These side effects may go away during treatment as your body adjusts to the medicine. However, check with your doctor if any of the following side effects continue or are bothersome:

More common
  Blurred vision
  Constipation
  Difficult urination
  Dizziness or lightheadedness, especially
    when getting up from a lying or sitting
    position
  Drowsiness
  Dry mouth
  Headache (mild)
  Increased appetite and weight gain
  Tiredness and weakness

Less common or rare
  Chills
  Decreased sexual ability
  Muscle twitching during sleep
  Restlessness
  Shakiness or trembling
  Trouble in sleeping
  Weakness

The above side effects are more likely to occur in elderly patients, who are usually more sensitive to the effects of monoamine oxidase inhibitor antidepressants.

Other side effects not listed above may also occur in some patients. If you notice any other effects, check with your doctor.

ANTIDEPRESSANTS, TRICYCLIC
(Systemic)

This information applies to the following medicines:

Amitriptyline (a-mee-TRIP-ti-leen)
Amoxapine (a-MOX-a-peen)
Clomipramine (cloe-MIP-ra-meen)
Desipramine (dess-IP-ra-meen)
Doxepin (DOX-e-pin)
Imipramine (im-IP-ra-meen)
Nortriptyline (nor-TRIP-ti-leen)
Protriptyline (proe-TRIP-ti-leen)
Trimipramine (trye-MIP-ra-meen)

Some commonly used brand names are:	Generic names:
Amitril Elavil Emitrip Endep Enovil SK-Amitriptyline	Amitriptyline†
Asendin	Amoxapine
Anafranil*	Clomipramine
Norpramin Pertofrane	Desipramine
Adapin Sinequan	Doxepin
Janimine SK-Pramine Tipramine Tofranil Tofranil-PM	Imipramine†
Aventyl Pamelor	Nortriptyline
Vivactil Triptil*	Protriptyline
Surmontil	Trimipramine

*Not available in the United States.
†Generic name product may also be available.

This medicine belongs to the group of medicines known as tricyclic antidepressants or "mood elevators." It is used to relieve mental depression and depression that sometimes occurs with anxiety.

One form of this medicine (imipramine) may be used to treat enuresis (bedwetting). Tricyclic antidepressants may also be used for other conditions as determined by your doctor.

These medicines are available only with your doctor's prescription.

Before Using This Medicine

In order to decide on the best treatment for your medical problem, your doctor should be told:

—if you have ever had an unusual or allergic reaction to any tricyclic antidepressant or maprotiline or trazodone.

—if you are on a low-salt, low-sugar, or any other special diet, or if you are allergic to any substance, such as sulfites or other preservatives or dyes. Most medicines contain more than their active ingredient, and many liquid medicines contain alcohol. Your doctor or pharmacist can help you avoid products that may cause a problem.

—if you are pregnant, or if you intend to become pregnant while taking this medicine. Studies have not been done in humans. However, there have been reports of newborns suffering from heart, breathing, and urinary problems when their mothers had taken tricyclic antidepressants immediately before delivery. Also, studies in animals have shown that some tricyclic antidepressants may cause unwanted effects in the fetus.

—if you are breast-feeding an infant. Although tricyclic antidepressants have not been shown to cause problems in humans, the chance always exists, since some of these medicines pass into breast milk.

—if you have any of the following medical problems:

Alcoholism
Asthma (history of)
Convulsions (seizures)
Difficult urination
Enlarged prostate
Glaucoma or increased eye pressure
Heart disease
High blood pressure
Kidney disease
Liver disease
Manic-depressive illness
Overactive thyroid
Schizophrenia
Stomach or intestinal problems

—if you are now taking *any* other medicines, including over-the-counter (OTC) or nonprescription medicine, especially the following:

Allergy medicine
Antihistamines
Barbiturates
Blood pressure medicine
Cold remedies
Hay fever medicine
Narcotics
Oral contraceptives (birth control pills)
Other medicine for depression
Pain medicine
Pimozide
Sedatives
Seizure medicine
Sleeping medicine
Thyroid medicine
Tranquilizers

—if you are now taking or have taken within the past 2 weeks monoamine oxidase (MAO) inhibitors such as:

Furazolidone
Isocarboxazid
Pargyline
Phenelzine
Procarbazine
Tranylcypromine

Proper Use of This Medicine

Take this medicine only as directed by your doctor, to benefit your condition as much as possible. Do not take more of it, do not take it more often, and do not take it for a longer period of time than your doctor ordered.

To lessen stomach upset, take this medicine with food, even for a daily bedtime dose, unless your doctor has told you to take it on an empty stomach.

For patients taking the oral liquid form of this medicine:

• This medicine is to be taken by mouth even though it may come in a dropper bottle. The amount you should take is to be measured with the specially marked dropper and diluted just before you take each dose. Dilute it with about ½ glass (4 ounces) of water, milk, citrus fruit juice, or prune juice. Do not mix this medicine with grape juice or carbonated beverages since these may decrease the medicine's activity.

• If your prescription is a liquid form but not in a dropper bottle and the directions on the bottle say to take by teaspoonful, it is not necessary to dilute it before using.

Sometimes this medicine must be taken for several weeks before you begin to feel better. Your doctor should check your progress at regular visits.

If you miss a dose of this medicine and your dosing schedule is:

More than one dose a day—Take the missed dose as soon as possible and then go back to your regular dosing schedule. However, if it is almost time for your next dose, skip it, and go back to your regular dosing schedule. Do not double doses.

One dose daily at bedtime—Do not take the missed dose in the morning since it may cause disturbing side effects during waking hours. Instead, check with your doctor.

How to store this medicine:

• Store away from heat and direct light.

• **Keep out of the reach of children** since overdose is especially dangerous in young children.

• Do not store in the bathroom medicine cabinet because the heat or moisture may cause the medicine to break down.

• Keep the liquid form of this medicine from freezing.

• Do not keep outdated medicine or medicine no longer needed. Flush the contents of the container down the toilet, unless otherwise directed.

Precautions While Using This Medicine

It is very important that your doctor check your progress at regular visits, in order to allow dosage adjustments and help reduce side effects.

Do not stop taking this medicine without first checking with your doctor. Your doctor may want you to reduce gradually the amount you are using before stopping completely. This may help prevent a possible worsening of your condition and reduce the possibility of withdrawal symptoms such as headache, nausea, and/or an overall feeling of discomfort.

Before having any kind of surgery (including dental surgery) or emergency treatment, tell the physician or dentist in charge that you are using this medicine.

This medicine will add to the effects of alcohol and other CNS depressants (medicines that slow down the nervous system, possibly causing drowsiness). Some examples of CNS depressants are antihistamines or medicine for hay fever, other allergies, or colds; sedatives, tranquilizers, or sleeping medicine; prescription pain medicine or narcotics; barbiturates; medicine for seizures; muscle relaxants; or anesthetics, including some dental anesthetics. **Check with your doctor before taking any of the above while you are taking this medicine.**

This medicine may cause some people to become drowsy or less alert than they are normally. **Make sure you know how you react to this medicine before you drive, use machines, or do other jobs that require you to be alert.**

Dizziness, lightheadedness, or fainting may occur, especially when you get up from a lying or sitting position. Getting up slowly may help. If this problem continues or gets worse, check with your doctor.

The effects of this medicine may last for 3 to 7 days after you have stopped taking it. Therefore, stated precautions must be observed during this time.

Side Effects of This Medicine

Along with its needed effects, a medicine may cause some unwanted effects. Although not all of these side effects appear very often, when they do occur they may require medical attention. **Stop taking this medicine and get emergency help immediately** if any of the following side effects occur:

Rare

Convulsions (seizures)
Difficult or unusually fast breathing
High body temperature with increased sweating
Loss of bladder control
Muscle stiffness (severe)
Unusual feeling of tiredness or weakness
Unusually fast heartbeat or irregular pulse

Signs of acute overdose

Confusion
Convulsions (seizures)
Drowsiness (severe)
Fever
Hallucinations
Restlessness and agitation
Shortness of breath or troubled breathing
Unusually fast, slow, or irregular heartbeat
Unusual tiredness or weakness
Vomiting

Check with your doctor as soon as possible if any of the following side effects occur:

Less common

Blurred vision
Confusion or delirium
Constipation (especially in the elderly)
Decreased sexual ability

Difficulty in speaking or swallowing (with amoxapine)
Eye pain
Fainting
Hallucinations (seeing, hearing, or feeling things that are not there)
Irregular heartbeat (pounding, racing, skipping)
Loss of balance control (with amoxapine)
Mask-like face (with amoxapine)
Nervousness or restlessness
Problems in urinating
Shakiness or trembling
Shuffling walk (with amoxapine)
Slowed movements (with amoxapine)
Stiffness of arms and legs (with amoxapine)
Trouble in sleeping
Uncontrolled movements of hands, mouth, tongue, arms, or legs (with amoxapine)
Unusually slow or fast pulse

Rare

Anxiety
Breast enlargement in both males and females (with amoxapine)
Convulsions (seizures)
Hair loss
Irritability
Increased sensitivity to sunlight
Muscle twitching
Skin rash and itching
Sore throat and fever
Swelling of face and tongue
Swelling of testicles (with amoxapine)
Weakness
Yellowing of eyes and skin

Other side effects may occur which usually do not require medical attention. These side effects may go away during treatment as your body adjusts to the medicine. However, check with your doctor if any of the following side effects continue or are bothersome:

More common

Dizziness
Drowsiness (rare with protriptyline)
Dry mouth
Headache
Increased appetite for sweets
Nausea

Tiredness or weakness (less common with
    protriptyline)
Unpleasant taste
Weight gain

Less common
    Diarrhea
    Excessive sweating
    Heartburn
    Trouble in sleeping (more common with
        protriptyline especially when taken
        late in the day)
    Vomiting

The above side effects, especially drowsiness, dizziness, confusion, vision problems, dry mouth, constipation, and problems in urinating are more likely to occur in elderly patients, who are usually more sensitive to the effects of tricyclic antidepressants.

Side effects in children taking this medicine for bedwetting usually disappear upon continued use. The most common of these are nervousness, sleeping problems, tiredness, and mild upset of the stomach. However, if these side effects continue or are bothersome, check with your doctor.

Certain side effects of this medicine may occur after you have stopped taking it. Check with your doctor if you notice any of the following effects:

For all tricyclic antidepressants
    Irritability
    Restlessness
    Trouble in sleeping with vivid dreams
    Headache
    Excitement
    Nausea, vomiting, or diarrhea

For amoxapine only
    Chewing movements
    Puffing of cheeks
    Rapid or worm-like movements of the
        tongue
    Unusual, uncontrolled movements of
        arms or legs

Other side effects not listed above also may occur in some patients. If you notice any other effects, check with your doctor.

ANTIDIABETICS, ORAL (Systemic)

This information applies to the following medicines:

Acetohexamide (a-set-oh-HEX-a-mide)
Chlorpropamide (klor-PROE-pa-mide)
Glipizide (GLIP-i-zide)
Glyburide (GLYE-byoo-ride)
Tolazamide (tole-AZ-a-mide)
Tolbutamide (tole-BYOO-ta-mide)

Some commonly used brand and other names are:	Generic names:
Dimelor* Dymelor	Acetohexamide
Apo-Chlorpropamide* Chloronase* Diabinese Glucamide Novopropamide*	Chlorpropamide†
Glucotrol	Glipizide
DiaBeta Euglucon* Glibenclamide Micronase	Glyburide
Ronase Tolinase	Tolazamide
Apo-Tolbutamide* Mobenol* Novobutamide* Oramide Orinase SK-Tolbutamide	Tolbutamide†

*Not available in the United States.
†Generic name product may also be available.

Oral antidiabetes medicines (hypoglycemics) are taken by mouth to help reduce the amount of sugar present in the blood. They are used to treat certain types of diabetes mellitus (sugar diabetes).

Chlorpropamide may also be used for other conditions as determined by your doctor.

Oral antidiabetes medicine can usually be used only by adults who develop diabetes after 30 years of age and who do not require insulin shots (or who usually do not require more than 20 Units of insulin a day) to control their condition. This type of diabetic patient is said to have non-insulin-dependent diabetes mellitus (or NIDDM), sometimes known as maturity-onset or Type II diabetes. Oral antidiabetes medicines do not help diabetic patients who have insulin-dependent diabetes mellitus (or IDDM), sometimes known as juvenile-onset or Type I diabetes.

Patients who are taking oral antidiabetes medicines may have to switch to insulin if they:

—develop diabetic coma or ketoacidosis.
—have a severe injury or burn.
—develop a severe infection.
—are to have major surgery.
—are pregnant.

The use of oral antidiabetes medicines has been reported to increase the risk of death from heart and blood vessel disease. A study (UGDP) compared the use of one of the oral medicines (tolbutamide) to the use of diet alone or diet plus insulin. Although only tolbutamide was studied, other oral antidiabetes medicines may cause a similar effect since they are related chemically and in the way they work. Before you begin treatment with this medicine, you and your doctor should talk about the good the medicine will do as well as the risks of using it. You should also find out about other possible ways to treat your diabetes such as by diet alone or by diet plus insulin.

Oral antidiabetes medicines are available only with your doctor's prescription.

Before Using This Medicine

Importance of diet—**Before prescribing medicine for your diabetes, your doctor will probably try to control your condition by prescribing a personal diet for you.** Such a diet is low in refined carbohydrates (foods such as sugar and candy used for quick energy). The daily number of calories in this diet should equal the number of calories used by your body each day. In addition, meals and snacks are arranged to meet the energy needs of your body at different times of the day.

Many diabetic patients are able to control their condition by carefully following their doctor's orders for proper diet and exercise. **Medicine is prescribed only when additional help is needed and is effective only when a schedule of diet and exercise is properly followed.**

Oral antidiabetes medicines are less effective if you are greatly overweight. It may be very important for you to go on a reducing diet. However, check with your doctor before going on any diet.

In order to decide on the best treatment for your medical problem, your doctor should be told:

—if you have ever had any unusual or allergic reaction to any oral antidiabetes medicine, or to sulfonamide-type (sulfa) medications, including thiazide diuretics.

—if you are on a low-salt, low-sugar, or any other special diet, or if you are allergic to any substance, such as sulfites or other preservatives or dyes. Most medicines contain more than their active ingredient. Your doctor or pharmacist can help you avoid products that may cause a problem.

—if you are pregnant or if you intend to become pregnant while taking this medicine. Oral antidiabetes medicines should not be used during pregnancy. Insulin is needed to maintain blood sugar levels as close to normal as possible. Poor control of blood sugar levels may cause birth defects or death of the fetus. In addition, use of oral antidiabetes medicines during pregnancy may cause the newborn baby to have low blood sugar levels. This may last for several days following birth.

—if you are breast-feeding an infant. Although these medicines have not been shown to cause problems in humans, the chance always exists since they pass into the breast milk in small amounts and could cause low blood sugar in the infant.

—if you have any of the following medical problems:

Adrenal disease
Infection (severe)
Kidney disease
Liver disease
Pituitary disease
Thyroid disease

—if you are taking chlorpropamide and have heart disease.

—if you are now taking any of the following medicines or types of medicine:

Adrenocorticoids
Anticoagulants (blood thinners)
Amphetamines
Aspirin or other salicylates
Beta-adrenergic blocking agents
  (atenolol, labetalol, metoprolol, nadolol, oxprenolol, pindolol, propranolol, sotalol, timolol)
Calcium channel blocking agents
  (diltiazem, nifedipine, verapamil)
Carbamazepine—with chlorpropamide only
Chloramphenicol
Clofibrate
Danazol
Disopyramide
Dextrothyroxine
Diuretics (water pills)
Epinephrine
Fenfluramine
Guanethidine
Inflammation medicine (for example, arthritis medicine)
Insulin
Ketoconazole
Mazindol
Medicine for diabetes insipidus (water diabetes)—with chlorpropamide only
Medicine for gout

Miconazole
Oral contraceptives (birth control pills)
Phenytoin (seizure medicine)
Probenecid
Rifampin
Sulfonamides (sulfa drugs)
Thyroid medicine

—if you are now taking or have taken within the past 2 weeks monoamine oxidase (MAO) inhibitors such as:

Furazolidone
Isocarboxazid
Pargyline
Phenelzine
Procarbazine
Tranylcypromine

Proper Use of This Medicine

Follow carefully the special diet your doctor gave you. This is the most important part of controlling your condition, and is necessary if the medicine is to work properly.

Take your oral antidiabetes medicine only as directed by your doctor. Do not take more or less of it than your doctor ordered, and take it at the same time each day. This will help to control your blood sugar levels.

If you miss a dose of this medicine, take it as soon as possible. However, if it is almost time for your next dose, skip the missed dose and go back to your regular dosing schedule. Do not double doses.

How to store this medicine:

• Store away from heat and direct light.

• **Keep out of the reach of children.**

• Do not store in the bathroom medicine cabinet because the heat or moisture may cause the medicine to break down.

• Do not keep outdated medicine or medicine no longer needed. Flush the contents of the container down the toilet, unless otherwise directed.

Precautions While Using This Medicine

Your doctor should check your progress at regular visits, especially during the first few weeks you take this medicine.

Test for sugar in your blood or urine as directed by your doctor. This is a convenient way to make sure your diabetes is being controlled and it provides an early warning when it is not.

Do not take any other medicine, unless prescribed or approved by your doctor. This especially includes over-the-counter (OTC) or nonprescription medicine such as that for colds, cough, asthma, hay fever, or appetite control.

Avoid alcoholic beverages until you have discussed their use with your doctor. Some patients who drink alcohol while taking this medicine may suffer stomach pain, nausea, vomiting, dizziness, pounding headache, sweating, or flushing (redness of face and skin). In addition, alcohol may produce hypoglycemia (low blood sugar).

While taking this medicine, use caution during exposure to the sun. Some people find their skin to be more sensitive to direct sunlight because of the medicine.

Eat or drink something containing sugar and check with your doctor right away if symptoms of low blood sugar (hypoglycemia) appear. Good sources of sugar are orange juice, corn syrup, honey, or sugar cubes or table sugar (dissolved in water).

- **Signs of low blood sugar are:**
    Anxiety
    Chills
    Cold sweats
    Confusion
    Cool pale skin
    Difficulty in concentration
    Drowsiness
    Excessive hunger

    Headache
    Nausea
    Nervousness
    Rapid heartbeat
    Shakiness
    Unsteady walk
    Unusual tiredness or weakness

- **These signs may occur if you:**
    —skip or delay meals.
    —exercise much more than usual.
    —cannot eat because of nausea and vomiting.
    —drink a significant amount of alcohol.

- **Instruct someone with you to take you to your doctor or to a hospital right away if you think you are going to pass out.** Even if these signs are corrected by sugar, it is very important to call your doctor or hospital emergency service right away. The blood sugar–lowering effects of this medicine may last for days and the signs may return often during this period of time.

Before having any kind of surgery (including dental surgery) or emergency treatment, tell the physician or dentist in charge that you are taking this medicine.

Your doctor may want you to carry an identification card or wear a bracelet or necklace stating that you are using this medicine.

Side Effects of This Medicine

Along with their needed effects, oral antidiabetes medicines may cause some unwanted effects. Along with the side effects described below, these medicines have been reported to increase the risks of heart and blood vessel disease. Even though these effects are rare, they must be kept in mind.

Although not all of these side effects appear very often, when they do occur they may require medical attention. Check with your doctor as soon as possible if any of the following side effects occur:

Rare

Dark urine
Fatigue
Itching of the skin
Light-colored stools
Sore throat and fever
Unusual bleeding or bruising
Weakness and fever
Yellowing of the eyes or skin

Signs of overdose (hypoglycemia)

Anxiety
Chills
Cold sweats
Confusion
Cool pale skin
Difficulty in concentration
Drowsiness
Excessive hunger
Headache
Nausea
Nervousness
Rapid heartbeat
Shakiness
Unsteady walk
Unusual tiredness or weakness

Other side effects may occur which usually do not require medical attention. These side effects may go away during treatment as your body adjusts to the medicine. However, check with your doctor if any of the following side effects continue or are bothersome:

More common

Diarrhea
Dizziness
Headache
Heartburn
Loss of appetite
Nausea and vomiting
Stomach pain or discomfort

Less common or rare

Increased sensitivity of skin to sun
Skin rash

For patients taking chlorpropamide:

• Some patients who take chlorpropamide may retain or keep more body water than usual. This may cause more problems in the elderly or in those patients who have heart disease. Check with your doctor as soon as possible if any of the following signs occur:

Breathing difficulty
Drowsiness
Muscle cramps
Seizures
Shortness of breath
Swelling or puffiness of face, hands, or ankles
Weakness

The above side effects are more likely to occur in elderly patients and patients with kidney disease, who are usually more sensitive to the effects of oral antidiabetes medicines.

Other side effects not listed above may also occur in some patients. If you notice any other effects, check with your doctor.

ANTIDYSKINETICS (Systemic)

This information applies to the following medicines:

Benztropine (BENZ-troe-peen)
Biperiden (bye-PER-i-den)
Ethopropazine (eth-oh-PROE-pa-zeen)
Procyclidine (proe-SYE-kli-deen)
Trihexyphenidyl (trye-hex-ee-FEN-i-dill)

This information does *not* apply to:

Amantadine	Haloperidol
Carbidopa and Levodopa	Levodopa
Diphenhydramine	

Some commonly used brand names are:	Generic names:
Apo-Benztropine*	
Bensylate*	
Cogentin	Benztropine
PMS Benztropine*	

Akineton	Biperiden
Parsidol Parsitan*	Ethopropazine
Kemadrin PMS Procyclidine* Procyclid*	Procyclidine
Aparkane* Apo-Trihex* Artane Artane Sequels Novohexidyl* Trihexane Trihexidyl Trihexy	Trihexyphenidyl†

*Not available in the United States.
†Generic name product may also be available.

This medicine belongs to the general class of medicines called antidyskinetics. It is used to treat Parkinson's disease, sometimes referred to as "shaking palsy." By improving muscle control and reducing stiffness, this medicine allows more normal movements of the body as the disease symptoms are reduced. It is also used to control the severe reactions to certain medicines such as reserpine (medicine to control high blood pressure) or phenothiazines, chlorprothixene, thiothixene, loxapine, and haloperidol (medicines for nervous, mental, and emotional conditions).

This medicine is available only with your doctor's prescription.

Before Using This Medicine

In order to decide on the best treatment for your medical problem, your doctor should be told:

—if you have ever had any unusual or allergic reaction to antidyskinetics.

—if you are on a low-salt, low-sugar, or any other special diet, or if you are allergic to any substance, such as sulfites or other preservatives or dyes. Most medicines contain more than their active ingredient, and many liquid medicines contain alcohol. Your doctor or pharmacist can help you avoid products that may cause a problem.

—if you are pregnant or if you intend to become pregnant while taking this medicine. Although antidyskinetics have not been shown to cause problems in humans, the chance always exists. Studies on birth defects with biperiden have not been done in either humans or animals.

—if you are breast-feeding an infant. Although antidyskinetics have not been shown to cause problems in humans, the chance always exists. Also, since these medicines tend to decrease the secretions of the body, it is possible that the flow of breast milk may be reduced in some patients.

—if you have any of the following medical problems:
 Difficult urination
 Enlarged prostate
 Glaucoma
 Heart or blood vessel disease
 High blood pressure
 Intestinal blockage
 Kidney disease
 Liver disease
 Myasthenia gravis
 Uncontrolled movements of hands, mouth, or tongue

—if you are taking any of the following medicines or types of medicine:
 Amantadine
 Antacids
 Antimuscarinics (medicine for abdominal or stomach spasms or cramps)
 Chlorpromazine
 Clonidine
 Cyclobenzaprine
 Guanabenz
 Haloperidol

Heart medicine
Medicine for diarrhea
Methyldopa
Metyrosine
Other medicine for Parkinson's disease

—if you are now taking central nervous system (CNS) depressants such as:

Anticonvulsants (seizure medicine)
Antihistamines or medicine for hay fever, other allergies, or colds
Barbiturates
Narcotics
Prescription pain medicine
Sedatives, tranquilizers, or sleeping medicine

—if you are now taking tricyclic antidepressants such as:

Amitriptyline
Amoxapine
Clomipramine
Desipramine
Doxepin
Imipramine
Nortriptyline
Protriptyline
Trimipramine

—if you are now taking or have taken within the past 2 weeks monoamine oxidase (MAO) inhibitors such as:

Furazolidone
Isocarboxazid
Pargyline
Phenelzine
Procarbazine
Tranylcypromine

Proper Use of This Medicine

Take this medicine only as directed by your doctor. Do not take more of it, do not take it more often, and do not take it for a longer period of time than your doctor ordered. To do so may increase the chance of side effects.

To lessen stomach upset, take this medicine with meals or immediately after meals, unless otherwise directed by your doctor.

If you miss a dose of this medicine, take it as soon as possible. If it is within 2 hours of your next dose, skip the missed dose and go back to your regular dosing schedule. Do not double doses.

How to store this medicine:

• Store away from heat and direct light.

• **Keep out of the reach of children.**

• Do not store in the bathroom medicine cabinet because the heat or moisture may cause the medicine to break down.

• Keep the liquid dosage form of this medicine from freezing.

• Do not keep outdated medicine or medicine no longer needed. Flush the contents of the container down the toilet, unless otherwise directed.

Precautions While Using This Medicine

Your doctor should check your progress at regular visits, especially for the first few months you take this medicine. This will allow your dosage to be changed as necessary to meet your needs.

Your doctor may want you to have your eyes examined by an ophthalmologist before and also sometime later during treatment.

Do not stop taking this medicine without first checking with your doctor. Your doctor may want you to reduce gradually the amount you are taking before stopping completely, in order to prevent side effects or making your condition worse.

This medicine will add to the effects of alcohol and other CNS depressants (medicines that slow down the nervous system, possibly causing drowsiness). Some examples of CNS depressants are antihistamines or medicine for hay fever, other allergies, or colds; sedatives, tranquilizers, or sleeping medicine; prescription pain medicine or narcotics; barbiturates; medicine for seizures; muscle relaxants; or anesthetics, including some dental anesthetics. **Check with your doctor before taking any of the above while you are using this medicine.**

Do not take this medicine within 1 hour of taking antacid or medicine for diarrhea. Taking them too close together will make this medicine less effective.

If you think you have taken an overdose, get emergency help at once. Taking an overdose of this medicine may lead to unconsciousness. Some signs of an overdose are clumsiness or unsteadiness; convulsions; severe drowsiness; hallucinations (seeing, hearing, or feeling things that are not there); shortness of breath or troubled breathing; unusual excitement, nervousness, restlessness, or irritability; unusually fast heartbeat; and unusual warmth, dryness, and flushing of skin.

This medicine may cause your eyes to become more sensitive to light than they are normally. Wearing sunglasses may help lessen the discomfort from bright light.

This medicine may cause some people to have blurred vision or to become drowsy, dizzy, or less alert than they are normally. **Make sure you know how you react to this medicine before you drive, use machines, or do other jobs that require you to be alert.**

Dizziness, lightheadedness, or fainting may occur, especially when you get up from a lying or sitting position. Getting up slowly may help. If the problem continues or gets worse, check with your doctor.

This medicine will often reduce your tolerance of heat, since it makes you sweat less, causing your body temperature to increase. **Use extra care not to become overheated during exercise or hot weather while you are taking this medicine as this could possibly result in heat stroke.** Also, hot baths or saunas may make you feel dizzy or faint while you are taking this medicine.

Your mouth, nose, and throat may feel very dry while you are taking this medicine. **To help relieve mouth dryness, chew sugarless gum or dissolve bits of ice in your mouth.**

Side Effects of This Medicine

Along with its needed effects, a medicine may cause some unwanted effects. Although not all of these side effects appear very often, when they do occur they may require medical attention. Check with your doctor as soon as possible if any of the following side effects occur:

Rare
   Confusion (more common in the elderly or with high doses)
   Eye pain
   Skin rash

Signs of overdose
   Clumsiness or unsteadiness
   Convulsions (seizures)
   Drowsiness (severe)
   Dryness of mouth, nose, or throat (severe)
   Hallucinations (seeing, hearing, or feeling things that are not there)
   Mood or mental changes
   Shortness of breath or troubled breathing
   Trouble in sleeping
   Unusually fast heartbeat
   Unusual warmth, dryness, and flushing of skin

Other side effects may occur which usually do not require medical attention. These side effects may go away during treatment as your body adjusts to the medicine. However, check with your doctor if

any of the following side effects continue or are bothersome:

More common
  Blurred vision
  Constipation
  Decrease in sweating
  Difficult or painful urination (especially in older men)
  Drowsiness
  Dryness of mouth, nose, or throat
  Headache
  Increased sensitivity of eyes to light
  Nausea or vomiting

Less common or rare
  Dizziness or lightheadedness when getting up from a lying or sitting position
  False sense of well-being (especially in the elderly or with high doses)
  Headache
  Muscle cramps
  Nervousness
  Numbness or weakness in hands or feet
  Soreness of mouth and tongue
  Stomach upset or pain
  Unusual excitement (more common with large doses of trihexyphenidyl)

The above side effects are more likely to occur in children since they are usually more sensitive to the effects of antidyskinetics.

Mental changes and confusion, disorientation, agitation, and hallucinations may be more likely to occur in elderly patients since they are usually more sensitive to the effects of antidyskinetics.

Other side effects not listed above may also occur in some patients. If you notice any other effects, check with your doctor.

ANTIHISTAMINES (Systemic)

This information applies to the following medicines:

Azatadine (a-ZA-ta-deen)
Bromodiphenhydramine (broe-moe-dye-fen-HYE-dra-meen)
Brompheniramine (brome-fen-EER-a-meen)
Carbinoxamine (kar-bi-NOX-a-meen)
Chlorpheniramine (klor-fen-EER-a-meen)
Clemastine (KLEM-as-teen)
Cyproheptadine (si-proe-HEP-ta-deen)
Dexchlorpheniramine (dex-klor-fen-EER-a-meen)
Dimenhydrinate (dye-men-HYE-dri-nate)
Diphenhydramine (dye-fen-HYE-dra-meen)
Diphenylpyraline (dye-fen-il-PEER-a-leen)
Doxylamine (dox-ILL-a-meen)
Phenindamine (fen-IN-da-meen)
Pyrilamine (peer-ILL-a-meen)
Terfenadine (ter-FEN-a-deen)
Tripelennamine (tri-pel-ENN-a-meen)
Triprolidine (trye-PROE-li-deen)

This information does *not* apply to Hydroxyzine, Promethazine, or Trimeprazine.

Some commonly used brand names and other names are:	Generic names:
Optimine	Azatadine
	Bromodiphen-hydramine*
Bromamine Brombay Bromphen Dimetane Dimetane Extentabs Dimetane-Ten Nasahist B Oraminic II Veltane	Brompheniramine†
Clistin	Carbinoxamine
Alermine Aller-Chlor Allerid-O.D. Chlo-Amine Chlor-100 Chlor-Mal Chlor-Niramine Chlorphen*	Chlorpheniramine†

Chlor-Pro	
Chlorspan	
Chlortab	
Chlor-Trimeton	
Chlor-Trimeton Repetabs	
Chlor-Tripolon*	
Hal-Chlor	Chlorphenira-
Histrey	mine†
Novopheniram*	
Phenetron	
Phenetron Lanacaps	
T.D. Alermine	
Teldrin	
Trymegen	

Tavist	Clemastine

Periactin	Cyproheptadine†
Vimicon*	

Polaramine	Dexchlorphenira-
Polaramine Repetabs	mine

Apo-Dimenhydrinate*	
Calm X	
Dimentabs	
Dinate	
Dommanate	
Dramamine	
Dramilin	
Dramocen	
Dramoject	
Dymenate	Dimenhydrinate†
Gravol*	
Hydrate	
Marmine	
Motion-Aid	
Nauseatol*	
Novodimenate*	
PMS-Dimenhydrinate*	
Reidamine	
Travamine*	
Wehamine	

Allerdryl*	
Bena-D	
Benadryl	
Benahist	
Bendylate	Diphenhydra-
Benoject-10	mine†
Benylin	
Compoz	
Diahist	
Dihydrex	
Diphen	

Diphenacen	
Diphenadril	
Fenylhist	
Fynex	
Hydril	
Hyrexin-50	
Insomnal*	
Noradryl	Diphenhydra-
Nordryl	mine†
Nytol with DPH	
Robalyn	
Sleep-Eze 3	
Sominex Formula 2	
Somnifere*	
Tusstat	
Twilite	
Valdrene	
Wehdryl	

Hispril	Diphenylpyraline

Unisom Nighttime	Doxylamine
Sleep Aid	

Nolahist	Phenindamine

Dormarex	
Nervine Nighttime	
Sleep-Aid	Pyrilamine†
Sominex	
Somnicaps	

Seldane	Terfenadine

PBZ	Tripelennamine†
PBZ-SR	

Actidil	Triprolidine†
Bayidyl	

*Not available in the United States.
†Generic name product may also be available.

Antihistamines are used to relieve or prevent the symptoms of hay fever and other types of allergy. They work by preventing the effects of a substance called histamine, which is produced by the body.

Some of the antihistamines are also used to prevent motion sickness, nausea, vomiting, and dizziness. In patients with Parkinson's disease, diphenhydramine may be used to decrease stiffness and tremors. In addition, since antihistamines may cause drowsiness as a side effect, some of them may be used to help people go to sleep.

Antihistamines may also be used for other conditions as determined by your doctor.

Some antihistamine preparations are available only with your doctor's prescription. Others are available without a prescription; however, your doctor may have special instructions on the proper dose of the medicine for your medical condition.

Before Using This Medicine

Before you use this medicine check with your doctor, nurse, or pharmacist:

—if you have ever had any unusual or allergic reaction to antihistamines.

—if you are on a low-salt, low-sugar, or any other special diet, or if you are allergic to any substance, such as sulfites or other preservatives or dyes. Most medicines contain more than their active ingredient, and many liquid medicines contain alcohol. Your doctor or pharmacist can help you avoid products that may cause a problem.

—if you are pregnant or if you intend to become pregnant while using this medicine. Although antihistamines have not been shown to cause problems in humans, the chance always exists since studies in animals have shown that some other antihistamines, such as meclizine and cyclizine, may cause birth defects. Studies have not been done in humans with terfenadine. However, studies in animals have shown that terfenadine, when given in doses several times the human dose, lowers the weight of the baby and increases the risk of death of the baby.

—if you are breast-feeding an infant. Small amounts of antihistamines pass into the breast milk. Use is not recommended since the chances are greater for most antihistamines to cause side effects, such as unusual excitement or irritability, in the infant. Also, since these medicines tend to decrease the secretions of the body, it is possible that the flow of breast milk may be reduced in some patients. It is not known yet whether terfenadine may cause these same side effects.

—if you have any of the following medical problems:
  Asthma attack
  Enlarged prostate
  Glaucoma
  Urinary tract blockage or difficult
    urination

—if you are now taking or receiving any of the following medicines or types of medicine:
  Amantadine
  Antimuscarinics (medicine for
    abdominal or stomach spasms or
    cramps)
  Aspirin or other salicylates
  Cisplatin
  Clonidine
  Guanabenz
  Haloperidol
  Maprotiline
  Methyldopa
  Metyrosine
  Paromomycin
  Procainamide
  Trazodone
  Vancomycin

—if you are now taking any central nervous system (CNS) depressants such as:
  Anticonvulsants (seizure medicine)
  Barbiturates
  Muscle relaxants
  Narcotics
  Other antihistamines or medicine for hay
    fever, other allergies, or colds
  Prescription pain medicine
  Sedatives, tranquilizers, or sleeping
    medicine

—if you are now taking tricyclic antidepressants such as:
  Amitriptyline
  Amoxapine
  Clomipramine

Desipramine
Doxepin
Imipramine
Nortriptyline
Protriptyline
Trimipramine

—if you are now taking or have taken within the past 2 weeks monoamine oxidase (MAO) inhibitors such as:

Furazolidone
Isocarboxazid
Pargyline
Phenelzine
Procarbazine
Tranylcypromine

Proper Use of This Medicine

Antihistamines are used to relieve or prevent the symptoms of your medical problem. Take them only as directed. Do not take more of them and do not take them more often than recommended on the label, unless otherwise directed by your doctor. To do so may increase the chance of side effects.

For patients taking this medicine by mouth:
• Take it with food or a glass of water or milk to lessen stomach irritation if necessary.
• If you are taking the extended-release tablet form of this medicine, swallow the tablets whole. Do not break, crush, or chew before swallowing.

For patients taking dimenhydrinate or diphenhydramine:
• If you are taking this medicine for motion sickness, take it at least 30 minutes or, even better, 1 to 2 hours before you begin to travel.

For patients using the suppository form of this medicine:
• How to insert suppository: First remove foil wrapper and moisten the suppository with water. Lie down on side and push the suppository well up into the rectum with finger. If the suppository is too soft to insert because of storage in a warm place, before removing the foil wrapper chill the suppository in the refrigerator for 30 minutes or run cold water over it.

For patients using the injection form of this medicine:
• If you will be giving yourself the injections, make sure you understand exactly how to give them. If you have any questions about this, check with your doctor, nurse, or pharmacist.

If you must take this medicine regularly and you miss a dose, take it as soon as possible. However, if it is almost time for your next dose, skip the missed dose and go back to your regular dosing schedule. Do not double doses.

How to store this medicine:
• Store away from heat and direct light.
• **Keep out of the reach of children**, since overdose may be very dangerous in children.
• Do not store in the bathroom medicine cabinet because the heat or moisture may cause the medicine to break down.
• Keep the liquid dosage form of this medicine from freezing.
• Do not keep outdated medicine or medicine no longer needed. Flush the contents of the container down the toilet, unless otherwise directed.

Precautions While Using This Medicine

Tell the doctor in charge that you are taking this medicine before you have any skin tests for allergies. The results of the test may be affected by this medicine.

When taking antihistamines on a regular basis, make sure your doctor knows if you are taking large amounts of aspirin at the same time (as in arthritis or rheumatism). Effects of too much aspirin, such as ringing in the ears, may be covered up by the antihistamine.

Antihistamines will add to the effects of alcohol and other CNS depressants (medicines that slow down the nervous system, possibly causing drowsiness). Some examples of CNS depressants are sedatives, tranquilizers, or sleeping medicine; prescription pain medicine or narcotics; barbiturates; medicine for seizures; muscle relaxants; or anesthetics, including some dental anesthetics. **Check with your doctor before taking any of the above while you are using this medicine.**

Antihistamines may cause some people to become drowsy or less alert than they are normally. Even if taken at bedtime, it may cause some people to feel drowsy or less alert on arising. Some antihistamines are more likely to cause drowsiness than others (terfenadine, for example, produces this effect rarely). **Make sure you know how you react to the antihistamine you are taking before you drive, use machines, or do other jobs that require you to be alert.**

For patients using dimenhydrinate or diphenhydramine:

• This medicine controls nausea and vomiting. For this reason, it may cover up the signs of overdose caused by other medicines or the symptoms of appendicitis. This will make it difficult for your doctor to diagnose these conditions. Make sure your doctor knows that you are taking this medicine if you have other symptoms of appendicitis such as stomach or lower abdominal pain, cramping, or soreness. Also, if you think you may have taken an overdose of any medicine, tell your doctor that you are taking this medicine.

Side Effects of This Medicine

Along with its needed effects, a medicine may cause some unwanted effects. Although not all of these side effects appear very often, when they do occur they may require medical attention. Check with your doctor as soon as possible if any of the following side effects occur:

Rare
    Sore throat and fever
    Unusual bleeding or bruising
    Unusual tiredness or weakness

Signs of overdose
    Clumsiness or unsteadiness
    Convulsions (seizures)
    Drowsiness (severe)
    Dryness of mouth, nose, or throat (severe)
    Feeling faint
    Flushing or redness of face
    Hallucinations (seeing, hearing, or feeling things that are not there)
    Shortness of breath or troubled breathing
    Trouble in sleeping

Other side effects may occur which usually do not require medical attention. These side effects may go away during treatment as your body adjusts to the medicine. However, check with your doctor or pharmacist if any of the following side effects continue or are bothersome:

More common—rare with terfenadine
    Drowsiness
    Thickening of bronchial secretions

Less common or rare
    Blurred vision or any change in vision
    Confusion
    Difficult or painful urination
    Dizziness
    Dryness of mouth, nose, or throat
    Increased sensitivity of skin to sun
    Loss of appetite (increased appetite with cyproheptadine)
    Nightmares
    Ringing or buzzing sound in ears
    Skin rash
    Stomach upset or stomach pain (more common with pyrilamine and tripelennamine)

Unusual excitement, nervousness, rest-
lessness, or irritability
Unusual increase in sweating
Unusually fast heartbeat

Use of antihistamines is not recommended
in premature or newborn infants. Serious side effects, such as convulsions (seizures) are more likely to occur in children and would be of greater risk to
these infants.

Children and elderly patients are usually
more sensitive to the effects of antihistamines. Confusion, difficult and painful urination, dizziness, drowsiness, feeling faint, or dryness of mouth, nose, or
throat may be more likely to occur in
elderly patients. Also, nightmares or unusual excitement, nervousness, restlessness, or irritability may be more likely to
occur in children and in elderly patients.

Other side effects not listed above may also
occur in some patients. If you notice any
other effects, check with your doctor or
pharmacist.

ANTIHISTAMINES AND
DECONGESTANTS (Systemic)

Note: For quick reference the following antihistamine and decongestant combinations
are numbered to match the corresponding
brand names.

This information applies to the following medicines:

1. Azatadine and Pseudoephedrine
2. Brompheniramine, Phenylephrine, and
   Phenylpropanolamine
2a. Brompheniramine and Phenylpropanolamine
3. Brompheniramine and Pseudoephedrine
4. Carbinoxamine and Pseudoephedrine
5. Chlorpheniramine and Pseudoephedrine
6. Chlorpheniramine, Pyrilamine, and Phenylpropanolamine
7. Chlorpheniramine, Tripelennamine, Phenylpropanolamine, and Phenylephrine
8. Clemastine and Phenylpropanolamine
9. Dexbrompheniramine and Pseudoephedrine
9a. Diphenhydramine and Pseudoephedrine
10. Phenindamine, Chlorpheniramine, and
    Phenylpropanolamine
11. Phenylephrine and Brompheniramine
12. Phenylephrine and Chlorpheniramine
13. Phenylephrine, Chlorpheniramine, and
    Pyrilamine
14. Phenylephrine, Phenylpropanolamine, and
    Chlorpheniramine
15. Phenylephrine, Phenylpropanolamine, Pyr-
    ilamine, and Chlorpheniramine
16. Phenylpropanolamine and Chlorphenir-
    amine
17. Phenylpropanolamine, Pheniramine, and
    Pyrilamine
18. Phenylpropanolamine, Phenylephrine, Phen-
    yltoloxamine, and Chlorpheniramine
19. Phenylpropanolamine, Phenyltoloxamine,
    Pyrilamine, and Pheniramine
20. Promethazine and Phenylephrine
21. Promethazine and Pseudoephedrine
22. Pseudoephedrine and Chlorcyclizine
23. Triprolidine and Pseudoephedrine

Some commonly used brand names:

Actacin[23]
Actagen[23]
Actamine[23]
Actifed[23]
Actihist[23]
Alamine[16]
Allerest[16]
Allerform[16]
Allerfrin[23]
Allergesic[16]
Allergine[16]
Allergy Relief
   Medicine[16]
Allerid-D.C.[5]
Amaril D[18]
Amaril D Spantab[18]
Anafed[5]
Anamine[5]
Anamine T.D.[5]
A.R.M.[16]
Bayaminic[16]
Bayhistine[16]
Benadryl
   Decongestant[9a]

Biphetap[2a]
Brexin L.A.[5]
Bromalix[2]
Bromfed[3]
Bromophen[2]
Bromophen T.D.[2]
Bromphen Compound
   T.D.[2]
Children's Allerest[16]
Chlorafed[5]
Chlorafed Timecelles[5]
Chlor-Rest[16]
Chlor-Trimeton
   Decongestant[5]
Chlor-Trimeton Decon-
   gestant Repetabs[5]
Codimal-L.A.[5]
Cold Factor 12[16]
Colrex Decongestant[7]
Coltab[12]
Condrin-LA[16]
Conex D.A.[16]
Contac[16]
Cophene No.2[14]

Co-Pyronil 2[5]
Cordamine-PA[2]
Corsym[16]
Cotrol-D[5]
Covanamine[15]
Decohist[12]
Deconade[16]
Deconamine[5]
Deconamine SR[5]
Decongestabs[18]
Dehist[14]
Demazin[12]
Demazin
  Repetabs[16]
Dimalix[2]
Dimetane
  Decongestant[11]
Dimetapp[2]
Dimetapp
  Extentabs[2]
Disophrol[9]
Disophrol
  Chronotabs[9]
Dristan 12-Hour[12]
Drixoral[3] [9]
Drize[16]
Duphrene[18]
Duralex[5]
Efedra P.A.[9]
E-Tapp[2]
Fedahist[5]
Fedahist
  Gyrocaps[5]
Fedrazil[22]
Fernhist[6]
Histabid
  Duracaps[16]
Histalet[5]
Histalet Forte[15]
Histamic[18]
Histarall[9]
Histaspan-Plus[12]
Histatab Plus[12]
Histatapp[2]
Histatapp TD[2]
Hista-Vadrin[14]
Histor-D[12]
Hournaze[5]
Isoclor[5]
Isoclor Timesules[5]
Kronofed-A
  Kronocaps[5]
Kronohist
  Kronocaps[6]
Midatap[2]

Naldecon[18]
Naldelate[18]
Napril Plateau[15]
Nasahist[14]
ND Clear T.D.[5]
ND-Hist[14]
Neotep
  Granucaps[12]
Nolamine[10]
Norafed[23]
Noraminic[16]
Normatane[2]
Novafed A[5]
Novahistine[12]
Novahistine LP[12]
Novahistine
  Melet[12]
Novamor[16]
Orahist[16]
Oraminic
  Spancaps[16]
Ornade
  Spansules[16]
Panadyl[17]
PediaCare 2[5]
Phenergan-D[21]
Phenergan VC[20]
Phenhist[16]
Poly-Histine-D[19]
Poly-Histine-DX[3]
Pseudodine[23]
Pseudo-Hist[5]
Pseudo-Mal[9]
Purebrom[2]
Purebrom
  Compound T.D.[2]
Quadra Hist[18]
Relemine[15]
Resaid T.D.[16]
Rhinolar-EX[16]
Rhinosyn[5]
Rhinosyn-PD[5]
Rinade B.I.D.[5]
Rofed[23]
Rondec[4]
Rondec-TR[4]
Rotapp[2]
Ru-Tuss II[16]
Ryna[5]
Rynatan[13]
Sinocon[18]
S-T Decongest[2]
Sudafed Plus[5]
Tagafed[23]
Tagatap[2]

Tamine[2]
Tamine SR[2]
Tavist-D[6]
Triacin[23]
Triafed[23]
Triaminic[16] [17]
Triaminic-12[16]
Triaminic
  Chewables[16]
Triaminic
  Juvelets[17]
Triaminic TR[17]
Trifed[23]
Tri-Fed[23]

Trinalin Repetabs[1]
Trind[16]
Tri-Nefrin[16]
Triphed[23]
Tri-Phen[2]
Tri-Phen-Chlor[18]
Triphenyl[16] [17]
Tripodrine[23]
Triposed[23]
Tudecon[18]
Tussanil[15]
Veltap[2]
Westapp[2]

Antihistamine and decongestant combinations are used to treat nasal congestion (stuffy nose) and other symptoms of colds and hay fever.

Antihistamines work by preventing the effects of a substance called histamine which is produced by the body. The decongestants, such as phenylpropanolamine (fen-ill-proe-pa-NOLE-a-meen) (also known as PPA), produce a narrowing of blood vessels. This leads to clearing of nasal congestion, but it may also cause an increase in blood pressure in patients who have high blood pressure.

Some of these combinations are available only with your doctor's prescription. Others are available without a prescription; however, your doctor may have special instructions on the proper dose of the medicine for your medical condition.

Before Using This Medicine

Before you use this medicine, check with your doctor, nurse, or pharmacist:

—if you have ever had any unusual or allergic reaction to antihistamines or to amphetamine, dextroamphetamine, ephedrine, epinephrine, isoproterenol, metaproterenol, methamphetamine, norepinephrine, phenylephrine, pseudoephedrine, PPA, or terbutaline.

—if you are on a low-salt, low-sugar, or any other special diet, or if you are allergic to any substance, such as sulfites or other preservatives or dyes. Most medicines contain more than their active ingredient, and many liquid medicines contain alcohol. Your doctor or pharmacist can help you avoid products that may cause a problem.

—if you are pregnant or if you intend to become pregnant while taking this medicine. Although antihistamines have not been shown to cause problems in humans, the chance always exists.

Studies on birth defects have not been done in either humans or animals with decongestants such as ephedrine, phenylephrine, or phenylpropanolamine. Studies on birth defects have not been done in humans with the decongestant pseudoephedrine; however, in animal studies pseudoephedrine did not cause birth defects but did cause a reduction in average weight, length, and rate of bone formation in the animal fetus.

Phenothiazines, such as promethazine (contained in one of these combination medicines), have been shown to cause jaundice and muscle tremors in a few newborn infants whose mothers received phenothiazines during pregnancy. To avoid these effects, medicines that contain promethazine should be stopped 1 or 2 weeks before the delivery date.

—if you are breast-feeding an infant. Small amounts of antihistamines and decongestants pass into the breast milk. Use is not recommended since the chances are greater for this medicine to cause side effects, such as unusual excitement or irritability, in the infant. Also, since antihistamines tend to decrease the secretions of the body, it is possible that the flow of breast milk may be reduced in some patients.

—if you have any of the following medical problems:
Asthma attack
Diabetes mellitus (sugar diabetes)
Enlarged prostate
Glaucoma

Heart or blood vessel disease
High blood pressure
Overactive thyroid
Urinary tract blockage or difficult urination

—if you are now taking any of the following medicines or types of medicine:
Amantadine
Antimuscarinics (medicine for abdominal or stomach spasms or cramps)
Aspirin or other salicylates
Cisplatin
Clonidine
Diet aids, phenylpropanolamine-containing (medicines used for appetite control)
Digitalis glycosides (heart medicine)
Doxapram
Guanabenz
Haloperidol
Maprotiline
Medicine for asthma or other breathing problems
Methyldopa
Metyrosine
Paromomycin
Procainamide
Reserpine
Trazodone
Vancomycin

—if you are taking one of the combinations containing ephedrine, phenylpropanolamine, or pseudoephedrine and are also taking:
Acebutolol
Aminophylline
Amphetamines
Appetite suppressants
Atenolol
Caffeine
Chlophedianol
Dyphylline
Labetalol
Methylphenidate
Metoprolol
Nadolol
Oxtriphylline
Pemoline
Pindolol
Propranolol
Theophylline
Timolol

—if you are taking one of the combinations containing phenylephrine or phenylpropanolamine and are also taking:

Guanadrel
Guanethidine

—if you are now taking any central nervous system (CNS) depressants such as:

Anticonvulsants (seizure medicine)
Barbiturates
Muscle relaxants
Narcotics
Other antihistamines or medicine for hay fever, other allergies, or colds
Prescription pain medicine
Sedatives, tranquilizers, or sleeping medicine

—if you are now taking tricyclic antidepressants such as:

Amitriptyline
Amoxapine
Clomipramine
Desipramine
Doxepin
Imipramine
Nortriptyline
Protriptyline
Trimipramine

—if you are now taking or have taken within the past 2 weeks monoamine oxidase (MAO) inhibitors such as:

Furazolidone
Isocarboxazid
Pargyline
Phenelzine
Procarbazine
Tranylcypromine

Proper Use of This Medicine

Take this medicine only as directed. Do not take more of it and do not take it more often than recommended on the label, unless otherwise directed by your doctor. To do so may increase the chance of side effects.

Take this medicine with food or a glass of water or milk to lessen stomach irritation, if necessary.

For patients taking the extended-release capsule or tablet form of this medicine:

• Swallow it whole.

• Do not crush, break, or chew before swallowing.

• If the capsule is too large to swallow, you may mix the contents of the capsule with applesauce, jelly, honey, or syrup and swallow without chewing.

If you must take this medicine regularly and you miss a dose, take it as soon as possible. However, if it is almost time for your next dose, skip the missed dose and go back to your regular dosing schedule. Do not double doses.

How to store this medicine:

• Store away from heat and direct light.

• **Keep out of the reach of children.**

• Do not store in the bathroom medicine cabinet because the heat or moisture may cause the medicine to break down.

• Keep the liquid dosage form of this medicine from freezing.

• Do not keep outdated medicine or medicine no longer needed. Flush the contents of the container down the toilet, unless otherwise directed.

Precautions While Using This Medicine

Tell the doctor in charge that you are taking this medicine before you have any skin tests for allergies. The results of the test may be affected by the antihistamine in this medicine.

When taking antihistamines (contained in this combination medicine) on a regular basis, make sure your doctor knows if you are taking large amounts of aspirin at the same time (as in arthritis or rheumatism). Effects of too much aspirin, such as ringing in the ears, may be covered up by the antihistamine.

The antihistamine in this medicine will add to the effects of alcohol and other CNS depressants (medicines that slow down the nervous system, possibly causing drowsiness). Some examples of CNS depressants are other antihistamines or medicine for hay fever, other allergies, or colds; sedatives, tranquilizers, or sleeping medicine; prescription pain medicine or narcotics; barbiturates; medicine for seizures; muscle relaxants; or anesthetics, including some dental anesthetics. **Check with your doctor before taking any of the above while you are taking this medicine.**

The antihistamine in this medicine may cause some people to become drowsy, dizzy, or less alert than they are normally. **Make sure you know how you react before you drive, use machines, or do other jobs that require you to be alert.**

The decongestant in this medicine may add to the central nervous system (CNS) stimulant and other effects of phenyl-propanolamine (PPA)-containing diet aids. **Do not use medicines for diet or appetite control while taking this medicine unless you have checked with your doctor.**

The decongestant in this medicine may cause some people to be nervous or restless or to have trouble in sleeping. If you have trouble in sleeping, **take the last dose of this medicine for each day a few hours before bedtime.** If you have any questions about this, check with your doctor.

Side Effects of This Medicine

Along with its needed effects, a medicine may cause some unwanted effects. Although not all of these side effects appear very often, when they do occur they may require medical attention. Check with your doctor as soon as possible if any of the following side effects occur:

Rare
  Sore throat and fever
  Tightness in chest
  Unusual bleeding or bruising
  Unusual tiredness or weakness

With high doses
  Mood or mental changes
  Unusually fast or irregular heartbeat

Signs of overdose
  Clumsiness or unsteadiness
  Convulsions (seizures)
  Drowsiness (severe)
  Dryness of mouth, nose, or throat (severe)
  Flushing or redness of face
  Hallucinations (seeing, hearing, or feeling things that are not there)
  Headache (continuing)
  Muscle spasms (especially of neck and back)
  Restlessness
  Shortness of breath or troubled breathing
  Shuffling walk
  Tic-like (jerky) movements of head and face
  Trembling and shaking of hands
  Unusually slow or fast heartbeat

Other side effects may occur which usually do not require medical attention. These side effects may go away during treatment as your body adjusts to the medicine. However, check with your doctor or pharmacist if any of the following side effects continue or are bothersome:

More common
  Drowsiness
  Thickening of the bronchial secretions

Less common—more common with high doses
  Blurred vision
  Confusion
  Difficult or painful urination
  Dizziness
  Dryness of mouth, nose, or throat
  Headache
  Loss of appetite
  Nightmares
  Pounding heartbeat

Ringing or buzzing sound in ears

Skin rash

Stomach upset or pain (more common with pyrilamine and tripelennamine)

Unusual excitement, nervousness, restlessness, or irritability

Use of this medicine is not recommended in premature or newborn infants. Serious side effects, such as convulsions (seizures) and unusually fast or irregular heartbeats, are more likely to occur in children and would be of greater risk to these infants.

Children and elderly patients are usually more sensitive to the effects of this medicine. Confusion, convulsions, difficult and painful urination, dizziness, drowsiness, or dryness of mouth may be more likely to occur in elderly patients. Nightmares or unusual excitement, nervousness, restlessness, or irritability may be more likely also to occur in children and in elderly patients.

Other side effects not listed above may also occur in some patients. If you notice any other effects, check with your doctor.

Some commonly used brand names are:	Generic names:
Dolobid	Diflunisal
Nalfon	Fenoprofen
Advil Amersol* Motrin Nuprin Rufen	Ibuprofen
Meclomen	Meclofenamate
Ponstan* Ponstel	Mefenamic Acid
Anaprox Apo-Naproxen* Naprosyn Naxen* Novonaprox*	Naproxen
Feldene	Piroxicam
Clinoril	Sulindac
Tolectin Tolectin DS	Tolmetin

*Not available in the United States.

ANTI-INFLAMMATORY ANALGESICS (Systemic)

This information applies to the following medicines:

Diflunisal (dye-FLOO-ni-sal)

Fenoprofen (fen-oh-PROE-fen)

Ibuprofen (eye-byoo-PROE-fen)

Meclofenamate (me-kloe-FEN-am-ate)

Mefenamic (me-fe-NAM-ik) Acid

Naproxen (na-PROX-en)

Piroxicam (peer-OX-i-kam)

Sulindac (sul-IN-dak)

Tolmetin (TOLE-met-in)

This information does *not* apply to aspirin or other salicylates, indomethacin, oxyphenbutazone, and phenylbutazone.

Anti-inflammatory analgesics are taken by mouth to relieve some symptoms caused by arthritis or rheumatism, such as inflammation, swelling, stiffness, and joint pain. However, this medicine does not cure arthritis and will help you only as long as you continue to take it.

Some of these medicines are also used to relieve other kinds of pain or to treat other painful conditions, such as:

—gout attacks;

—bursitis;

—tendinitis;

—sprains, strains, or other injuries; or

—menstrual cramps.

Ibuprofen is also used to reduce fever.

Anti-inflammatory analgesics may also be used for treating other conditions as determined by your doctor.

Although ibuprofen may be used instead of aspirin to treat many of the same medical problems, it must not be used by people who are allergic to aspirin.

The 200-mg strength of ibuprofen is available without a prescription. However, your physician or dentist may have special instructions on the proper dose of ibuprofen for your medical condition.

Other anti-inflammatory analgesics and other strengths of ibuprofen are available only with your physician's or dentist's prescription.

Before Using This Medicine

Before you take this medicine, your physician or dentist should be told:

—if you have ever had any unusual or allergic reaction, such as skin rash, hives, or itching or breathing problems (wheezing or asthma), to any of the anti-inflammatory analgesics or to any of the following medicines:

Aspirin or other salicylates
Indomethacin
Oxyphenbutazone
Phenylbutazone
Zomepirac

—if you are on a low-salt, low-sugar, or any other special diet, or if you are allergic to any substance, such as sulfites or other preservatives or dyes. Most medicines contain more than their active ingredient. Your doctor or pharmacist can help you avoid products that may cause a problem.

—if you are pregnant or if you intend to become pregnant while taking this medicine. Studies on birth defects with these medicines have not been done in humans. However, if taken regularly during the last few months of pregnancy, there is a chance that these medicines may cause unwanted effects on the heart or blood flow in the fetus or newborn infant. Also, studies in animals have shown that these medicines, if taken late in pregnancy, may increase the length of pregnancy, prolong labor, or cause other problems during delivery.

Studies in animals have not shown that fenoprofen, ibuprofen, naproxen, piroxicam, or tolmetin causes birth defects. Diflunisal causes birth defects of the spine and ribs in rabbits, but not in mice or rats. Meclofenamate causes unwanted effects on the formation of bones and other unwanted effects in animals. Sulindac causes a lowering of the newborn's weight and, in some animal studies, unwanted effects on the development of bones and organs. Studies on birth defects with mefenamic acid have not been done in animals.

—if you are breast-feeding an infant. Although these medicines have not been shown to cause problems in humans, the chance always exists. Diflunisal, fenoprofen, mefenamic acid, and naproxen pass into the breast milk. Sulindac and tolmetin may pass into the breast milk. Ibuprofen probably does not pass into the breast milk. It is not known whether meclofenamate or piroxicam pass into human breast milk. However, use of meclofenamate by nursing mothers is not recommended because animal studies have shown that it causes unwanted effects on the infant's development. Also, studies in animals have shown that piroxicam may decrease the amount of milk.

—if you have any of the following medical problems:

Asthma
Bleeding problems
Colitis, stomach ulcer, or other stomach problems
Heart disease

High blood pressure
Kidney disease or history of
Liver disease

—if you regularly take acetaminophen
or aspirin or other salicylates.

—if you are now taking or using any of
the following medicines or types of medicine:

Adrenocorticoids (cortisone-like
  medicine)
Anticoagulants, including heparin (blood
  thinners)
Antidiabetics, oral (diabetes medicine
  taken by mouth)
Antihypertensives (high blood pressure
  medicine)
APC and codeine
Dimethyl sulfoxide (DMSO)
Dipyridamole
Diuretics (medicine to increase the
  amount of urine or to treat high blood
  pressure)
Inflammation medicine (for example,
  other arthritis medicine)
Lithium
Nifedipine or verapamil
Phenobarbital
Probenecid

Proper Use of This Medicine

**For safe and effective use of this medicine,
do not take more of it, do not take it more
often, and do not take it for a longer
period of time than ordered by your physician or dentist or directed on the ibuprofen package label.** Taking too much
of any of these medicines may increase
the chance of unwanted effects.

**When used for severe or continuing arthritis,
this medicine must be taken regularly as
ordered by your doctor** in order for it to
help you. These medicines usually begin
to work within one week, but in severe
cases up to two weeks or even longer
may pass before you begin to feel better.
Also, several weeks may pass before you
feel the full effects of the medicine.

To lessen stomach upset, anti-inflammatory
analgesics may be taken with food or
antacids. This is especially important
when taking mefenamic acid or piroxicam. However, your doctor may want
you to take other anti-inflammatory analgesics 30 minutes before meals or 2
hours after meals so that they will get
into the blood more quickly. If stomach
upset (indigestion, nausea, vomiting,
stomach pain, or diarrhea) continues or
if you have any questions about how you
should be taking this medicine, check
with your doctor, nurse, or pharmacist.

**Take this medicine with a full glass (8
ounces) of water.** Also, do not lie down
for about 15 to 30 minutes after taking
it. This helps to prevent irritation that
may lead to trouble in swallowing.

For patients taking mefenamic acid:

• **Do not take mefenamic acid for more
than 7 days at a time** unless your doctor
tells you to do so. To do so may increase
the chance of side effects.

• **Always take mefenamic acid with food
or antacids.**

For patients taking diflunisal: Swallow
these tablets whole. Do not break, crush,
or chew before swallowing.

If your doctor has ordered you to take this
medicine according to a regular schedule and you miss a dose, take it as soon as
you remember. However, if it is almost
time for your next dose, skip the missed
dose and go back to your regular dosing
schedule. Do not double doses.

How to store this medicine:

• Store away from heat and direct light.

• **Keep out of the reach of children.**

• Do not store in the bathroom medicine
cabinet because the heat or moisture
may cause the medicine to break down.

• Do not keep outdated medicine or medicine no longer needed. Flush the contents of the container down the toilet, unless otherwise directed.

Precautions While Using This Medicine

If you will be taking this medicine for a long time, as for arthritis or rheumatism, your doctor should check your progress at regular visits.

Stomach problems may be more likely to occur if you take two or more anti-inflammatory analgesics regularly (for example, every day) or drink alcoholic beverages while being treated with this medicine. Aspirin or other salicylates, indomethacin, oxyphenbutazone, and phenylbutazone are also anti-inflammatory analgesics that may cause problems if taken regularly with any of these medicines. Therefore, **do not take other anti-inflammatory analgesics regularly or drink alcoholic beverages while taking this medicine,** unless otherwise directed by your doctor.

Too much use of acetaminophen together with an anti-inflammatory analgesic may increase the chance of kidney problems. Therefore, do not regularly take acetaminophen together with this medicine, unless your physician or dentist has directed you to do so.

Before having any kind of surgery (including dental surgery), tell the physician or dentist in charge that you are taking this medicine.

This medicine may cause some people to become drowsy, dizzy, lightheaded, or less alert than they are normally. **Make sure you know how you react to this medicine before you drive, use machinery, or do other jobs that require you to be alert.**

Anti-inflammatory analgesics may cause a serious type of allergic reaction called anaphylaxis. Although this is rare, it may occur more often in patients who are allergic to aspirin or to any other anti-inflammatory analgesic. **Anaphylaxis requires immediate medical attention.** Some signs of this reaction are very pale, gray, or blue color of the skin of the face; very fast but irregular heartbeat or pulse; very fast or irregular breathing or gasping for breath; fainting; and swellings on the skin. If these effects occur, get emergency help at once. Ask someone to drive you to the the nearest hospital emergency room. Do not try to drive yourself. If this is not possible, call an ambulance, lie down, cover yourself to keep warm, and prop your feet higher than your head. Stay in that position until help arrives.

For patients taking ibuprofen without a prescription:

• Check with your physician or dentist:
—if your symptoms do not improve or if they get worse.
—if you are using this medicine to bring down a fever and the fever lasts more than 3 days or returns.
—if the painful area becomes red or swollen.

For patients taking mefenamic acid: If diarrhea occurs while you are using this medicine, **stop taking it and check with your doctor immediately. Do not take it again without first checking with your doctor,** because severe diarrhea may occur each time you take it.

Check with your doctor immediately if chills, fever, muscle aches or pains, or other influenza-like symptoms occur shortly before, or together with, a skin rash. Very rarely, these effects may be the first signs of a serious reaction to this medicine.

Side Effects of This Medicine

Along with its needed effects, a medicine may cause some unwanted effects. Although not all of these side effects appear very often, when they do occur they may require medical attention. **Stop taking this medicine and check with your doctor immediately** if any of the following side effects occur:

Rare

Convulsions (seizures)
Shortness of breath, troubled breathing, wheezing, or pain or tightness in chest
Sudden decrease in amount of urine

Also, check with your doctor as soon as possible if any of the following side effects occur:

More common

Skin rash

Less common or rare

Abdominal or stomach pain (severe)
Bleeding sores on lips
Bloody or black tarry stools
Bloody or cloudy urine
Blurred vision or any change in vision
Chills and/or fever
Confusion or mental depression
Decreased hearing or ringing or buzzing in ears
Difficult or painful urination
Frequent urge to urinate
Hives or itching of skin
Muscle weakness
Redness, tenderness, burning, or peeling of skin
Sores, ulcers, or white spots in mouth
Swelling of face
Swelling of feet or lower legs
Thickened or scaly skin
Unexplained sore throat and fever
Unusual bleeding or bruising
Unusual tiredness or weakness
Unusual weight gain
Vomiting of blood or material that looks like coffee grounds
Yellowing of eyes or skin

Other side effects may occur which usually do not require medical attention. These side effects may go away during treatment as your body adjusts to the medicine. However, check with your doctor if any of the following side effects continue or are bothersome:

More common

Diarrhea (if taking mefenamic acid, stop taking the medicine and check with your doctor immediately)
Dizziness, drowsiness, or lightheadedness
Headache
Heartburn or indigestion
Nausea or vomiting
Stomach pain or discomfort (mild to moderate)

Less common or rare

Bloated feeling, gas, or constipation
Decreased appetite
General feeling of discomfort or illness
Irritation or soreness of mouth
Irritation or swelling of eyes
Nervousness or trembling
Numbness, tingling, pain, or weakness in hands or feet
Trouble in sleeping
Unexplained nosebleeds
Unusually fast or pounding heartbeat
Unusual sweating

Although not all of the side effects listed above have been reported for all of these medicines, they have been reported for at least one of them. However, since all anti-inflammatory analgesics are very similar, it is possible that any of the above side effects may occur with any of these medicines.

Some of the above side effects may be especially likely to occur in the elderly, who are usually more sensitive to the effects of these medicines.

Other side effects not listed above may also occur in some patients. If you notice any other effects, check with your doctor.

APPETITE SUPPRESSANTS
(Systemic)

This information applies to the following medicines:

Benzphetamine (benz-FET-a-meen)
Diethylpropion (dye-eth-il-PROE-pee-on)
Mazindol (MAY-zin-dole)
Phendimetrazine (fen-dye-MET-ra-zeen)
Phenmetrazine (fen-MET-ra-zeen)
Phentermine (FEN-ter-meen)

This information does not apply to fenfluramine.

Some commonly used brand names are:	Generic names:
Didrex	Benzphetamine

Nobesine-75*	
Regibon*	
Tenuate	
Tenuate Dospan	Diethylpropion†
Tepanil	
Tepanil Ten-Tab	

Mazanor	Mazindol
Sanorex	

Adipost	
Adphen	
Anorex	
Bacarate	
Bontril PDM	
Bontril Slow Release	
Di-AP-Trol	
Dyrexan-OD	
Hyrex-105	
Melfiat	
Melfiat-105 Unicelles	
Metra	
Obalan	
Obeval	
Phenzine	
Plegine	Phendimetrazine†
Prelu-2	
Slyn-LL	
Sprx-1	
Sprx-3	
Sprx-105	
Statobex	
Statobex-G	
Trimcaps	
Trimstat	
Trimtabs	
Wehless	

Wehless Timecelles-105	
Weightrol	
X-Trozine	Phendimetrazine†
X-Trozine LA	

Preludin	Phenmetrazine

Adipex-P	
Dapex-37.5	
Fastin	
Ionamin	
Obe-Nix	
Obephen	
Obermine	
Obestin-30	
Oby-Trim	Phentermine†
Parmine	
Phentamine	
Phentrol	
Phentrol 2	
Phentrol 4	
Phentrol 5	
Teramine	
Tora	
Unifast Unicelles	
Wilpowr	

*Not available in the United States.
†Generic name product also available.

Appetite suppressants are used in the short-term (a few weeks) treatment of obesity. For a few weeks (6 to 12), these medicines in combination with dieting, exercise, and changes in eating habits can help patients lose weight. However, since their appetite-reducing effect is only temporary, they are useful only for the first few weeks of dieting until new eating habits are established. They are not effective for continuous use in diet control.

These medicines are available only with your doctor's prescription.

Before Using This Medicine

In order to decide on the best treatment for your medical problem, your doctor should be told:

—if you have ever had any unusual or allergic reaction to amphetamine, dextroamphetamine, ephedrine, epinephrine, isoproterenol, metaproterenol, methamphetamine, norepinephrine, phenylephrine, phenylpropanolamine, pseudoephedrine, or terbutaline.

—if you are on a low-salt, low-sugar, or any other special diet, or if you are allergic to any substance, such as sulfites or other preservatives or dyes. Most medicines contain more than their active ingredient. Your doctor or pharmacist can help you avoid products that may cause a problem.

—if you are pregnant or if you intend to become pregnant while taking this medicine. Although benzphetamine, phendimetrazine, and phentermine have not been shown to cause birth defects or other problems in humans, the chance always exists.

Studies in animals have shown that other appetite suppressants, such as mazindol, and related medicines such as amphetamines (no longer recommended for appetite control), may cause birth defects or other toxic or harmful effects when taken in large doses during pregnancy. Also, studies in animals have shown that mazindol increases the chance of death in the newborn.

Phenmetrazine has been reported to cause birth defects in humans, although this has not been proven. However, it has not been shown to cause birth defects in animal studies. Studies in animals have also shown that phenmetrazine may lessen the chance of becoming pregnant and when taken during pregnancy causes a decrease in the baby's body weight at weaning.

Diethylpropion has not been shown to cause birth defects or other problems in human and animal studies.

—if you are breast-feeding an infant. Although appetite suppressants have not been shown to cause problems in humans, the chance always exists.

—if you have any of the following medical problems:
Diabetes mellitus (sugar diabetes)
Epilepsy
Glaucoma
Heart or blood vessel disease
High blood pressure
Mental illness (severe)
Overactive thyroid

—if you are planning to have surgery of any kind.

—if you are now taking any of the following medicines or types of medicine:
Guanethidine
Phenothiazines

—if you are now taking medicine for asthma or other breathing problems (for example, epinephrine, isoproterenol).

—if you are now taking central nervous system (CNS) stimulants such as:
Amphetamines
Caffeine
Medicine for narcolepsy (uncontrolled desire for sleep or sudden attacks of sleep at irregular intervals)
Other medicine for appetite control

—if you are using mazindol and are also taking medicine for sugar diabetes.

—if you are now taking or have taken within the past 2 weeks monoamine oxidase (MAO) inhibitors such as:
Furazolidone
Isocarboxazid
Pargyline
Phenelzine
Procarbazine
Tranylcypromine

Proper Use of This Medicine

Take this medicine only as directed by your doctor. Do not take more of it, do not take it more often, and do not take it for a longer period of time than your doctor ordered. If too much is taken, it may become habit-forming.

If you think this medicine is not working as well after you have taken it for a few weeks, **do not increase the dose.** Instead, check with your doctor.

If you are taking the short-acting form of this medicine:

• Take the last dose for each day about 4 to 6 hours before bedtime to help prevent trouble in sleeping.

If you are taking the long-acting form of this medicine:

• Take the daily dose about 10 to 14 hours before bedtime to help prevent trouble in sleeping.

• These capsules or tablets are to be swallowed whole. Do not break, crush, or chew before swallowing.

If you are taking mazindol:

• To help prevent trouble in sleeping, if you are taking this medicine in a:

—*1-mg tablet,* take the last dose for each day about 4 to 6 hours before bedtime.

—*2-mg tablet,* take the dose once each day about 10 to 14 hours before bedtime.

How to store this medicine:

• Store away from heat and direct light.

• **Keep out of the reach of children.**

• Do not store in the bathroom medicine cabinet because the heat or moisture may cause the medicine to break down.

• Do not keep outdated medicine or medicine no longer needed. Flush the contents of the container down the toilet, unless otherwise directed.

Precautions While Using This Medicine

Your doctor should check your progress at regular visits in order to make sure that this medicine does not cause unwanted effects.

Dryness of the mouth may occur while you are taking this medicine. Sucking on hard sugarless candy or ice chips or chewing sugarless gum may help relieve the dry mouth.

This medicine may cause some people to feel a false sense of well-being or to become dizzy, lightheaded, drowsy, or less alert than they are normally. **Make sure you know how you react to this medicine before you drive, use machines, or do other jobs that require you to be alert.**

If you will be taking this medicine in large doses for a long period of time, do not stop taking it without first checking with your doctor. Your doctor may want you to reduce gradually the amount you are taking before stopping completely.

Side Effects of This Medicine

Along with its needed effects, a medicine may cause some unwanted effects. Although not all of these side effects appear very often, when they do occur they may require medical attention. Check with your doctor as soon as possible if any of the following side effects occur:

Rare
    Mood or mental changes
    Skin rash or hives

Other side effects may occur which usually do not require medical attention. These side effects may go away during treatment as your body adjusts to the medicine. However, check with your doctor if any of the following side effects continue or are bothersome:

More common
    False sense of well-being (less common with mazindol and phentermine)
    Irritability

Nervousness
Restlessness
Trouble in sleeping

Note: After such stimulant effects have
worn off, drowsiness, trembling, unusual tiredness or weakness, or mental depression may occur.

Less common
Blurred vision
Changes in sexual desire or decreased
  sexual ability
Constipation (more common with
  mazindol)
Diarrhea
Difficult or painful urination
Dizziness or lightheadedness
Dryness of mouth (more common with
  mazindol)
Frequent urge to urinate or increased
  urination
Headache
Nausea or vomiting
Stomach cramps or pain
Unpleasant taste
Unusually fast, pounding, or irregular
  heartbeat
Unusual sweating

Although not all of the side effects listed
above have been reported for all of these
medicines, they have been reported for
at least one of them. However, since all
of the appetite suppressants are very
similar, any of the above side effects
may occur with any of these medicines.

After you stop using this medicine, your
body may need time to adjust. The
length of time this takes depends on the
amount of medicine you were using and
how long you used it. During this period
of time check with your doctor if you
notice any of the following side effects:
Mental depression
Nausea or vomiting
Stomach cramps or pain
Trembling
Unusual tiredness or weakness

Other side effects not listed above may also
occur in some patients. If you notice any
other effects, check with your doctor.

BACLOFEN (Systemic)
A commonly used brand name is Lioresal.

Baclofen (BAK-loe-fen) is a medicine
used to help relax certain muscles in your
body. It relieves the spasms, cramping, and
tightness of muscles caused by medical
problems such as multiple sclerosis or certain injuries to the spine. Baclofen does not
cure these problems, but it may allow other
treatment, such as physical therapy, to be
more helpful in improving your condition.
Baclofen acts on the central nervous system
(CNS) to produce its muscle relaxant effects. Its actions on the CNS may also
cause some of the medicine's side effects.
Baclofen may also be used to relieve other
conditions as determined by your doctor.

This medicine is available only with
your doctor's prescription.

Before Using This Medicine

In order to decide on the best treatment for
your medical problem, your doctor
should be told:

—if you have ever had any unusual or
allergic reaction to baclofen.

—if you are on a low-salt, low-sugar, or
any other special diet, or if you are allergic to any substance, such as sulfites or

other preservatives. Most medicines contain more than their active ingredient.

—if you are pregnant or if you intend to become pregnant while taking this medicine. Studies on birth defects with baclofen have not been done in humans. However, studies in animals have shown that baclofen, when given in doses several times the human dose, increases the chance of hernias in the fetus, incomplete or slow development of bones, and lower birth weight.

—if you are breast-feeding an infant. It is not known whether baclofen passes into the breast milk. Although this medicine has not been shown to cause problems in humans, the chance always exists.

—if you have any of the following medical problems:

> Diabetes mellitus (sugar diabetes)
> Epilepsy
> Kidney disease
> Mental or emotional problems
> Stroke or other brain disease

—if you are taking any of the following medicines or types of medicine:

> Antidiabetics, oral (diabetes medicine you take by mouth)
> Insulin

—if you are now taking other central nervous system (CNS) depressants, such as:

> Anticonvulsants (seizure medicine)
> Antihistamines or medicine for hay fever, other allergies, or colds
> Barbiturates
> Narcotics
> Other muscle relaxants
> Pain medicine (prescription)
> Sedatives, tranquilizers, or sleeping medicine
> Tricyclic antidepressants (medicine for depression)

—if you are now taking or have taken within the past 2 weeks monoamine oxidase (MAO) inhibitors such as:

> Furazolidone
> Isocarboxazid
> Pargyline
> Phenelzine
> Procarbazine
> Tranylcypromine

Proper Use of This Medicine

If you miss a dose of this medicine, and you remember within an hour or so of the missed dose, take it as soon as you remember. However, if you do not remember until later, skip the missed dose and go back to your regular dosing schedule. Do not double doses.

How to store this medicine:

- Store away from heat and direct light.
- **Keep out of the reach of children.**
- Do not store in the bathroom medicine cabinet because the heat or moisture may cause the medicine to break down.
- Do not keep outdated medicine or medicine no longer needed. Flush the contents of the container down the toilet, unless otherwise directed.

Precautions While Using This Medicine

Do not suddenly stop taking this medicine. Unwanted effects may occur if the medicine is stopped suddenly. Check with your doctor for the best way to reduce gradually the amount you are taking before stopping completely.

This medicine will add to the effects of alcohol and other CNS depressants (medicines that slow down the nervous system, possibly causing drowsiness). Some examples of CNS depressants are antihistamines or medicine for hay fever, other allergies, or colds; sedatives, tranquilizers, or sleeping medicine; prescription pain medicine or narcotics; barbiturates; medicine for seizures; tricyclic antidepressants (medicine for depression); other muscle relaxants; or anesthetics, including some dental anesthetics. **Check with your doctor before taking any of the above while you are using baclofen.**

This medicine may cause drowsiness, dizziness, vision problems, or clumsiness or unsteadiness in some people. **Make sure you know how you react to this medicine before you drive, use machines, or do other jobs that require you to be alert, wellcoordinated, and able to see well.**

For diabetics—This medicine may cause your blood sugar levels to rise. If you notice a change in the results of your urine sugar test or if you have any questions about this, check with your doctor.

Side Effects of This Medicine

Along with its needed effects, a medicine may cause some unwanted effects. Although not all of these side effects appear very often, when they do occur they may require medical attention. Check with your doctor as soon as possible if any of the following side effects occur:

Rare

Bloody or dark urine
Chest pain
Fainting
Hallucinations (seeing or hearing things that are not there)
Mental depression or other mood changes
Ringing or buzzing in the ears
Skin rash or itching

Signs of overdose

Blurred or double vision or any change in vision
Convulsions (seizures)
Shortness of breath or unusually slow or troubled breathing
Unusual muscle weakness (severe)
Vomiting

Other side effects may occur which usually do not require medical attention. These side effects may go away during treatment as your body adjusts to the medicine. However, check with your doctor if any of the following side effects continue or are bothersome:

More common

Dizziness or lightheadedness
Drowsiness
Mental confusion
Nausea
Unusual weakness, especially muscle weakness

Less common or rare

Abdominal or stomach pain or discomfort
Clumsiness, unsteadiness, trembling, or other problems with muscle control
Constipation
Diarrhea
False sense of well-being
Difficult or painful urination or decrease in amount of urine
Frequent urge to urinate or uncontrolled urination
Headache
Loss of appetite
Muscle pain
Numbness or tingling in hands or feet
Sexual problems in males
Slurred speech or other speech problems
Stuffy nose
Swelling of ankles
Trouble in sleeping
Unexplained muscle stiffness
Unusual excitement
Unusually low blood pressure
Unusual pounding heartbeat
Unusual tiredness
Unusual weight gain

Some side effects may occur after you have stopped taking this medicine, especially if you stop taking it suddenly. **Check with your doctor immediately** if any of the following effects occur:

Convulsions (seizures)
Hallucinations (seeing or hearing things that are not there)
Increase in muscle spasm, cramping, or tightness
Mood or mental changes
Unusual nervousness or restlessness

Some side effects may be more likely to occur in elderly patients, who are usually more sensitive to the effects of baclofen. These include hallucinations, mental confusion or depression, other mood or mental changes, and severe drowsiness.

Other side effects not listed above may also occur in some patients. If you notice any other effects, check with your doctor.

BARBITURATES (Systemic)

This information applies to the following medicines:

Amobarbital (am-oh-BAR-bi-tal)
Aprobarbital (a-proe-BAR-bi-tal)
Butabarbital (byoo-ta-BAR-bi-tal)
Mephobarbital (me-foe-BAR-bi-tal)
Metharbital (meth-AR-bi-tal)
Pentobarbital (pen-toe-BAR-bi-tal)
Phenobarbital (fee-noe-BAR-bi-tal)
Secobarbital (see-koe-BAR-bi-tal)
Secobarbital and Amobarbital (see-koe-BAR-bi-tal and am-oh-BAR-bi-tal)
Talbutal (TAL-byoo-tal)

Some commonly used brand names are:	Generic names:
Amytal	Amobarbital†
Alurate	Aprobarbital
Butalan Butatran Buticaps Butisol Day-Barb* Neo-Barb* Sarisol No. 2	Butabarbital†
Mebaral	Mephobarbital
Gemonil	Metharbital
Nembutal	Pentobarbital†
Barbita Gardenal* Luminal PBR/12 Sedadrops SK-Phenobarbital Solfoton	Phenobarbital†
Seconal Seral*	Secobarbital†
Tuinal	Secobarbital and Amobarbital
Lotusate	Talbutal

*Not available in the United States.
†Generic name product may also be available.

Barbiturates (bar-BI-tyoo-rates) belong to the group of medicines called central nervous system (CNS) depressants (medicines that slow down the nervous system). They act on the brain and CNS to produce effects which may be helpful or harmful. This depends on the individual patient's condition and response and the amount of medicine taken.

Barbiturates are taken by mouth, given by injection, or used rectally. They may be used to treat insomnia (sleeplessness) by helping patients fall asleep. Also, they may be used to relieve anxiety or tension. Some of the barbiturates are used as anticonvulsants to help control convulsions or seizures in certain disorders or diseases, such as epilepsy. Barbiturates may also be used for other conditions as determined by your doctor.

If barbiturates are used regularly (for example, every day) for insomnia, they usually are not effective for longer than 2 weeks. Also, if too much of a barbiturate is used, it may become habit-forming.

These medicines are available only with your doctor's prescription.

Before Using This Medicine

In order to decide on the best treatment for your medical problem, your doctor should be told:

—if you have ever had any unusual or allergic reaction to barbiturates.

—if you are on a low-salt, low-sugar, or any other special diet, or if you are allergic to any substance, such as sulfites or other preservatives or dyes. Most medicines contain more than their active ingredient, and many liquid medicines contain alcohol. Your doctor or pharmacist can help you avoid products that may cause a problem.

—if you are pregnant or if you intend to become pregnant while using this medicine, since barbiturates have been shown to increase the chance of birth defects in humans. However, this medicine may be needed in serious diseases or other situations which threaten the mother's life. Be sure you have discussed this and the following information with your doctor:

• taking barbiturates regularly during the last 3 months of pregnancy may cause the baby to become dependent on the medicine. This may lead to withdrawal side effects in the baby after birth.

• barbiturates taken for epilepsy during pregnancy may cause bleeding problems in the newborn infant.

• one study in humans has suggested that barbiturates taken during pregnancy may increase the chance of brain tumors in the baby.

• barbiturates taken for anesthesia during labor and delivery may reduce the force and frequency of contractions of the uterus; this may prolong labor and delay delivery.

• use of barbiturates during labor may cause breathing problems in the newborn infant.

—if you are breast-feeding an infant. Barbiturates pass into the breast milk and may cause drowsiness, unusually slow heartbeat, shortness of breath, or troubled breathing in infants of nursing mothers taking this medicine.

—if you have any of the following medical problems:
Anemia (severe)
Asthma (history of), emphysema, or other chronic lung disease
Diabetes mellitus (sugar diabetes)
Hyperactivity (in children)
Kidney disease
Liver disease
Mental depression
Overactive thyroid
Pain
Porphyria (or history of)
Underactive adrenal gland

—if you are now taking or receiving any of the following medicines or types of medicine:
Acetaminophen
Acetazolamide
Adrenocorticoids (cortisone-like medicines)
Aminophylline
Anticoagulants, oral (blood thinners you take by mouth)
Antihypertensives (high blood pressure medicine)
Ascorbic acid (vitamin C)
Bumetanide
Carbamazepine
Chlorprothixene
Contraceptives containing estrogens, oral (birth-control pills)
Corticotropin
Cyclophosphamide
Cyclosporine
Dacarbazine
Dichlorphenamide
Digitalis
Digitoxin
Diltiazem
Disopyramide
Divalproex sodium
Doxycycline
Dyphylline
Estramustine
Estrogens

Ethotoin
Fenoprofen
Griseofulvin
Haloperidol
Leucovorin
Levothyroxine
Loxapine
Maprotiline
Mephenytoin
Methazolamide
Methylphenidate
Nifedipine
Oxtriphylline
Phenytoin
Posterior pituitary
Primidone
Quinidine
Theophylline
Thiothixene
Valproic acid
Verapamil
Vitamin D

—if you are now taking any central nervous system (CNS) depressants such as:

Anticonvulsants (seizure medicine)
Antihistamines or medicine for hay fever, other allergies, or colds
Muscle relaxants
Narcotics
Other barbiturates
Prescription pain medicine
Sedatives, tranquilizers, or sleeping medicine

—if you are now taking any tricylic antidepressants (medicine for depression) such as:

Amitriptyline
Amoxapine
Desipramine
Doxepin
Imipramine
Nortriptyline
Protriptyline
Trimipramine

—if you are now taking or have taken within the past 2 weeks monoamine oxidase (MAO) inhibitors such as:

Furazolidone
Isocarboxazid
Pargyline
Phenelzine
Procarbazine
Tranylcypromine

Proper Use of This Medicine

Use this medicine only as directed by your doctor. Do not use more of it, do not use it more often, and do not use it for a longer period of time than your doctor ordered. If too much is used, it may become habit-forming (causing mental or physical dependence).

If you think this medicine is not working as well after you have taken it for a few weeks, **do not increase the dose.** To do so may increase the chance of your becoming dependent on the medicine. Instead, check with your doctor.

If you are taking this medicine for epilepsy, it must be taken every day in regularly spaced doses as ordered by your doctor in order for it to control your seizures. This is necessary to keep a constant amount of medicine in the blood. To help keep this amount constant, do not miss any doses.

If you are taking this medicine regularly (for example, every day as in epilepsy) and you do miss a dose, take it as soon as possible. However, if it is almost time for your next dose, skip the missed dose and go back to your regular dosing schedule. Do not double doses.

For patients taking the *extended-release capsule or tablet* form of this medicine:

• These capsules or tablets are to be swallowed whole. Do not break, crush, or chew before swallowing.

For patients taking the *pediatric drop* form of this medicine:

• Do not use if solution is cloudy.

• This medicine is to be taken by mouth even though it may come in a dropper bottle. Measure the correct amount with the specially marked dropper. Each dose may be taken straight or mixed with water, milk, or fruit juices. Be sure to drink all of the liquid in order to get the full dose of medicine.

For patients using the *rectal suppository* form of this medicine:

• How to insert suppository: First remove the foil wrapper and moisten the suppository with water. Lie down on side and push the suppository well up into rectum with finger.

How to store this medicine:

• Store away from heat and direct light.

• **Keep out of the reach of children** since overdose is especially dangerous in children.

• Do not store in the bathroom medicine cabinet because the heat or moisture may cause the medicine to break down.

• Store the suppository form of this medicine in the refrigerator.

• Keep the liquid form of this medicine from freezing.

• Do not keep outdated medicine or medicine no longer needed. Flush the contents of the container down the toilet, unless otherwise directed.

Precautions While Using This Medicine

If you will be using this medicine regularly for a long period of time:

• Your doctor should check your progress at regular visits.

• Do not stop using it without first checking with your doctor. Your doctor may want you to reduce gradually the amount you are using before stopping completely.

This medicine will add to the effects of alcohol and other CNS depressants (medicines that slow down the nervous system, possibly causing drowsiness). Some examples of CNS depressants are antihistamines or medicine for hay fever, other allergies, or colds; sedatives, tranquilizers, or sleeping medicine; prescription pain medicine or narcotics; barbiturates; medicine for seizures; muscle relaxants; or anesthetics, including some dental anesthetics. **Check with your doctor before taking any of the above while you are using this medicine.**

If you have been using this medicine for a long period of time and you think that you may have become mentally or physically dependent on it, check with your doctor. Some signs of mental or physical dependence on barbiturates are:

—a strong desire or need to continue taking the medicine.

—a need to increase the dose to receive the effects of the medicine.

—withdrawal side effects (for example, anxiety or unusual restlessness, convulsions or seizures, feeling faint, nausea or vomiting, trembling of hands, trouble in sleeping) occurring after the medicine is stopped.

If you think you may have taken an overdose, get emergency help at once. Taking an overdose of a barbiturate or taking alcohol or other CNS depressants with the barbiturate may lead to unconsciousness and possibly death. Some signs of an overdose are severe drowsiness, mental confusion, severe weakness, shortness of breath or unusually slow or troubled breathing, slurred speech, staggering, and unusually slow heartbeat.

This medicine may cause some people to become dizzy, lightheaded, drowsy, or less alert than they are normally. Even if taken at bedtime, it may cause some people to feel drowsy or less alert on arising. **Make sure you know how you react to this medicine before you drive, use machines, or do other jobs that require you to be alert.**

Side Effects of This Medicine

Studies in animals (mice and rats) have shown that phenobarbital causes cancer when given for the lifetime of the animal; however, there is no evidence to show that phenobarbital causes cancer in humans.

Along with its needed effects, a medicine may cause some unwanted effects. Although not all of these side effects appear very often, when they do occur they may require medical attention. **Check with your doctor immediately** if any of the following side effects occur:

Rare

Bleeding sores on lips
Chest pain
Muscle or joint pain
Red, thickened, or scaly skin
Skin rash or hives
Sore throat and/or fever
Sores, ulcers, or white spots in mouth
(painful)
Swelling of eyelids, face, or lips
Wheezing or tightness in chest

Also, check with your doctor as soon as possible if any of the following side effects occur:

Less common

Confusion
Mental depression
Unusual excitement

Rare

Hallucinations (seeing, hearing, or feeling things that are not there)
Unusual bleeding or bruising
Unusual tiredness or weakness

With long-term or chronic use

Bone pain, tenderness, or aching
Loss of appetite
Muscle weakness
Unusual weight loss
Yellowing of eyes or skin

Possible signs of overdose

Confusion (severe)
Drowsiness (severe)
Poor judgment
Shortness of breath or unusually slow or
troubled breathing
Slurred speech
Staggering
Trouble in sleeping

Unusual irritability (continuing)
Unusually slow heartbeat
Unusual movements of the eyes
Weakness (severe)

Other side effects may occur which usually do not require medical attention. These side effects may go away during treatment as your body adjusts to the medicine. However, check with your doctor if any of the following side effects continue or are bothersome:

More common

Clumsiness or unsteadiness
Dizziness or lightheadedness
Drowsiness
"Hangover" effect

Less common

Anxiety or nervousness
Constipation
Feeling faint
Headache
Nausea or vomiting
Nightmares or trouble in sleeping
Unusual irritability

Unusual excitement may be more likely to occur in children and in elderly or very ill patients. Also, confusion and mental depression may be more likely to occur in elderly or very ill patients.

After you stop using this medicine, your body may need time to adjust. If you took this medicine in high doses or for a long period of time, this may take up to about 15 days. During this period of time check with your doctor if any of the following side effects occur (usually occur within 8 to 16 hours after medicine is stopped):

Anxiety or unusual restlessness
Convulsions or seizures
Dizziness or lightheadedness
Feeling faint
Hallucinations (seeing, hearing, or feeling things that are not there)
Muscle twitching
Nausea or vomiting
Trembling of hands

Trouble in sleeping, increased dreaming, or nightmares
Unusual weakness
Vision problems

Other side effects not listed above may also occur in some patients. If you notice any other effects, check with your doctor.

BELLADONNA ALKALOIDS
(Systemic)

This information applies to the following medicines:

Atropine (A-troe-peen)
Belladonna (bell-a-DON-a)
Hyoscyamine (hye-oh-SYE-a-meen)
Hyoscyamine and Scopolamine (skoe-POL-a-meen)
Scopolamine

Some commonly used brand names are:	Generic names:
Lyopine Vari-Dose	Atropine†
	Belladonna†
Cystospaz	Hyoscyamine
Anaspaz Bellaspaz Cystospaz-M Levsin Levsinex Timecaps Neoquess	Hyoscyamine Sulfate
Bellafoline	Hyoscyamine and Scopolamine
Transderm-Scōp Triptone	Scopolamine†

†Generic name product may also be available.

Belladonna alkaloids belong to the group of medicines known as antimuscarinics. They are taken by mouth or given by injection. Scopolamine is used also by transdermal disk (a small patch that is applied to the skin).

Belladonna alkaloids are used to relieve cramps or spasms of the stomach, intestines, and bladder. Some are used in the treatment of peptic ulcer together with antacids or other medicine. Others are used to prevent nausea and vomiting and motion sickness. In patients with Parkinson's disease, belladonna alkaloids may be used to decrease stiffness and tremors.

In surgery, some of the belladonna alkaloids are given by injection before anesthesia to help relax you and to decrease secretions, such as saliva. During anesthesia and surgery, atropine, hyoscyamine, and scopolamine are used to help keep the heartbeat normal. Atropine is given also by injection to help relax the stomach and intestines for certain types of examinations. In addition, atropine and hyoscyamine are used to treat poisoning caused by medicines such as neostigmine and physostigmine, and by certain types of mushrooms. Atropine is used also for poisoning by "nerve" gases or organic phosphorous pesticides (for example, demeton [Systox], diazinon, malathion, parathion, and ronnel [Trolene]).

Belladonna alkaloids are available only with your doctor's prescription.

Before Using This Medicine

In order to decide on the best treatment for your medical problem, your doctor should be told:

—if you have ever had any unusual or allergic reaction to any of the belladonna alkaloids (atropine, belladonna, hyoscyamine, and scopolamine).

—if you are on a low-salt, low-sugar, or any other special diet, or if you are allergic to any substance, such as sulfites or other preservatives or dyes. Most medicines contain more than their active ingredient, and many liquid medicines contain alcohol. Your doctor or pharmacist can help you avoid products that may cause a problem.

—if you are pregnant or if you intend to become pregnant while using this medicine. Studies with atropine have not been done in humans. However, atropine has not been shown to cause birth defects or other problems in animal studies.

Studies with belladonna, hyoscyamine, or scopolamine have not been done in either humans or animals. Atropine and hyoscyamine have been reported to increase the heartbeat of the fetus when given during pregnancy by injection into a vein.

When scopolamine is given before labor begins, it may cause in the newborn infant an unusually slow heartbeat, shortness of breath, or troubled breathing, and may also increase the possibility of bleeding.

—if you are breast-feeding an infant. Although the belladonna alkaloids have not been shown to cause problems in humans, the chance always exists. Small amounts of atropine, hyoscyamine, and scopolamine may pass into the breast milk. Also, since the belladonna alkaloids tend to decrease the secretions of the body, it is possible that the flow of breast milk may be reduced in some patients.

—if you have any of the following medical problems:

Bleeding problems (severe)
Brain damage (in children)
Colitis (severe)
Down's syndrome (mongolism)
Dry mouth (severe and continuing)
Enlarged prostate
Fever
Glaucoma (or predisposition to)
Heart disease
Hernia (hiatal)
High blood pressure
Intestinal blockage or other intestinal
    problems
Kidney disease
Liver disease
Lung disease (chronic)
Myasthenia gravis

Overactive thyroid
Spastic paralysis (in children)
Toxemia of pregnancy
Urinary tract blockage or difficult
    urination

—if you are taking *any* other medicines including over-the-counter (OTC) or nonprescription medicines (for example, antacids or diarrhea medicine). Many medicines change the way belladonna alkaloids affect your body. Also, the effect of other medicines may be reduced by belladonna alkaloids.

—if you are taking any of the belladonna alkaloids and are also taking central nervous system (CNS) depressants such as:

Antihistamines or medicine for hay fever,
    other allergies, or colds
Muscle relaxants
Narcotics
Prescription pain medicine
Sedatives, tranquilizers, or sleeping
    medicine

—if you are now taking tricyclic antidepressants such as:

Amitriptyline
Amoxapine
Clomipramine
Desipramine
Doxepin
Imipramine
Nortriptyline
Protriptyline
Trimipramine

—if you are taking any of the belladonna alkaloids and are also taking or have taken within the past 2 weeks monoamine oxidase (MAO) inhibitors such as:

Furazolidone
Isocarboxazid
Pargyline
Phenelzine
Procarbazine
Tranylcypromine

—if you are taking scopolamine and are also taking anticonvulsants (seizure medicine) or barbiturates.

Proper Use of This Medicine

Take this medicine only as directed. Do not take more of it, do not take it more often, and do not take it for a longer period of time than your doctor ordered. To do so may increase the chance of side effects.

For patients taking any of the belladonna alkaloids by mouth:
• Take this medicine 30 minutes to 1 hour before meals unless otherwise directed by your doctor.

For patients using the transdermal disk form of scopolamine:
• This medicine usually comes with patient directions. Read them carefully before using this medicine.

• Wash and dry hands thoroughly before and after handling.

• Apply to the hairless area of the skin behind the ear. Do not place over any cuts or irritations.

If you miss a dose of this medicine, take it as soon as possible. However, if it is almost time for your next dose, skip the missed dose and go back to your regular dosing schedule. Do not double doses.

How to store this medicine:
• Store away from heat and direct light.

• **Keep out of the reach of children** since overdose is especially dangerous in young children.

• Do not store in the bathroom medicine cabinet because the heat or moisture may cause the medicine to break down.

• Keep the liquid form of this medicine from freezing.

• Do not keep outdated medicine or medicine no longer needed. Flush the contents of the container down the toilet, unless otherwise directed.

Precautions While Using This Medicine

If you think you may have taken an overdose, get emergency help at once. Taking an overdose of any of the belladonna alkaloids or taking scopolamine with alcohol or other CNS depressants may lead to unconsciousness and possibly death. Some signs of overdose are clumsiness or unsteadiness; dizziness; severe drowsiness; fever; hallucinations (seeing, hearing, or feeling things that are not there); confusion; shortness of breath or troubled breathing; slurred speech; unusual excitement, nervousness, restlessness, or irritability; unusually fast heartbeat; and unusual warmth, dryness, and flushing of skin.

Belladonna alkaloids may make you sweat less, causing your body temperature to increase. **Use extra care not to become overheated during exercise or hot weather while you are taking this medicine,** since overheating may result in heat stroke.

This medicine may cause some people to have blurred vision. **Make sure your vision is clear before you drive or do other jobs that require you to see well.** This medicine may also cause your eyes to become more sensitive to light than they are normally. Wearing sunglasses may help lessen the discomfort from bright light.

Your mouth, nose, and throat may feel very dry while you are taking this medicine. To help relieve mouth dryness, chew sugarless gum or dissolve bits of ice in your mouth.

For patients taking any of the belladonna alkaloids by mouth:
• Do not take this medicine within 1 hour of taking antacids or medicine for diarrhea. Taking them too close together may prevent belladonna alkaloids from working as well.

For patients taking scopolamine:

• This medicine will add to the effects of alcohol and other CNS depressants (medicines that slow down the nervous system, possibly causing drowsiness). Some examples of CNS depressants are antihistamines or medicine for hay fever, other allergies, or colds; sedatives, tranquilizers, or sleeping medicine; prescription pain medicine or narcotics; barbiturates; medicine for seizures; muscle relaxants; or anesthetics, including some dental anesthetics. **Check with your doctor before taking any of the above while you are using this medicine.**

• This medicine may cause some people to become dizzy or drowsy. **Make sure you know how you react to this medicine before you drive, use machines, or do other jobs that require you to be alert.**

Side Effects of This Medicine

Along with its needed effects, a medicine may cause some unwanted effects. Although not all of these side effects appear very often, when they do occur they may require medical attention. Check with your doctor as soon as possible if any of the following side effects occur:

Rare
> Eye pain
> Skin rash or hives

Signs of overdose
> Blurred vision (continuing) or changes in near vision
> Clumsiness or unsteadiness
> Confusion
> Convulsions (seizures)
> Dizziness
> Drowsiness (severe)
> Dryness of mouth, nose, or throat (severe)
> Fever
> Hallucinations (seeing, hearing, or feeling things that are not there)
> Shortness of breath or troubled breathing
> Slurred speech
> Unusual excitement, nervousness, restlessness, or irritability
> Unusually fast heartbeat
> Unusual warmth, dryness, and flushing of skin

Other side effects may occur which usually do not require medical attention. These side effects may go away during treatment as your body adjusts to the medicine. However, check with your doctor if any of the following side effects continue or are bothersome:

More common
> Constipation (less common with hyoscyamine)
> Decrease in sweating
> Dryness of mouth, nose, throat, or skin

Less common or rare
> Bloated feeling
> Blurred vision
> Decreased flow of breast milk
> Difficult urination (may require medical attention if patient has enlarged prostate)
> Difficulty in swallowing
> Drowsiness (more common with high doses and with scopolamine when given by mouth or by injection)
> False sense of well-being (for scopolamine only)
> Headache
> Increased sensitivity of eyes to light
> Loss of memory (for scopolamine only)
> Nausea or vomiting
> Trouble in sleeping (for scopolamine only)
> Unusual tiredness or weakness

For patients using scopolamine:

• After you stop using scopolamine, your body may need time to adjust. The length of time this takes depends on the amount of scopolamine you were using and how long you used it. During this period of time check with your doctor if you notice any of the following side effects:

> Anxiety
> Irritability
> Nightmares
> Trouble in sleeping

For patients using the transdermal disk of scopolamine:

• While using the disk or even after removing it, your eyes may become more sensitive to light than usual. You may also notice the pupil in one eye is larger than the other. Check with your doctor if this side effect continues or is bothersome.

In infants and children, especially those with spastic paralysis or brain damage, this medicine may be more likely to cause severe side effects. Fever or unusual warmth, dryness, and flushing of skin are more likely to occur in children. Also, when it is given to children during hot weather, a rapid increase in body temperature may occur.

Children and elderly patients are usually more sensitive to the effects of the belladonna alkaloids. Confusion, constipation, difficult urination, drowsiness, dryness of mouth, nose, throat, or skin may be more likely to occur in elderly patients. Also, unusual excitement, nervousness, restlessness, or irritability may be more likely to occur in children and in elderly patients.

Other side effects not listed above may also occur in some patients. If you notice any other effects, check with your doctor.

BELLADONNA ALKALOIDS AND BARBITURATES (Systemic)

This information applies to the following medicines:

Atropine (A-troe-peen), Hyoscyamine (hye-oh-SYE-a-meen), Scopolamine (skoe-POL-a-meen), and Butabarbital (byoo-ta-BAR-bi-tal)

Atropine, Hyoscyamine, Scopolamine, and Phenobarbital (fee-noe-BAR-bi-tal)

Atropine and Phenobarbital

Belladonna and Amobarbital (am-oh-BAR-bi-tal)

Belladonna and Butabarbital

Belladonna and Phenobarbital

Hyoscyamine and Phenobarbital

Some commonly used brand names are:	Generic names:
Palbar No. 2	Atropine, Hyoscyamime, Scopolamine, and Butabarbital
Barbidonna Barophen Bay-Ase Bellalphen Bellastal Donnapine Donna-Sed Donnatal Donnatal Extentabs Donphen Hybephen Hyosophen Kinesed Malatal Palbar Relaxadon Seds Spaslin Spasmolin Spasmophen Spasquid Susano Vanatal Vanodonnal	Atropine, Hyoscyamine, Scopolamine, and Phenobarbital
Antrocol	Atropine and Phenobarbital
Amobell	Belladonna and Amobarbital
Butibel	Belladonna and Butabarbital
Belap Bellkatal Chardonna-2 Pheno-Bella	Belladonna and Phenobarbital†

Anaspaz PB	
Levsinex with Pheno-barbital Timecaps	Hyoscyamine and
Levsin-PB	Phenobarbital
Levsin with Phenobar-bital	

†Generic name product may also be available.

Belladonna alkaloids and barbiturates are combination medicines used to relieve cramping and spasms of the stomach and intestines. They are used also to decrease the amount of acid formed in the stomach.

These medicines are available only with your doctor's prescription.

For information about the precautions and side effects of the medicines in this combination, see:

Belladonna Alkaloids (Systemic)
Barbiturates (Systemic)

Combination products are designed for specific uses. These uses may not be the same as the uses of the individual ingredients. Therefore, some of the information provided in the individual listings may not be relevant to the combination product. If questions arise, check with your doctor, nurse, or pharmacist.

BENZODIAZEPINES (Systemic)

This information applies to the following medicines:

Alprazolam (al-PRAZ-oh-lam)
Chlordiazepoxide (klor-dye-az-e-POX-ide)
Clonazepam (kloe-NA-ze-pam)
Clorazepate (klor-AZ-e-pate)
Diazepam (dye-AZ-e-pam)
Flurazepam (flure-AZ-e-pam)
Halazepam (hal-AZ-e-pam)
Lorazepam (lor-AZ-e-pam)
Oxazepam (ox-AZ-e-pam)
Prazepam (PRAZ-e-pam)
Temazepam (tem-AZ-e-pam)
Triazolam (trye-AY-zoe-lam)

Some commonly used brand names are:	Generic names:
Xanax	Alprazolam

Apo-Chlordiazepoxide*	
Libritabs	
Librium	
Lipoxide	
Medilium*	
Murcil	Chlordiazepoxide†
Novopoxide*	
Reposans	
Sereen	
SK-Lygen	
Solium*	

Clonopin	Clonazepam
Rivotril*	

Tranxene	Clorazepate
Tranxene-SD	

Apo-Diazepam*	
E-Pam*	
Meval*	
Neo-Calme*	
Novodipam*	
Rival*	Diazepam†
Stress-Pam*	
Valium	
Valrelease	
Vivol*	

Apo-Flurazepam*	Flurazepam
Dalmane	
Novoflupam*	

Paxipam	Halazepam

Ativan	Lorazepam†

Apo-Oxazepam*	
Ox-Pam*	Oxazepam
Serax	
Zapex*	

Centrax	Prazepam

Restoril	Temazepam

Halcion	Triazolam

*Not available in the United States.
†Generic name product may also be available.

Benzodiazepines (ben-zoe-dye-AZ-e-peens) belong to the group of medicines called central nervous system (CNS) depressants (medicines that slow down the nervous system). They are taken by mouth or given by injection. Some are used to relieve nervousness or tension. Others are used in the treatment of insomnia or sleeplessness. However, if used regularly (for example, every day) for insomnia or sleeplessness, they are usually not effective for more than a few weeks. Also, one of the benzodiazepines, diazepam, is used to relax muscles or relieve muscle spasm. Clonazepam, clorazepate and diazepam are also used to treat certain convulsive disorders, such as epilepsy. The benzodiazepines may also be used for other conditions as determined by your doctor.

Benzodiazepines should not be used for nervousness or tension caused by the stress of everyday life.

These medicines are available only with your doctor's prescription.

Before Using This Medicine

In order to decide on the best treatment for your medical problem, your doctor should be told:

—if you have ever had any unusual or allergic reaction to benzodiazepines.

—if you are on a low-salt, low-sugar, or any other special diet, or if you are allergic to any substance, such as sulfites or other preservatives or dyes. Most medicines contain more than their active ingredient. Your doctor or pharmacist can help you avoid products that may cause a problem.

—if you are pregnant or if you intend to become pregnant while using this medicine. Chlordiazepoxide and diazepam have been reported to increase the chance of birth defects when used during the first 3 months of pregnancy. Although similar problems have not been reported with the other benzodiazepines, the chance always exists since all of the benzodiazepines are related. Also, studies in animals have shown that clonazepam, lorazepam, and temazepam cause birth defects or other problems, including death of the animal fetus.

In addition, too much use of benzodiazepines during pregnancy may cause the baby to become dependent on the medicine. This may lead to withdrawal side effects after birth. Also, use of benzodiazepines during pregnancy, especially during the last weeks, may cause drowsiness, unusually slow heartbeat, shortness of breath, or troubled breathing in the newborn infant.

Benzodiazepines given just before or during labor may cause weakness in the newborn infant. When diazepam is given in high doses (especially by injection) within 15 hours before delivery, it may cause breathing problems, muscle weakness, difficulty in feeding, and body temperature problems in the newborn infant.

—if you are breast-feeding an infant. Benzodiazepines may pass into the breast milk and cause drowsiness, unusually slow heartbeat, shortness of breath, or troubled breathing in infants of mothers taking this medicine.

—if you have any of the following medical problems:

Emphysema, asthma, bronchitis, or other chronic lung disease
Epilepsy or history of convulsions (seizures)
Hyperactivity (in children)
Kidney disease
Liver disease
Mental depression
Mental illness (severe)
Myasthenia gravis
Porphyria

—if you are taking any of the benzodiazepines and are also taking any of the following medicines or types of medicine:

    Alseroxylon
    Carbamazepine
    Cimetidine
    Clonidine
    Deserpidine
    Guanabenz
    Levodopa
    Methyldopa
    Metyrosine
    Rauwolfia serpentina
    Reserpine

—if you are taking any of the benzodiazepines and are also taking other central nervous system (CNS) depressants such as:

    Antihistamines or medicine for hay fever, other allergies, or colds
    Barbiturates
    Muscle relaxants
    Narcotics
    Other anticonvulsants (seizure medicine)
    Other sedatives, tranquilizers, or sleeping medicine
    Prescription pain medicine

—if you are taking any of the benzodiazepines and are also taking tricyclic antidepressants (medicine for depression) such as:

    Amitriptyline
    Amoxapine
    Desipramine
    Doxepin
    Imipramine
    Nortriptyline
    Protriptyline
    Trimipramine

—if you are taking any of the benzodiazepines and are also taking or have taken within the past 2 weeks monoamine oxidase (MAO) inhibitors such as:

    Furazolidone
    Isocarboxazid
    Pargyline
    Phenelzine
    Procarbazine
    Tranylcypromine

—if you are taking chlordiazepoxide, clorazepate, or diazepam and are also taking antacids.

—if you are taking clonazepam and are also taking valproic acid.

—if you are taking diazepam and are also taking isoniazid or rifampin.

—if you are taking triazolam and are also taking isoniazid.

Proper Use of This Medicine

Take this medicine only as directed by your doctor. Do not take more of it, do not take it more often, and do not take it for a longer period of time than your doctor ordered. If too much is taken, it may become habit-forming (causing mental or physical dependence).

If you think this medicine is not working as well after you have taken it for a few weeks, **do not increase the dose.** Instead, check with your doctor.

If you are taking this medicine regularly (for example, every day as for epilepsy) and you miss a dose, take it right away if you remember within an hour or so of the missed dose. However, if you do not remember until later, skip the missed dose and go back to your regular dosing schedule. Do not double doses.

For patients taking the extended-release form of diazepam:
    • Swallow capsules whole.
    • Do not crush, break, or chew before swallowing.

For patients taking this medicine for epilepsy or other convulsive disorder:
    • **In order for this medicine to control your convulsions (seizures), it must be taken every day in regularly spaced doses as ordered by your doctor.** This is necessary to keep a constant amount of the medicine in the blood. To help keep this amount constant, do not miss any doses.

For patients taking flurazepam:

• **When you begin to take this medicine, your sleeping problem will improve somewhat the first night. However, 2 or 3 nights may pass before you receive the full effects of this medicine.**

How to store this medicine:

• Store away from heat and direct light.

• **Keep out of the reach of children** since overdose may be especially dangerous in children.

• Do not store in the bathroom medicine cabinet because the heat or moisture may cause the medicine to break down.

• Do not keep outdated medicine or medicine no longer needed. Flush the contents of the container down the toilet, unless otherwise directed.

Precautions While Using This Medicine

If you will be taking this medicine regularly for a long period of time:

• Your doctor should check your progress at regular visits in order to make sure that this medicine does not cause unwanted effects. If you are taking clonazepam, this is also important during the first few months of treatment.

• If you are taking this medicine for nervousness or tension or for insomnia (sleeplessness), check with your doctor at least every 4 months to make sure you need to continue taking this medicine. However, if you are taking flurazepam, temazepam, or triazolam, check with your doctor every month.

If you will be taking this medicine in large doses or for a long period of time, do not stop taking it without first checking with your doctor. Your doctor may want you to reduce gradually the amount you are taking before stopping completely. Stopping this medicine suddenly may cause withdrawal side effects. Also, if you are taking this medicine for epilepsy or other convulsive disorder, stopping this medicine suddenly may cause convulsions (seizures).

This medicine will add to the effects of alcohol and other CNS depressants (medicines that slow down the nervous system, possibly causing drowsiness). Some examples of CNS depressants are antihistamines or medicine for hay fever, other allergies, or colds; sedatives, tranquilizers, or sleeping medicine; prescription pain medicine or narcotics; barbiturates; medicine for seizures; muscle relaxants; or anesthetics, including some dental anesthetics. This effect may last for a few days after you stop taking this medicine. **Check with your doctor before taking any of the above while you are taking this medicine.**

If you think you may have taken an overdose, get emergency help at once. Taking an overdose of a benzodiazepine or taking alcohol or other CNS depressants with the benzodiazepine may lead to unconsciousness and possibly death. Some signs of an overdose are continuing slurred speech or confusion, severe drowsiness, severe weakness, and staggering.

This medicine may cause some people, especially older ones, to become drowsy, dizzy, lightheaded, clumsy or unsteady, or less alert than they are normally. Even if taken at bedtime, it may cause some people to feel drowsy or less alert on arising. **Make sure you know how you react to this medicine before you drive, use machines, or do other jobs that require you to be alert.**

For patients taking this medicine for epilepsy or other convulsive disorder:

• Your doctor may want you to carry a medical identification card or bracelet stating that you are taking this medicine.

Side Effects of This Medicine

When clonazepam is used for long periods of time in children, it may cause unwanted effects on physical and mental development. These effects may not be noticed until after many years. Before this medicine is given to children for long periods of time, you should discuss the use of it with your doctor.

Along with its needed effects, a medicine may cause some unwanted effects. Although not all of these side effects appear very often, when they do occur they may require medical attention. Check with your doctor as soon as possible if any of the following side effects occur:

Less common or rare

Behavior problems, including difficulty in concentrating and outbursts of anger, especially in children
Confusion or mental depression
Hallucinations (seeing, hearing, or feeling things that are not there)
Muscle weakness
Skin rash or itching
Sore throat and fever
Trouble in sleeping
Ulcers or sores in mouth or throat (continuing)
Uncontrolled movements of body, including the eyes
Unusual bleeding or bruising
Unusual excitement, nervousness, or irritability
Unusual tiredness or weakness
Yellowing of eyes or skin

Possible signs of overdose

Confusion (continuing)
Drowsiness (severe)
Shakiness
Slurred speech (continuing)
Staggering
Unusually slow heartbeat, shortness of breath, or troubled breathing
Weakness (severe)

Other side effects may occur which usually do not require medical attention. These side effects may go away during treatment as your body adjusts to the medicine. However, check with your doctor if any of the following side effects continue or are bothersome:

More common

Clumsiness or unsteadiness
Dizziness or lightheadedness
Drowsiness

Less common

Abdominal or stomach cramps or pain
Blurred vision or other changes in vision
Constipation
Diarrhea
False sense of well-being
Headache
Increased bronchial secretions or watering of mouth
Nausea or vomiting
Problems with urination
Slurred speech
Unusual dryness of mouth or increase in thirst
Unusual tiredness or weakness

Although not all of the side effects listed above have been reported for all of these medicines, they have been reported for at least one of them. However, since all of the benzodiazepines are very similar, any of the above side effects may occur with any of these medicines.

Most of the above side effects are more likely to occur in children, especially the very young, and in elderly patients. These patients are usually more sensitive to the effects of benzodiazepines.

After you stop using this medicine, your body may need time to adjust. If you took this medicine in high doses or for a long time, this may take up to 3 weeks. During this period of time check with your doctor if you notice any of the following side effects:

More common

Trouble in sleeping
Unusual irritability
Unusual nervousness

Less common or rare

Abdominal or stomach cramps
Confusion
Convulsions (seizures)

Muscle cramps
Nausea or vomiting
Trembling
Unusual sweating

For patients having diazepam or lorazepam injected:

• Check with your doctor if any of the following side effects occur: redness, swelling, or pain at the place of injection.

Other side effects not listed above may also occur in some patients. If you notice any other effects, check with your doctor.

BETA-ADRENERGIC BLOCKING AGENTS (Systemic)

This information applies to the following medicines:

Acebutolol (a-se-BYOO-toe-lole)
Atenolol (a-TEN-oh-lole)
Labetalol (la-BET-a-lole)
Metoprolol (me-TOE-proe-lole)
Nadolol (NAY-doe-lole)
Oxprenolol (ox-PREN-oh-lole)
Pindolol (PIN-doe-lole)
Propranolol (proe-PRAN-oh-lole)
Timolol (TYE-moe-lole)

Some commonly used brand names are:	Generic names:
Sectral	Acebutolol
Tenormin	Atenolol
Normodyne Trandate	Labetalol
Betaloc* Lopressor	Metoprolol
Corgard	Nadolol
Slow-Trasicor* Trasicor*	Oxprenolol*

Visken	Pindolol
Detensol* Inderal Inderal LA	Propranolol
Blocadren	Timolol

*Not available in the United States.

These medicines belong to a group of medicines known as beta-adrenergic blocking agents, beta-blocking agents, or more commonly, beta-blockers. Beta-blockers are used in the treatment of high blood pressure. Some beta-blockers are also used in the relief of angina (heart pain) and in heart attack patients to help prevent additional heart attacks. Beta-blockers have also been found useful in a number of other conditions such as correcting irregular heartbeats and preventing migraine headaches. They may also be used for other conditions as determined by your doctor.

Beta-blockers work by affecting the response to some nerve impulses in certain parts of the body. As a result, they increase the supply of blood and oxygen to the heart while reducing its workload. They also help the heart to beat more regularly.

Beta-adrenergic blocking agents are available only with your doctor's prescription.

Before Using This Medicine

In order to decide on the best treatment for your medical problem, your doctor should be told:

—if you have ever had any unusual or allergic reaction to beta-blocker medicine.

—if you are on a low-salt, low-sugar, or any other special diet, or if you are allergic to any substance, such as sulfites or other preservatives or dyes. Most medicines contain more than their active ingredient. Your doctor or pharmacist can help you avoid products that may cause a problem.

—if you are pregnant or if you intend to become pregnant while using this medicine. Although adequate studies have not been done in humans, use of some beta-blockers during pregnancy has been associated with breathing problems and a lower heart rate in the newborn infant. However, some reports have shown no unwanted effects on the newborn infant. Animal studies have shown some beta-blockers to cause problems in pregnancy when used in doses many times the usual human dose.

—if you are breast-feeding an infant. Although this medicine has not been shown to cause problems in humans, the chance always exists, since most beta-blockers pass into the breast milk.

—if you have any of the following medical problems:

  Allergy, history of (asthma, eczema, hay
    fever, hives)
  Bradycardia (unusually slow heartbeat)
  Bronchitis
  Diabetes mellitus (sugar diabetes)
  Emphysema
  Heart or blood vessel disease
  Kidney disease
  Liver disease
  Mental depression (or history of)
  Myasthenia gravis (a muscle disease)
  Overactive thyroid
  Pheochromocytoma (PCC; for labetalol
    only)

—if you are now taking any of the following medicines or types of medicine:

  Albuterol
  Aminophylline
  Amphetamines
  Antidiabetic agents, oral (diabetes medi-
    cine you take by mouth)
  Cimetidine
  Clonidine
  Digitalis glycosides (heart medicine)
  Diltiazem
  Diuretics (water pills) or other antihyper-
    tensives (high blood pressure
    medicines)

  Dyphylline
  Ephedrine
  Epinephrine
  Inflammation medicines, including
    ibuprofen and aspirin in large doses
  Insulin
  Isoproterenol
  Nifedipine
  Nitroglycerin—for labetalol only
  Oxtriphylline
  Phenothiazines
  Phenoxybenzamine—for labetalol only
  Phentolamine—for labetalol only
  Phenylephrine
  Phenytoin
  Reserpine
  Theophylline
  Verapamil

—if you are now taking or have taken within the past 2 weeks monoamine oxidase (MAO) inhibitors such as:

  Isocarboxazid
  Pargyline
  Phenelzine
  Procarbazine
  Tranylcypromine

—if you smoke.

Proper Use of This Medicine

For patients taking the extended-release capsule or tablet form of this medicine:

• Swallow the capsule or tablet whole.

• Do not crush, break, or chew before swallowing.

Ask your doctor about checking your pulse rate before and after taking beta-blocking agents. Then, while you are taking this medicine, check your pulse regularly. If it is much slower than your usual rate (or less than 50 beats per minute), check with your doctor. A pulse rate that is too slow may cause circulation problems.

In order to help remember to take your medicine, try to get into the habit of taking it at the same time each day.

For patients taking this medicine for high blood pressure:

• **Importance of diet**—When prescribing medicine for your condition, your doctor may also prescribe a personal diet for you. Such a diet may be low in sodium (salt). **Most people eat much more sodium than they need. Too much sodium in the diet may increase blood pressure.** Some foods that contain large amounts of sodium include canned soup, pickles, ketchup, green and ripe olives, relish, frankfurters, soy sauce, and carbonated beverages. Your doctor may want you to limit the amounts of these and other high-sodium foods in your diet. **Medicine is usually more effective when such a diet is properly followed.**

Also, it may be very important for you to go on a reducing diet. However, check with your doctor before going on any diet.

• Many patients who have high blood pressure will not notice any signs of the problem. In fact, many may feel normal. It is very important that you take your medicine exactly as directed. Also, keep your doctor's appointments even if you feel well.

• Remember that this medicine will not cure your high blood pressure but it does control it. Therefore, you must continue to take it as directed if you expect to lower your blood pressure and keep it down. **You may have to take medicine for the rest of your life.** If high blood pressure is not treated, it can cause serious problems such as heart failure, blood vessel disease, stroke, or kidney disease.

Do not miss any doses. This is especially important when you are taking only one dose per day. Some conditions may become worse when this medicine is not taken regularly.

If you do miss a dose of this medicine, take it as soon as possible. However, if it is within 4 hours of your next dose (8 hours when using atenolol, labetalol, nadolol, or extended-release oxprenolol or propranolol), skip the missed dose and go back to your regular dosing schedule. Do not double doses.

How to store this medicine:

• Store away from heat and direct light.

• **Keep out of the reach of children.**

• Do not store in the bathroom medicine cabinet because the heat or moisture may cause the medicine to break down.

• Do not keep outdated medicine or medicine no longer needed. Flush the contents of the container down the toilet, unless otherwise directed.

Precautions While Using This Medicine

It is important that your doctor check your progress at regular visits. This will allow the dosage to be changed if needed and to make sure the medicine is working for you.

Do not stop taking this medicine without first checking with your doctor. Your doctor may want you to reduce gradually the amount you are taking before stopping completely. Some conditions may become worse when the medicine is stopped suddenly, and danger of heart attack is increased in some patients.

Make sure that you have enough medicine on hand to last through weekends, holidays, or vacations. You may want to carry an extra prescription in your billfold or purse in case of an emergency. You could than have it filled if you run out while you are away from home.

Your doctor may want you to carry a medical identification card stating that you are taking this medicine.

Before having any kind of surgery (including dental surgery) or emergency treatment, tell the physician or dentist in charge that you are taking this medicine.

Diabetics—This medicine may cause your blood sugar levels to fall. Also, this medicine may cover up signs of hypoglycemia (low blood sugar), such as change in pulse rate or increased blood pressure.

This medicine may cause some people to become dizzy, drowsy, lightheaded, or less alert than they are normally. Make sure you know how you react to this medicine before you drive, use machines, or do other jobs that require you to be alert. If the problem continues or gets worse, check with your doctor.

Beta-blockers will often make you more sensitive to cold. They tend to decrease blood circulation in the skin, fingers, and toes. Dress warmly during cold weather and be careful during prolonged exposure to cold, such as in winter sports.

Chest pain resulting from exercise or physical exertion is usually reduced or prevented by this medicine. This may tempt a patient to be overly active. Make sure you discuss with your doctor a safe amount of exercise for your medical problem.

For patients taking this medicine for high blood pressure:
• Do not take other medicines unless they have been discussed with your doctor. This especially includes over-the-counter (nonprescription) medicines for appetite control, asthma, colds, cough, hay fever, or sinus problems since they may tend to increase your blood pressure.

For patients taking labetalol by mouth:
• Dizziness, lightheadedness, or fainting may occur, especially when you get up from a lying or sitting position. This is more likely to occur when you first start taking labetalol or when the dose is increased. Getting up slowly may help. When you get up from lying down, sit on the edge of the bed with your feet dangling for 1 to 2 minutes. Then stand up slowly. If the problem continues or gets worse, check with your doctor.

• The dizziness, lightheadedness, or fainting is also more likely to occur if you drink alcohol, stand for long periods of time, exercise, or if the weather is hot. While you are taking this medicine, be careful in the amount of alcohol you drink. Also, use extra care during exercise or hot weather or if you must stand for long periods of time.

For patients receiving labetalol by injection:
• It is very important that you lie down flat while receiving labetalol and for up to 3 hours afterward. If you try to get up too soon, you may become dizzy or faint. Do not try to sit or stand until your doctor tells you to do so.

Side Effects of This Medicine

Along with its needed effects, a medicine may cause some unwanted effects. Although not all of these side effects appear very often, when they do occur they may require medical attention. Check with your doctor as soon as possible if any of the following side effects occur:

Less common
    Breathing difficulty and/or wheezing
    Chest pain
    Cold hands and feet
    Confusion, especially in elderly
    Hallucinations (seeing, hearing, or feeling things that are not there)
    Irregular heartbeat
    Mental depression
    Skin rash

Swelling of ankles, feet, and/or lower legs
Unusually slow pulse (especially less than
50 beats per minute)—more common
with nadolol and propranolol; rare
with labetalol

Rare

Back pain or joint pain—more common
with labetalol and pindolol
Fever and sore throat
Unusual bleeding and bruising

*Possible signs of overdose in the order in
which they occur*

Unusually slow heartbeat
Dizziness (severe) or fainting
Unusually fast or irregular heartbeat
Difficulty in breathing
Bluish-colored fingernails or palms of
hands
Convulsions (seizures)

Other side effects may occur which usually
do not require medical attention. These
side effects may go away during treatment as your body adjusts to the medicine. However, check with your doctor if
any of the following side effects continue or are bothersome:

More common

Dizziness or lightheadedness
Drowsiness (slight)
Trouble in sleeping
Unusual tiredness or weakness

Less common

Anxiety and/or nervousness
Changes in taste—for labetalol only
Constipation
Decreased sexual ability
Diarrhea
Dry, sore eyes
Headache
Itching of skin
Nausea or vomiting
Nightmares and vivid dreams
Numbness and/or tingling of fingers
and/or toes
Numbness and/or tingling of skin,
especially on scalp—for labetalol only
Stomach discomfort
Stuffy nose
Unusually frequent urination—for
acebutolol only

Although not all of the side effects listed
above have been reported for all of these
medicines, they have been reported for
at least one of them. Since all of the
beta-adrenergic blocking agents are
very similar, any of the above side effects may occur with any of these medicines. However, they may be more or
less common with some agents than with
others.

After you have been taking a beta-blocker
for a while, it may cause unpleasant or
even harmful effects if you stop taking it
too suddenly. After you stop taking this
medicine or while you are gradually reducing the amount you are taking,
check with your doctor right away if any
of the following occur:

Chest pain
Headache—for labetalol only
General feeling of body discomfort or
weakness—for labetalol only
Shortness of breath (sudden)
Sweating
Trembling—for labetalol only
Unusually fast or irregular heartbeat

Some of the above side effects are more
likely to occur in the elderly, who are
usually more sensitive to the effects of
beta-blockers.

You may notice a tingling feeling on your
scalp when you first begin to take labetalol. This is to be expected and usually
goes away after you have been taking
labetalol for a while.

Other side effects not listed above may also
occur in some patients. If you notice any
other effects, check with your doctor.

BETA-ADRENERGIC BLOCKING AGENTS AND THIAZIDE DIURETICS (Systemic)

This information applies to the following medicines:

Atenolol (a-TEN-oh-lole) and Chlorthalidone (klor-THAL-i-doan)

Metoprolol (me-TOE-proe-lole) and Hydrochlorothiazide (hye-droe-klor-oh-THYE-a-zide)

Nadolol (NAY-doe-lole) and Bendroflumethiazide (ben-droe-floo-meth-EYE-a-zide)

Pindolol (PIN-doe-lole) and Hydrochlorothiazide

Propranolol (proe-PRAN-oh-lole) and Hydrochlorothiazide

Timolol (TYE-moe-lole) and Hydrochlorothiazide

Some commonly used brand names are:	Generic names:
Tenoretic	Atenolol and Chlorthalidone
Lopressor HCT	Metoprolol and Hydrochlorothiazide
Corzide	Nadolol and Bendroflumethiazide
Viskazide*	Pindolol and Hydrochlorothiazide*
Inderide	Propranolol and Hydrochlorothiazide
Timolide	Timolol and Hydrochlorothiazide

* Not available in the United States.

Beta-blocker and thiazide diuretic combinations belong to the group of medicines known as antihypertensives (blood pressure medicine). Both ingredients of the combination control high blood pressure, but work in different ways. Beta-blockers (atenolol, metoprolol, nadolol, pindolol, propranolol, and timolol) reduce the workload on the heart as well as having other effects. Thiazide diuretics (bendroflumethiazide, chlorthalidone, and hydrochlorothiazide) reduce the amount of fluid pressure in the body by increasing the flow of urine.

High blood pressure adds to the workload of the heart and arteries. If it continues for a long time, they may not function properly. This can damage the blood vessels of the brain, heart, and kidneys resulting in a stroke, heart attack, or kidney failure. These problems may be avoided if blood pressure is controlled.

Beta-blocker and thiazide diuretic combinations are available only with your doctor's prescription.

For information about the precautions and side effects of the medicines in this combination, see:

Beta-adrenergic Blocking Agents (Systemic)

Diuretics, Thiazide (Systemic)

Combination products are designed for specific uses. These uses may not be the same as the uses of the individual ingredients. Therefore, some of the information provided in the individual listings may not be relevant to the combination product. If questions arise, check with your doctor, nurse, or pharmacist.

BETAXOLOL (Ophthalmic)

A commonly used brand name is Betoptic.

Betaxolol (be-TAX-oh-lol) is used in the eye to treat certain types of glaucoma. It works by lowering the pressure in the eye.

This medicine is available only with your doctor's prescription.

Before Using This Medicine

In order to decide on the best treatment for your medical problem, your doctor should be told:

—if you have ever had any unusual or allergic reaction to betaxolol or other beta blockers (such as acebutolol, atenolol, labetalol, metoprolol, nadolol, oxprenolol, pindolol, sotalol, or timolol).

—if you are allergic to any substance, such as preservatives. Most medicines contain more than their active ingredient. Your doctor or pharmacist can help you avoid products that may cause a problem.

—if you are pregnant or if you intend to become pregnant while using this medicine, since ophthalmic betaxolol may be absorbed into the body. Studies on birth defects have not been done in humans. However, studies in animals have not shown that betaxolol causes birth defects.

—if you are breast-feeding an infant, since ophthalmic betaxolol may be absorbed into the body. Although it is not known whether ophthalmic betaxolol passes into the breast milk and this medicine has not been shown to cause problems in humans, the chance always exists.

—if you have any of the following medical problems:

Diabetes mellitus (sugar diabetes)
Heart disease
Lung disease
Overactive thyroid

—if you are now using any of the following medicines or types of medicine:

Acebutolol
Atenolol
Chlorprothixene
Ephedrine
Epinephrine
Haloperidol
Isoproterenol
Labetalol
Levobunolol
Metoprolol
Nadolol
Oxprenolol
Phenothiazines (tranquilizers)
Pindolol
Propranolol
Reserpine
Sotalol
Thiothixene
Timolol

Proper Use of This Medicine

How to apply betaxolol eye drops: First, wash your hands. With the middle finger, apply pressure to the inside corner of the eye (and continue to apply pressure for 1 or 2 minutes after the medicine has been placed in the eye). Tilt the head back and with the index finger of the same hand, pull the lower eyelid away from the eye to form a pouch. Drop the medicine into the pouch and gently close the eyes. Do not blink. Keep the eyes closed for 1 or 2 minutes to allow the medicine to be absorbed.

To prevent contamination of the eye drops, do not touch the applicator tip to any surface (including the eye) and keep the container tightly closed.

Use this medicine only as directed. Do not use more of it and do not use it more often than your doctor ordered. To do so may increase the chance of too much medicine being absorbed into the body and the chance of side effects.

If you miss a dose of this medicine, apply it as soon as possible. However, if it is almost time for your next dose, skip the missed dose and apply your next dose at the regularly scheduled time. Then continue with your regular dosing schedule.

How to store this medicine:

• Store away from heat and direct light.

• **Keep out of the reach of children.**

• Keep the medicine from freezing.

• Do not keep outdated medicine or medicine no longer needed. Flush the contents of the container down the toilet, unless otherwise directed.

Precautions While Using This Medicine

Your doctor should check your eye pressure at regular visits in order to make certain that your glaucoma is being controlled.

Before having any kind of surgery (including dental surgery) or emergency treatment, tell the physician or dentist in charge that you are using this medicine.

Diabetics—**This medicine may cover up some signs of hypoglycemia (low blood sugar),** such as increase in pulse rate or trembling. However, other signs of low blood sugar, such as sweating, are not affected. If you have any questions about this, check with your doctor.

Side Effects of This Medicine

Along with its needed effects, a medicine may cause some unwanted effects. Although not all of these side effects appear very often, when they do occur they may require medical attention. Check with your doctor as soon as possible if any of the following side effects occur:

Rare
> Irritation or inflammation of eye

Signs of too much medicine being absorbed into the body
> Confusion or mental depression
> Trouble in sleeping
> Unusually slow heartbeat
> Unusual tiredness or weakness
> Wheezing or troubled breathing

Other side effects may occur which usually do not require medical attention. These side effects may go away during treatment as your body adjusts to the medicine. However, check with your doctor if any of the following side effects continue or are bothersome:

Less common or rare
> Increased sensitivity of eye to light
> Stinging or unusual watering of eye

Other side effects not listed above may also occur in some patients. If you notice any other effects, check with your doctor.

BITOLTEROL (Systemic)

A commonly used brand name is Tornalate.

Bitolterol (bye-TOLE-ter-ole) belongs to the group of medicines called bronchodilators (medicines that open up the bronchial tubes or air passages of the lungs). It is taken by oral inhalation to treat the symptoms of bronchial asthma and other lung diseases. Bitolterol relieves wheezing, shortness of breath, and troubled breathing by increasing the flow of air through the bronchial tubes.

Bitolterol is available only with your doctor's prescription.

Before Using This Medicine

In order to decide on the best treatment for your medical problem, your doctor should be told:

—if you have ever had any unusual or allergic reaction to bitolterol or other inhalation aerosol medicines.

—if you are pregnant or if you intend to become pregnant while using this medicine. Studies in humans have not been done. However, some studies in animals have shown that bitolterol causes birth defects when it is given in doses many times the usual human dose.

—if you are breast-feeding an infant. Although it is not known whether bitolterol passes into the breast milk and this medicine has not been shown to cause problems in humans, the chance always exists.

—if you have any of the following medical problems:

Convulsive (seizure) disorders
Diabetes mellitus (sugar diabetes)
Heart or blood vessel disease
High blood pressure
Overactive thyroid

—if you are now taking any other oral inhalation aerosol for asthma or breathing problems.

Proper Use of This Medicine

Bitolterol usually comes with patient directions. Read them carefully before using this medicine.

It is very important that you use this medicine only as directed. Do not use more of it and do not use it more often than your doctor ordered. To do so may increase the chance of serious side effects. Inhalation aerosol medicines similar to bitolterol have been reported to cause death when too much of the medicine was used.

Keep the spray away from the eyes because it may cause irritation.

If you are using bitolterol regularly and you miss a dose, use it as soon as possible. Then use any remaining doses for that day at regularly spaced intervals. Do not double doses.

How to store this medicine:

• Store away from heat and direct sunlight.

• **Keep out of the reach of children.**

• Do not store in the bathroom medicine cabinet because the heat or moisture may cause the medicine to break down.

• Keep the medicine from freezing.

• Do not puncture, break, or burn container, even if it is empty.

• Do not keep outdated medicine or medicine no longer needed.

Precautions While Using This Medicine

Check with your doctor at once if you still have trouble breathing after using a dose of this medicine or if your condition gets worse.

If you are also using the inhalation aerosol form of an adrenocorticoid (cortisone-like medicine, such as beclomethasone, dexamethasone, flunisolide, or triamcinolone), **allow 15 minutes between using the bitolterol and an adrenocorticoid,** unless otherwise directed by your doctor. This will help to reduce the possibility of side effects.

Side Effects of This Medicine

Along with its needed effects, a medicine may cause some unwanted effects. Although not all of these side effects appear very often, when they do occur they may require medical attention. Check with your doctor as soon as possible if any of the following side effects occur:

Rare

Chest discomfort
Increase in blood pressure
Increase in wheezing or difficulty in breathing
Irregular heartbeat
Unusual excitement or restlessness

Signs of overdose

Chest discomfort (severe)
Dizziness or lightheadedness (severe)
Headache (continuing or severe)
Increase in blood pressure (severe)
Trembling (severe)
Unusually fast or pounding heartbeat (continuing)

Other side effects may occur which usually do not require medical attention. These

side effects may go away during treatment as your body adjusts to the medicine. However, check with your doctor if any of the following side effects continue or are bothersome:

More common
  Nervousness
  Throat irritation
  Trembling
Less common or rare
  Coughing
  Dizziness or lightheadedness
  Headache
  Nausea
  Pounding heartbeat
  Trouble in sleeping
  Unusually fast heartbeat

Other side effects not listed above may also occur in some patients. If you notice any other effects, check with your doctor.

BUTALBITAL AND ASPIRIN
(Systemic)

Some commonly used brand names are:	Generic names:
Axotal	Butalbital and Aspirin

Buff-A-Comp	
Butal Compound	
Fiorinal	
Isollyl (Improved)	Butalbital,
Lanorinal	Aspirin, and
Marnal	Caffeine†
Protension	
Tenstan	

†Generic name product may also be available.

Butalbital (byoo-TAL-bi-tal) and aspirin (AS-pir-in) is a combined pain reliever and relaxant. It is used to treat tension headaches. Butalbital belongs to the group of medicines called barbiturates. Barbiturates act in the central nervous system (CNS) to produce their effects. When butalbital is used for a long time, your body may get used to it so that larger amounts are needed to produce its effects. This is called tolerance to the medicine. Also, butalbital may become habit-forming (causing mental or physical dependence) when it is used for a long time or in large doses. Physical dependence may lead to withdrawal side effects when you stop taking the medicine.

Butalbital and aspirin combination is available only with your doctor's prescription.

Before Using This Medicine

In order to decide on the best treatment for your medical problem, your doctor should be told:

—if you have ever had any unusual reaction to barbiturates, caffeine, or aspirin or other salicylates including diflunisal or methyl salicylate (oil of wintergreen), or to any of the following medicines:

  Fenoprofen
  Ibuprofen
  Indomethacin
  Meclofenamate
  Mefenamic acid
  Naproxen
  Oxyphenbutazone
  Phenylbutazone
  Piroxicam
  Sulindac
  Tolmetin
  Zomepirac

—if you are on a low-salt, low-sugar, or any other special diet, or if you are allergic to any substance, such as sulfites or other preservatives. Most medicines contain more than their active ingredient. Your doctor or pharmacist can help you avoid products that may cause a problem.

—if you are pregnant or if you intend to become pregnant while using this medicine.

For butalbital

Barbiturates such as butalbital have been shown to increase the chance of birth defects in humans. Also, one study in humans has suggested that barbiturates taken during pregnancy may increase the chance of brain tumors in the baby.

Taking a barbiturate regularly during the last 3 months of pregnancy may cause the fetus to become dependent on the medicine. This may lead to withdrawal side effects in the newborn baby. In addition, butalbital may cause breathing problems in the newborn baby if taken just before or during delivery.

For aspirin

Although studies in humans have not shown that aspirin causes birth defects, it has caused birth defects in animal studies.

Some reports have suggested that too much use of aspirin late in pregnancy may cause a decrease in the newborn's weight and possible death of the fetus or newborn infant. However, the mothers in these reports had been taking much larger amounts of aspirin than are usually recommended. Studies of mothers taking aspirin in the doses that are usually recommended did not show these unwanted effects.

There is a chance that regular use of aspirin late in pregnancy may cause unwanted effects on the heart or blood flow in the fetus or in the newborn infant. Also, use of aspirin during the last 2 weeks of pregnancy may cause bleeding problems in the fetus before or during delivery or in the newborn infant. In addition, too much use of aspirin during the last 3 months of pregnancy may increase the length of pregnancy, prolong labor, cause other problems during delivery, or cause severe bleeding in the mother before, during, or after delivery.

For caffeine

Studies in humans have not shown that caffeine causes birth defects. However, studies in animals have shown that caffeine causes birth defects when given in very large doses (amounts equal to the amount of caffeine present in 12 to 24 cups of coffee a day).

—if you are breast-feeding an infant. Although this combination medicine has not been shown to cause problems, the chance always exists, especially if the medicine is taken for a long time or in large amounts. Barbiturates (such as butalbital), aspirin, and caffeine pass into the breast milk.

—if you have any of the following medical problems:
> Anemia
> Asthma, allergies, and nasal polyps (history of)
> Emphysema, asthma, or chronic lung disease
> Gout
> Heart disease (severe)
> Hemophilia or other bleeding problems
> Hyperactivity (in children)
> Hypoprothrombinemia
> Kidney disease
> Liver disease
> Mental depression
> Overactive thyroid
> Porphyria (or history of)
> Stomach ulcer or other stomach problems
> Underactive adrenal gland
> Vitamin K deficiency

—if you are now taking **any** medicine, including over-the-counter (OTC) or nonprescription medicines (such as acetaminophen or laxatives), especially:
> Adrenocorticoids (cortisone-like medicine)
> Anti-inflammatory analgesics, such as diflunisal, fenoprofen, ibuprofen, indomethacin, meclofenamate, mefenamic acid, naproxen, oxyphenbutazone, phenylbutazone, piroxicam, sulindac, or tolmetin
> Anticoagulants (blood thinners)
> Antidiabetics, oral (diabetes medicine you take by mouth)
> Contraceptives, oral, containing estrogens (birth control pills)
> Corticotropin

Digitalis glycosides (heart medicine)
Estramustine
Estrogens
Heparin
Levothyroxine
Methotrexate
Probenecid
Quinidine
Sulfinpyrazone
Valproic acid
Vancomycin

—if you regularly take large amounts of antacids.

—if you are now using central nervous system (CNS) depressants such as:

Anticonvulsants (seizure medicine)
Antihistamines or medicine for hay fever, other allergies, or colds
Muscle relaxants
Narcotics
Other barbiturates
Other prescription pain medicine
Sedatives, tranquilizers, or sleeping medicine
Tricyclic antidepressants (medicine for depression)

—if you are now taking or have taken within the past 2 weeks monoamine oxidase (MAO) inhibitors such as:

Furazolidone
Isocarboxazid
Pargyline
Phenelzine
Procarbazine
Tranylcypromine

Proper Use of This Medicine

Take this medicine only as directed by your doctor. Do not take more of it, do not take it more often, and do not take it for a longer period of time than your doctor ordered. If too much butalbital is taken, it may become habit-forming (causing mental or physical dependence) or lead to medical problems because of an overdose. Also, taking too much aspirin may cause stomach problems or lead to medical problems because of an overdose.

Take this medicine with food or a full glas (8 ounces) of water to lessen stomac irritation.

Do not take this medicine if it has a stron vinegar-like odor, since this means th aspirin in it is breaking down. If yc have any questions about this, chec with your doctor or pharmacist.

If your doctor has ordered you to take th medicine according to a regular sche ule and you miss a dose, take it as soon you remember. However, if it is almo time for your next dose, skip the misse dose and go back to your regular dosir schedule. Do not double doses.

How to store this medicine:

• Store away from heat and direct ligh

• **Keep out of the reach of children b** cause overdose is very dangerous young children.

• Do not store in the bathroom medicin cabinet because the heat or moistur may cause the medicine to break dow

• Do not keep outdated medicine or mer icine no longer needed. Flush the cor tents of the container down the toile unless otherwise directed.

Precautions While Using This Medicin

If you will be taking this medicine for a lor period of time (for example, for severa months at a time), your doctor shoul check your progress at regular visits.

Check the labels of all over-the-counte (OTC), nonprescription, and prescriptio medicines you now take. If any contain barbiturate, aspirin, or other salicylate including diflunisal, be especially car ful, since taking them while taking th medicine may lead to overdose. If yo have any questions about this, chec with your doctor or pharmacist.

The butalbital in this medicine will add to the effects of alcohol and other CNS depressants (medicines that slow down the nervous system, possibly causing drowsiness). Some examples of CNS depressants are antihistamines or medicine for hay fever, other allergies, or colds; sedatives, tranquilizers, or sleeping medicine; other prescription pain medicine or narcotics; other barbiturates; medicine for seizures; tricyclic antidepressants (medicine for depression); muscle relaxants; or anesthetics, including some dental anesthetics. Also, stomach problems may be more likely to occur if you drink alcoholic beverages while you are taking aspirin. **Check with your doctor before taking any of the above while you are using this medicine.**

Too much use of acetaminophen together with this combination medicine may increase the chance of kidney or liver problems. Therefore, do not regularly take acetaminophen together with this medicine, unless directed to do so by your doctor.

This medicine may cause some people to become drowsy, dizzy, or lightheaded. **Make sure you know how you react to this medicine before you drive, use machines, or do other jobs that require you to be alert and clearheaded.**

Before having any kind of surgery (including dental surgery) or emergency treatment, tell the physician or dentist in charge that you are taking this medicine.

Do not take this medicine for 5 days before any surgery, including dental surgery, unless otherwise directed by your doctor. Taking aspirin during this time may cause bleeding problems.

For diabetics—The aspirin in this medicine may cause false urine sugar test results when taken regularly. Occasional use of aspirin usually will not affect urine sugar tests. If you have any questions about this, check with your doctor, nurse, or pharmacist, especially if your diabetes is not well controlled.

If you have been taking large amounts of this medicine, or if you have been taking it regularly for several weeks or more, **do not suddenly stop using it without first checking with your doctor.** Your doctor may want you to reduce gradually the amount you are taking before stopping completely, in order to lessen the chance of withdrawal side effects.

If you think you or someone else in your home may have taken an overdose of this medicine, get emergency help at once. Taking an overdose of this medicine or taking alcohol or CNS depressants with this medicine may lead to unconsciousness or death. Signs of overdose of this medicine include convulsions or seizures; hearing loss; mental confusion; ringing or buzzing in the ear; severe excitement, nervousness, or restlessness; severe dizziness; severe drowsiness; shortness of breath or troubled breathing; and severe weakness.

Side Effects of This Medicine

Along with its needed effects, a medicine may cause some unwanted effects. Although not all of these side effects appear very often, when they do occur they may require medical attention. **Check with your doctor immediately** if any of the following side effects occur:

Less common or rare
   Shortness of breath, troubled breathing, tightness in chest, or wheezing

Signs of overdose
   Any loss of hearing
   Bloody urine
   Convulsions (seizures)
   Diarrhea (severe or continuing)
   Dizziness or lightheadedness (severe)
   Drowsiness (severe)

Hallucinations (seeing, hearing, or feeling things that are not there)
Headache (severe or continuing)
Nausea or vomiting (continuing)
Nervousness, excitement, or confusion (severe)
Poor judgment
Ringing or buzzing in ear (continuing)
Slurred speech
Staggering
Trouble in sleeping
Uncontrollable flapping movements of the hands, especially in elderly patients
Unusual irritability (continuing)
Unexplained fever
Unusual increase in sweating
Unusually slow heartbeat
Unusually slow or irregular breathing
Unusual movements of the eyes
Unusual thirst
Vision problems
Weakness (severe)

Also, check with your doctor as soon as possible if any of the following side effects occur:
More common
Nausea or vomiting
Stomach pain
Less common or rare
Bloody or black tarry stools
Mental confusion or depression
Skin rash, hives, or itching
Sore throat and fever
Swelling of eyelids, face, or lips
Unusual bleeding or bruising
Unusual excitement
Unusual tiredness or weakness
Vomiting of blood or material that looks like coffee grounds
Yellowing of eyes or skin

Other side effects may occur which usually do not require medical attention. These side effects may go away during treatment as your body adjusts to the medicine. However, check with your doctor if any of the following side effects continue or are bothersome:
More common
Clumsiness or unsteadiness
Dizziness or lightheadedness
Drowsiness

"Hangover" effect
Heartburn or indigestion
Less common or rare
Anxiety or nervousness
Constipation
Feeling faint
Headache
Nightmares
Trouble in sleeping
Unusual irritability

Some of the above side effects are more likely to occur in children, especially those who have lost large amounts of body fluid because of vomiting, diarrhea, or sweating, and in elderly patients (60 years of age or older) or very ill patients. These patients are usually more sensitive to the effects of butalbital and aspirin.

After you stop using this medicine, your body may need time to adjust. The length of time this takes depends on the amount of medicine you were using and how long you used it. During this period of time check with your doctor if you notice any of the following side effects:
Anxiety or unusual restlessness
Convulsions or seizures
Dizziness or lightheadedness
Feeling faint
Hallucinations (seeing, hearing, or feeling things that are not there)
Muscle twitching
Nausea or vomiting
Trembling of hands
Trouble in sleeping, increased dreaming, or nightmares
Unusual nervousness, restlessness, or irritability
Unusual weakness
Vision problems

Other side effects not listed above may also occur in some patients. If you notice any other effects, check with your doctor.

BUTALBITAL, ASPIRIN, AND CODEINE (Systemic)

Some commonly used brand names are Buff-A-Comp #3, Fiorinal with Codeine, and Isollyl with Codeine.

Butalbital (byoo-TAL-bi-tal), aspirin (AS-pir-in), and codeine (KOE-deen) is a combination medicine used to relieve pain. This combination medicine may provide better pain relief than either aspirin or codeine used alone. In some cases, relief of pain may come at lower doses of each medicine. This combination medicine also contains caffeine (KAF-een).

Codeine is a narcotic analgesic (nar-KOT-ik an-al-JEE-zik) which acts in the central nervous system (CNS) to relieve pain. Many of its side effects are also caused by actions in the CNS. Butalbital belongs to the group of medicines called barbiturates. Barbiturates also act in the CNS to produce their effects. When you use butalbital or codeine for a long time, your body may get used to these medicines so that larger amounts are needed to produce their effects. This is called tolerance to the medicine. Also, butalbital and codeine may become habit-forming (causing mental or physical dependence) when they are used for a long time or in large doses. Physical dependence may lead to withdrawal symptoms when you stop taking the medicine.

Aspirin is not a narcotic and does not cause physical dependence. However, it may cause other unwanted effects if too much is taken.

This combination medicine is available only with your doctor's prescription.

For information about the precautions and side effects of the medicines in this combination, see:

Butalbital and Aspirin (Systemic)
Narcotic Analgesics (Systemic)

Combination products are designed for specific uses. These uses may not be the same as the uses of the individual ingredients. Therefore, some of the information provided in the individual listings may not be relevant to the combination product. If questions arise, check with your doctor, nurse, or pharmacist.

CALCIUM CARBONATE (Systemic)

Some commonly used brand names are:

Alka-2	Equilet
Alka-Mints	Mallamint
Amitone	Os-Cal 500
BioCal	Pama No.1
Calcilac	Titracid
Calglycine	Titralac
Cal-Sup	Trialka
Caltrate 600	Tums
Chooz	Tums E-X
Dicarbosil	

Generic name product may also be available.

Note: Some products are not marketed for all potential uses of calcium carbonate. For example, some may be recommended only as a dietary supplement.

Calcium carbonate (KAL-see-um KAR-boe-nate) is taken by mouth to relieve heartburn or acid stomach by neutralizing excess stomach acid. When used for this purpose, it is said to belong to the group of medicines called antacids. It may be used to treat the symptoms of stomach or duodenal ulcers. Calcium carbonate may also be used to prevent or treat hypocalcemia (not enough calcium in the blood). In addition, it may be used as a dietary supplement for patients who are unable to get enough calcium in their regular diet or have a need for more calcium, when recommended by their doctor.

Calcium carbonate is available without a prescription; however, your doctor may have special instructions on the proper use and dose for your medical problem.

Before Using This Medicine

Antacids should not be given to young children (up to 6 years of age) unless prescribed by their doctor. Since children cannot usually describe their symptoms very well, a doctor should check the child before giving this medicine. This is to prevent an unknown condition from getting worse and to avoid causing unwanted effects in the child.

In order to decide on the best treatment for your medical problem, your doctor should be told:

—if you are on a low-salt, low-sugar, or any other special diet, or if you are allergic to any substance, such as sulfites or other preservatives or dyes. Most medicines contain more than their active ingredient, and many liquid medicines contain alcohol. Your doctor or pharmacist can help you avoid products that may cause a problem.

—if you are pregnant or if you intend to become pregnant while taking this medicine. Studies have not been done in either animals or humans; however, there are reports of antacids causing side effects in babies whose mothers took antacids for a long period of time, especially in high doses.

—if you are breast-feeding an infant. Calcium carbonate has not been shown to cause problems in humans.

—if you have any of the following medical problems:
Appendicitis (severe cramps in stomach or lower abdomen)
Black, tarry stools
Constipation
Heart disease
Hemorrhoids
High blood pressure
Kidney disease
Kidney stones
Peptic ulcer disease
Sarcoidosis
Underactive parathyroid glands

—if you are now taking or receiving any of the following medicines or types of medicine:
Amphetamines
Antacids, other
Anticoagulants, oral (blood thinners you take by mouth)
Antidyskinetics (medicine for Parkinson's disease)
Antimuscarinics (medicine for abdominal or stomach spasms or cramps)
Aspirin or other salicylates
Benzodiazepines
Bisacodyl
Calcitonin
Cellulose sodium phosphate
Cimetidine
Diflunisal
Diuretics (water pills)
Iron preparations
Ketoconazole
Levodopa
Loxapine
Mecamylamine
Methenamine
Pancrelipase
Potassium phosphate
Quinidine
Ranitidine
Sodium bicarbonate
Sodium fluoride
Sodium phosphate
Sodium polystyrene sulfonate resin (SPSR)
Sucralfate
Tetracyclines
Thioxanthenes
Vitamin D

—if you are now taking any other medicine by mouth.

Proper Use of This Medicine

For safe and effective use of calcium carbonate:

• Follow your doctor's instructions if this medicine was prescribed.

• Follow the manufacturer's package directions if you are treating yourself.

If you are taking the chewable tablet form of this medicine, chew the tablets well before swallowing. This is to allow the medicine to work faster and be more effective.

For patients taking this medicine as an antacid for a stomach or duodenal ulcer:

• **Take it exactly as directed and for the full time of treatment as ordered by your doctor** to obtain maximum relief of your symptoms.

• Take it 1 to 3 hours after meals and at bedtime for best results, unless otherwise directed by your doctor.

For patients taking this medicine for hypocalcemia or as a dietary supplement:

• **Take it 1 to 1½ hours after meals** unless otherwise directed by your doctor.

If you are taking this medicine on a regular schedule and you miss a dose, take it as soon as possible. However, if it is almost time for your next dose, skip the missed dose and go back to your regular dosing schedule. Do not double doses.

How to store this medicine:

• Store away from heat and direct light.

• **Keep out of the reach of children.**

• Do not store in the bathroom medicine cabinet because the heat or moisture may cause the medicine to break down.

• Keep the liquid form of this medicine from freezing.

• Do not keep outdated medicine or medicine no longer needed. Flush the contents of the container down the toilet, unless otherwise directed.

Precautions While Using This Medicine

If this medicine has been ordered by your doctor and if you will be taking it in large doses or for a long period of time, your doctor should check your progress at regular visits. This is to make sure the medicine does not cause unwanted effects.

Do not take this medicine if you have any signs of appendicitis (such as stomach or lower abdominal pain, cramping, bloating, soreness, nausea, or vomiting). Instead, check with your doctor as soon as possible.

Do not take calcium carbonate within 1 to 2 hours of taking other medicine by mouth. To do so may keep the other medicine from working as well.

Patients on a sodium-restricted diet—The *liquid form* of this medicine may contain a large amount of sodium. If you have any questions about this, check with your doctor or pharmacist.

For patients taking this medicine as an antacid:

• **Do not take with large amounts of milk or milk products or with other antacids.** To do so may increase the chance of milk-alkali syndrome with side effects such as continuing headache, loss of appetite, nausea or vomiting, or unusual tiredness or weakness.

• **Do not take for more than 2 weeks** or if the problem comes back often. Instead, check with your doctor. Antacids should be used only for occasional relief, unless otherwise directed by your doctor.

For patients taking this medicine for hypocalcemia or as a dietary supplement:

• **Do not eat certain foods such as spinach, rhubarb, bran, and whole-grain cereals.** To do so may keep this medicine from working as well.

Side Effects of This Medicine

Along with its needed effects, a medicine may cause some unwanted effects. Although the following side effects occur very rarely when calcium carbonate is taken as recommended, they may be more likely to occur if:

—too much medicine is taken.

—it is taken in large doses.

—it is taken for a long period of time in high doses.

—it is taken by patients with kidney disease.

Check with your doctor as soon as possible if any of the following side effects occur:

Constipation (severe and continuing)
Cramping
Difficult or painful urination
Frequent urge to urinate
Headache (continuing)
Loss of appetite (continuing)
Mood or mental changes
Muscle pain or twitching
Nausea or vomiting
Nervousness or restlessness
Stomach or lower abdominal pain (severe)
Unpleasant taste in mouth
Unusually slow breathing
Unusual tiredness or weakness

Other side effects may occur which usually do not require medical attention. These side effects may go away during treatment as your body adjusts to the medicine. However, check with your doctor if any of the following side effects continue or are bothersome:

More common
Belching
Chalky taste
Swelling of stomach or gas

Less common
Constipation (mild)

Severe constipation may occur more frequently in elderly persons, who usually do not absorb calcium carbonate as well.

Other side effects not listed above may also occur in some patients. If you notice any other effects, check with your doctor.

CALCIUM CHANNEL BLOCKING AGENTS (Systemic)

This information applies to the following medicines:

Diltiazem (dil-TYE-a-zem)
Nifedipine (nye-FED-i-peen)
Verapamil (ver-AP-a-mil)

Some commonly used brand names are:	Generic names:
Cardizem	Diltiazem
Adalat Procardia	Nifedipine
Calan Isoptin	Verapamil

Diltiazem, nifedipine, and verapamil belong to the group of medicines called calcium channel blockers. They are taken by mouth or given by injection to relieve and control angina (chest pain).

Calcium channel blocking agents affect the movement of calcium into the cells of the heart and blood vessels. As a result, they relax blood vessels and increase the supply of blood and oxygen to the heart while reducing its work load.

Calcium channel blocking agents may also be used for other conditions as determined by your doctor.

These medicines are available only with your doctor's prescription.

Before Using This Medicine

In order to decide on the best treatment for your medical problem, your doctor should be told:

—if you have ever had any unusual or allergic reaction to diltiazem, nifedipine, or verapamil.

—if you are on a low-salt, low-sugar, or any other special diet, or if you are allergic to any substance, such as sulfites or other preservatives or dyes. Most medicines contain more than their active ingredient. Your doctor or pharmacist can help you avoid products that may cause a problem.

—if you are pregnant or if you intend to become pregnant while using this medicine. Studies in humans have not been done. However, studies in animals have shown that large doses of calcium channel blockers cause birth defects, prolonged pregnancy, poor bone development, and stillbirth.

—if you are breast-feeding an infant. Although these medicines have not been shown to cause problems in humans, the chance always exists since they may pass into breast milk.

—if you have any of the following medical problems:

Kidney disease
Liver disease
Other heart or blood vessel disorders

—if you are now taking any of the following medicines or types of medicine:

Anticoagulants, oral (blood thinners you take by mouth)
Aspirin or other salicylates
Barbiturates
Beta-adrenergic blocking agents (acebutolol, atenolol, labetalol, metoprolol, nadolol, oxprenolol, pindolol, propranolol, sotalol, timolol)

Cimetidine
Digitalis glycosides (heart medicine)
Diuretics (water pills)
Disopyramide
Hydantoin anticonvulsants (seizure medicine)
Inflammation medicines, especially indomethacin
Narcotics or other prescription pain medicine
Other antihypertensives (high blood pressure medicines)
Quinidine
Quinine
Sulfinpyrazone

Proper Use of This Medicine

Take this medicine exactly as directed even if you feel well and do not notice any signs of chest pain. Do not take more of this medicine and do not take it more often than your doctor ordered. Do not miss any doses.

If you do miss a dose of this medicine, take it as soon as possible. However, if it is almost time for your next dose, skip the missed dose and go back to your regular dosing schedule. Do not double doses.

How to store this medicine:

• Store away from heat and direct light.

• **Keep out of the reach of children.**

• Do not store in the bathroom medicine cabinet because the heat or moisture may cause the medicine to break down.

• Do not keep outdated medicine or medicine no longer needed. Flush the contents of the container down the toilet, unless otherwise directed.

Precautions While Using This Medicine

It is important that your doctor check your progress at regular visits. This will allow your doctor to change the dosage if needed and to make sure the medicine is working properly.

If you have been using this medicine regularly for several weeks, do not suddenly stop using it. Stopping suddenly may bring on attacks of angina. Check with your doctor for the best way to reduce gradually the amount you are taking before stopping completely.

Dizziness, lightheadedness, or a fainting feeling may occur, especially when you get up quickly from a lying or sitting position. Getting up slowly may help. **Also, drinking alcohol may make these effects worse and may cause a serious drop in blood pressure.** Check with your doctor before drinking alcoholic beverages while you are taking this medicine.

Chest pain resulting from exercise or physical exertion is usually reduced or prevented by this medicine. This may tempt you to be overly active. **Make sure you discuss with your doctor a safe amount of exercise for your medical problem.**

After taking a dose of this medicine you may get a headache that lasts for a short time. This effect is more common if you are taking nifedipine. This should become less noticeable after you have taken this medicine for a while. If this effect continues or if the headaches are severe, check with your doctor.

For patients taking diltiazem or verapamil:
• **Ask your doctor how to count your pulse rate. Then, while you are taking this medicine, check your pulse regularly.** If it is much slower than your usual rate, or less than 50 per minute, check with your doctor. A pulse rate that is too slow may cause circulation problems.

Side Effects of This Medicine

Along with its needed effects, a medicine may cause some unwanted effects. Although not all of these side effects appear very often, when they do occur they may require medical attention. Check with your doctor as soon as possible if any of the following side effects occur:

Less common
  Breathing difficulty, coughing, or wheezing
  Irregular or unusually fast, pounding heartbeat
  Skin rash
  Swelling of ankles, feet, or lower legs (more common with nifedipine)
  Unusually slow heartbeat (less than 50 beats per minute—diltiazem and verapamil only)

Rare
  Fainting

Reported for nifedipine only (rare)
  Chest pain (may appear about 30 minutes after nifedipine is taken)

Other side effects may occur which usually do not require medical attention. These side effects may go away during treatment as your body adjusts to the medicine. However, check with your doctor if any of the following side effects continue or are bothersome:

More common
  Flushing and feeling of warmth (rare with diltiazem or verapamil)

Less common or rare
  Constipation
  Dizziness or lightheadedness (more common with nifedipine)
  Headache (more common with nifedipine)
  Nausea (more common with nifedipine)
  Nervousness or mood changes
  Shakiness or weakness
  Stomach cramps
  Stuffy nose
  Unusual tiredness

Although not all of the side effects listed above have been reported for all of these medicines, they have been reported for at least one of them. Since all of the calcium channel blockers are similar, any of the above side effects may occur with any of these medicines. However, they may be more common with some of these medicines than with others.

Other side effects not listed above may also occur in some patients. If you notice any other effects, check with your doctor.

CAPTOPRIL (Systemic)

A commonly used brand name is Capoten.

Captopril (KAP-toe-pril) belongs to the general class of medicines called antihypertensives. It is used to treat high blood pressure. High blood pressure adds to the workload of the heart and arteries. If it continues for a long time, they may not function properly. This can damage the blood vessels of the brain, heart, and kidneys resulting in a stroke, heart attack, or kidney failure. These problems may be avoided if blood pressure is controlled.

Captopril is also used to treat congestive heart failure.

The exact way that captopril works is not known. It blocks an enzyme in the blood that causes blood vessels to tighten. As a result, it probably relaxes blood vessels, which lowers blood pressure and increases the supply of blood and oxygen to the heart.

Captopril is available only with your doctor's prescription.

Before Using This Medicine

In order to decide on the best treatment for your medical problem, your doctor should be told:

—if you have ever had any unusual or allergic reaction to captopril.

—if you are on a low-salt, low-sugar, or any other special diet, or if you are allergic to any substance, such as sulfites or other preservatives or dyes. Most medicines contain more than their active ingredient. Your doctor or pharmacist can help you avoid products that may cause a problem.

—if you are pregnant or if you intend to become pregnant while using this medicine. Studies in rabbits and rats at doses up to 400 times the recommended human dose have shown that captopril causes an increase in deaths of the fetus and newborn. However, captopril has not been shown to cause birth defects in hamsters, rats, or rabbits. Studies have not been done in humans.

—if you are breast-feeding an infant. Although captopril has not been shown to cause problems, the chance always exists.

—if you have any of the following medical problems:

Heart or blood vessel disease
Kidney disease
Systemic lupus erythematosus (SLE)

—if you have recently had a heart attack or stroke.

—if you are now taking any of the following medicines or types of medicine:

Azathioprine
Cancer medicines
Chloramphenicol
Colchicine
Diuretics (water pills)
Flucytosine
Inflammation medicines, especially indomethacin
Other antihypertensives (high blood pressure medicine)
Oxyphenbutazone
Penicillamine
Phenylbutazone
Potassium supplements
Primaquine
Pyrimethamine
Salt substitutes
Trimethoprim

Proper Use of This Medicine

In order to help remember to take your medicine, try to get into the habit of taking it at the same time each day.

This medicine is best taken on an empty stomach 1 hour before meals, unless otherwise directed by your doctor.

For patients taking captopril for high blood pressure:

• Importance of diet—When prescribing medicine for your condition, your doctor may also prescribe a personal diet for you. Such a diet may be low in sodium (salt). Most people eat much more sodium than they need and too much sodium in the diet may increase blood pressure. Some foods that contain large amounts of sodium include canned soup, pickles, ketchup, green and ripe olives, relish, frankfurters, soy sauce, and carbonated beverages. Your doctor may want you to limit the amounts of these and other high-sodium foods in your diet. Medicine is usually more effective when such a diet is properly followed.

Also, it may be very important for you to go on a reducing diet. However, check with your doctor before going on any diet.

• Many patients who have high blood pressure will not notice any signs of the problem. In fact, many may feel normal. It is very important that you **take your medicine exactly as directed** and that you keep your doctor's appointments even if you feel well.

• Remember that captopril will not cure your high blood pressure but it does help control it. Therefore, you must continue to take it as directed if you expect to lower your blood pressure and keep it down. **You may have to take medicine for the rest of your life.** If high blood pressure is not treated, it can cause serious problems such as heart failure, blood vessel disease, stroke, or kidney disease.

If you miss a dose of this medicine, take it as soon as possible. However, if it is almost time for your next dose, skip the missed dose and go back to your regular dosing schedule. Do not double doses.

How to store this medicine:

• Store away from heat and direct light.

• **Keep out of the reach of children.**

• Do not store in the bathroom medicine cabinet because the heat or moisture may cause the medicine to break down.

• Do not keep outdated medicine or medicine no longer needed. Flush the contents of the container down the toilet, unless otherwise directed.

Precautions While Using This Medicine

It is important that your doctor check your progress at regular visits in order to make sure that this medicine is working properly and check for unwanted effects.

Dizziness, lightheadedness, or fainting may occur if you exercise or if the weather is hot. Use extra care during exercise or hot weather.

Check with your doctor right away if you become sick while taking captopril, especially with severe or continuing nausea and vomiting or diarrhea. These conditions may cause you to lose too much water.

Chest pain resulting from exercise or physical exertion is usually reduced or prevented by captopril. This may tempt a patient to be overly active. **Make sure you discuss with your doctor a safe amount of exercise for your medical problem.**

Since salt substitutes and low-salt milk may contain potassium, do not use them unless told to do so by your doctor.

Before having any kind of surgery (including dental surgery) or emergency treatment, tell the physician or dentist in charge that you are taking captopril.

For patients taking captopril for high blood pressure:

- **Do not take other medicines unless they have been discussed with your doctor.** This especially includes over-the-counter (nonprescription) medicines for appetite control, asthma, colds, cough, hay fever, or sinus problems, since they may tend to increase your blood pressure.

Side Effects of This Medicine

Along with its needed effects, a medicine may cause some unwanted effects. Although not all of these side effects appear very often, when they do occur they may require medical attention. Check with your doctor **immediately** if the following side effects occur:

Rare

Fever and chills or sore throat

Check with your doctor as soon as possible if the following side effects occur:

More common

Skin rash, with or without itching or fever

Less common

Chest pain

Dizziness, lightheadedness, or fainting

Swelling of face, mouth, hands, or feet

Unusually fast or irregular heartbeat

Other side effects may occur which usually do not require medical attention. These side effects may go away during treatment as your body adjusts to the medicine. However, check with your doctor if the following side effect continues or is bothersome:

More common

Loss of taste

Dizziness and lightheadedness are more likely to occur in the elderly, who are more sensitive to the effects of captopril.

Other side effects not listed above may also occur in some patients. If you notice any other effects, check with your doctor.

CAPTOPRIL AND HYDROCHLOROTHIAZIDE
(Systemic)

A commonly used brand name is Capozide.

The combination of captopril (KAP-toe-pril) and hydrochlorothiazide (hye-droe-klor-oh-THYE-a-zide) belongs to the general class of medicines called antihypertensives. It is used to treat high blood pressure.

High blood pressure adds to the workload of the heart and arteries. If it continues for a long time, they may not function properly. This can damage the vessels of the brain, heart, and kidney resulting in a stroke, heart attack, or kidney failure. These problems may be avoided if blood pressure is controlled.

Captopril blocks an enzyme in the blood that causes blood vessels to tighten. As a result, it probably relaxes blood vessels, which lowers blood pressure and increases the supply of blood and oxygen to the heart. Hydrochlorothiazide helps reduce the amount of water in the body by increasing the flow of urine; this also helps to lower blood pressure.

This medicine is available only with your doctor's prescription.

For information about the precautions and side effects of the medicines in this combination, see:

Captopril (Systemic)

Diuretics, Thiazide (Systemic)

Combination products are designed for specific uses. These uses may not be the same as the uses of the individual ingredients. Therefore, some of the information provided in the individual listings may not be relevant to the combination product. If questions arise, check with your doctor, nurse, or pharmacist.

CARBAMAZEPINE (Systemic)

Some commonly used brand names are Apo-Car-
bamazepine*, Mazepine*, and Tegretol.

---

* Not available in the United States.

Carbamazepine (kar-ba-MAZ-e-peen)
is used as an anticonvulsant to control some
types of convulsions (seizures) in the treatment of epilepsy. It is also used to relieve
pain due to trigeminal neuralgia or glosso-
pharyngeal neuralgia and other specific
kinds of pain. It must not be used for other
aches or pains.

This medicine may also be used for other conditions as determined by your doctor.

Carbamazepine is available only with
your doctor's prescription.

Before Using This Medicine

In order to decide on the best treatment for
your medical problem, your doctor
should be told:

—if you have ever had any unusual or
allergic reaction to carbamazepine or to
any of the tricyclic antidepressants,
such as amitriptyline, amoxapine, clomipramine, desipramine, doxepin, imipramine, nortriptyline, protriptyline, or
trimipramine.

—if you are on a low-salt, low-sugar, or
any other special diet, or if you are allergic to any substance, such as sulfites or
other preservatives or dyes. Most medicines contain more than their active ingredient. Your doctor or pharmacist can
help you avoid products that may cause
a problem.

—if any medicine you have taken has
ever caused an allergy or reaction that
affected your blood.

—if you are pregnant or if you intend to
become pregnant while taking this medicine. Studies on birth defects with carbamazepine have not been done in humans. However, birth defects have been
reported in some infants when the mothers took other medicines for epilepsy
during pregnancy. Also, studies in animals have shown that carbamazepine
causes birth defects when given in large
doses. Therefore, the use of carbamazepine during pregnancy should be discussed with your doctor.

—if you are breast-feeding an infant.
Carbamazepine passes into the breast
milk and in some cases the baby may
receive enough of it to cause unwanted
effects. In animal studies, carbamazepine has caused unwanted effects on the
growth and appearance of the nursing
infants. Therefore, the use of this medicine while you are breast-feeding an infant should first be discussed with your
doctor.

—if you have any of the following medi-
cal problems:
Alcoholism
Anemia or other blood problems
Diabetes mellitus (sugar diabetes)
Glaucoma
Heart or blood vessel disease
Kidney disease
Liver disease
Problems with urination

—if you are now taking any of the fol-
lowing medicines or types of medicine:
Acetaminophen
Anticoagulants, oral (blood thinners
taken by mouth)
Barbiturates
Benzodiazepines
Chlorpropamide
Clofibrate
Contraceptives, oral (birth control pills)
Digitalis (heart medicine)
Disopyramide
Doxycycline
Erythromycin

Estrogens
Levothyroxine
Lithium
Medicine for diabetes insipidus (water diabetes)
Nomifensine
Other anticonvulsants (seizure medicine)
Pimozide
Propoxyphene
Quinidine
Sedatives, tranquilizers, or sleeping medicine
Troleandomycin

—if you are now taking tricyclic anti-depressants (medicine for depression) such as:

Amitriptyline
Amoxapine
Clomipramine
Desipramine
Doxepin
Imipramine
Nortriptyline
Protriptylne
Trimipramine

—if you are now taking or have taken within the past 2 weeks monoamine oxidase (MAO) inhibitors such as:

Furazolidone
Isocarboxazid
Pargyline
Phenelzine
Procarbazine
Tranylcypromine

Proper Use of This Medicine

Carbamazepine is **not** an ordinary pain reliever. It should be used only when a doctor prescribes it for certain kinds of pain. **Do not take carbamazepine for any other aches or pains.**

It is very important that you take this medicine exactly as directed by your doctor in order to obtain the best results and lessen the chance of serious side effects.

Carbamazepine may be taken with meals to lessen the chance of stomach upset (nausea and vomiting).

If you miss a dose of this medicine, take it as soon as possible. However, if it is almost time for your next dose, skip the missed dose and go back to your regular dosing schedule. Do not double doses. However, if you miss more than one dose a day, check with your doctor.

How to store this medicine:

• Store away from heat and direct light.

• **Keep out of the reach of children.**

• Do not store in the bathroom medicine cabinet because the heat or moisture may cause the medicine to break down.

• Do not keep outdated medicine or medicine no longer needed. Flush the contents of the container down the toilet, unless otherwise directed.

Precautions While Using This Medicine

It is very important that your doctor check your progress at regular visits. Your doctor may want to do certain tests to see if you are receiving the right amount of medicine or if certain side effects may be occurring without your knowing it. Also, the amount you are taking may have to be changed often..

If you are taking this medicine for epilepsy:

• **Do not suddenly stop taking this medicine without first checking with your doctor.** It is usually best to reduce gradually the amount of carbamazepine you are taking before stopping completely in order to keep your seizures under control. However, carbamazepine must be stopped at once if certain side effects occur (see *Side Effects of This Medicine*). Your doctor may have special instructions for you to follow if this is necessary.

This medicine may cause some people to become drowsy, dizzy, lightheaded, or less alert than they are normally. It may also cause blurred vision, weakness, or loss of muscle control in some people. **Be sure you know how you react to this medicine before you drive, use machines, or do other jobs that require you to be alert and well-coordinated.**

Some people who take carbamazepine may become more sensitive to sunlight than they are normally. When you first begin taking this medicine, avoid too much sun or use of a sunlamp, or use a sun screen until you know how you react, especially if you tend to burn easily. If you have a severe reaction, check with your doctor.

Your mouth may become dry while you are taking this medicine. Sucking on sugarless hard candy or ice chips or chewing sugarless gum may help relieve the dry mouth.

Diabetics—Carbamazepine may affect urine sugar levels. While you are using this medicine, be especially careful in testing for sugar in your urine. If you have any questions about this, check with your doctor.

Before having any kind of surgery (including dental surgery) or emergency treatment, tell the physician or dentist in charge that you are taking this medicine.

Your doctor may want you to carry a medical identification card or bracelet stating that you are taking this medicine.

Side Effects of This Medicine

Carbamazepine has been shown to cause tumors in animals. It is not known whether this medicine may cause tumors or cancer in humans.

Along with its needed effects, a medicine may cause some unwanted effects. Although not all of these side effects appear very often, when they do occur they may require medical attention. **Stop taking this medicine and check with your doctor immediately if any of the following side effects occur:**

> Sores or ulcers in the mouth
> Sore throat and fever
> Unusual bleeding or bruising
> Unusual tiredness or weakness

Also, **check with your doctor immediately if** any of the following side effects occur:

Rare

> Darkening of urine
> Pain, tenderness, swelling, or bluish color in leg or foot
> Pale stools
> Yellowing of eyes and skin

Signs of overdose

> Convulsions
> Dizziness, severe
> Drowsiness, severe
> Irregular, slow, or shallow breathing
> Trembling
> Unusually fast heartbeat

In addition, check with your doctor as soon as possible if any of the following side effects occur:

More common

> Blurred vision or double vision

Less common

> Hives, itching, or skin rash
> Mental confusion, especially in the elderly

Rare

> Continuous back-and-forth eye movements
> Difficulty in speaking or slurred speech
> Fainting
> Frequent urination
> Irregular, pounding, or unusually slow heartbeat
> Mental depression with restlessness and nervousness or other mood or mental changes
> Numbness, tingling, pain, or weakness in hands and feet
> Pain in chest
> Ringing or buzzing sound in the ears
> Sudden decrease in amount of urine
> Swelling of feet or lower legs
> Swollen glands

Troubled breathing
Unusual, uncontrolled body movements
Visual hallucinations (seeing things that
are not there)

Other side effects may occur which usually
do not require medical attention. These
side effects may go away during treatment as your body adjusts to the medicine. However, check with your doctor if
any of the following side effects continue or are bothersome:

More common

Clumsiness or unsteadiness
Dizziness
Drowsiness
Lightheadedness
Nausea
Vomiting

Less common or rare

Aching joints or muscles
Constipation
Diarrhea
Dryness of mouth
Headache
Increased sensitivity of skin to sunlight
Irritation of tongue
Loss of appetite
Loss of hair
Sexual problems in males
Stomach pain or discomfort
Unusual increase in sweating

Mental confusion; restlessness and nervousness; irregular, pounding, or unusually
slow heartbeat; and pain in the chest are
more likely to occur in elderly patients,
who may be more sensitive to some of
the effects of carbamazepine.

Other side effects not listed above may also
occur in some patients. If you notice any
other effects, check with your doctor.

CEPHALOSPORINS (Systemic)

This information applies to the following medicines:

Cefaclor (SEF-a-klor)
Cefadroxil (sef-a-DROX-ill)
Cefamandole (sef-a-MAN-dole)
Cefazolin (sef-A-zoe-lin)
Cefonicid (sef-FON-i-sid)
Cefoperazone (sef-oh-PER-a-zone)
Ceforanide (se-FOR-a-nide)
Cefotaxime (sef-oh-TAKS-eem)
Cefoxitin (se-FOX-i-tin)
Ceftazidime (sef-TAY-zi-deem)
Ceftizoxime (sef-ti-ZOX-eem)
Ceftriaxone (sef-try-AX-one)
Cefuroxime (se-fyoor-OX-eem)
Cephalexin (sef-a-LEX-in)
Cephalothin (sef-A-loe-thin)
Cephapirin (sef-a-PYE-rin)
Cephradine (SEF-ra-deen)
Moxalactam (MOX-a-lak-tam)

Some commonly used brand names and other names are:	Generic names:
Ceclor	Cefaclor
Duricef Ultracef	Cefadroxil
Mandol	Cefamandole
Ancef Kefzol	Cefazolin
Monocid	Cefonicid
Cefobid Cefobine*	Cefoperazone
Precef	Ceforanide
Claforan	Cefotaxime
Mefoxin	Cefoxitin
Fortaz	Ceftazidime
Cefizox	Ceftizoxime
Rocephin	Ceftriaxone

Zinacef	Cefuroxime
Ceporex* Keflex Novolexin*	Cephalexin
Ceporacin* Keflin Neutral Seffin	Cephalothin†
Cefadyl	Cephapirin
Anspor Velosef	Cephradine
Lamoxactam Latamoxef Moxam Oxalactam*	Moxalactam

*Not available in the United States.
†Generic name product may also be available.

Cephalosporins (sef-a-loe-SPOR-ins) belong to the general family of medicines called antibiotics. Antibiotics are medicines used in the treatment of infections caused by bacteria. They work by killing bacteria or preventing their growth. Cephalosporins will not work for colds, flu, or other virus infections.

Cephalosporins are taken by mouth or given by injection to treat infections in many different parts of the body. They are sometimes given with other antibiotics. Some cephalosporins are also given by injection to prevent infections before, during, and after surgery.

Cephalosporins are available only with your doctor's prescription.

Before Using This Medicine

In order to decide on the best treatment for your medical problem, your doctor should be told:

—if you have ever had any unusual or severe allergic reaction to any of the cephalosporins, penicillins, penicillin-like medicines, or penicillamine.

—if you are on a low-salt, low-sugar, or any other special diet, or if you are allergic to any substance, such as sulfites or other preservatives or dyes. Most medicines contain more than their active ingredient, and many liquid medicines contain alcohol. Your doctor or pharmacist can help you avoid products that may cause a problem.

—if you are pregnant or if you intend to become pregnant while taking this medicine. Studies have not been done in humans. However, most cephalosporins have not been shown to cause birth defects or other problems in animal studies. Studies in rats and mice have shown that moxalactam causes a decrease in the animal's ability to live after birth. Moxalactam has not been shown to cause birth defects or other problems in rats and mice given up to 20 times the usual human dose.

—if you are breast-feeding an infant. Most cephalosporins pass into human breast milk, usually in small amounts. Although cephalosporins have not been shown to cause problems in humans, the chance always exists.

—if you have any of the following medical problems:

Bleeding problems, history of (cefamandole, cefoperazone, and moxalactam only)
Kidney disease
Liver disease (cefoperazone only)
Stomach or intestinal disease, history of (especially colitis, including colitis caused by antibiotics, or enteritis)

—if you are taking any of the following medicines or types of medicine:

Diarrhea medicine
Probenecid (except with ceforanide or ceftazidime)

—if you are receiving cefamandole, cefoperazone, or moxalactam and are also taking any of the following medicines or types of medicine:

Alcohol-containing medicine
Anticoagulants (blood thinners)
Aspirin or other salicylates

Diflunisal
Dipyridamole
Divalproex
Fenoprofen
Heparin
Ibuprofen
Indomethacin
Meclofenamate
Mefenamic acid
Naproxen
Oxyphenbutazone
Phenylbutazone
Piroxicam
Plicamycin
Streptokinase
Sulfinpyrazone
Sulindac
Tolmetin
Urokinase
Valproic acid

—if you are receiving cephalothin and are also receiving any of the following medicines or types of medicine:

Aminoglycosides (by injection) (medicine for serious infection), such as amikacin, gentamicin, kanamycin, neomycin, netilmicin, streptomycin, tobramycin
Bumetanide
Carmustine
Ethacrynic acid
Furosemide
Streptozocin

Proper Use of This Medicine

Cephalosporins may be taken on a full or empty stomach. However, if this medicine upsets your stomach, it may be taken with food.

For patients taking the oral liquid form of this medicine:

• This medicine is to be taken by mouth even though it may come in a dropper bottle. If this medicine does not come in a dropper bottle, use a specially marked measuring spoon or other device to measure each dose accurately since the average household teaspoon may not hold the right amount of liquid.

• Do not use after the expiration date on the label since the medicine may not work as well. Check with your pharmacist if you have any questions about this.

To help clear up your infection completely, **keep taking this medicine for the full time of treatment** even if you begin to feel better after a few days. **If you have a "strep" infection, you should keep taking this medicine for at least 10 days. This is especially important in "strep" infections since serious heart problems could develop later if your infection is not cleared up completely.** Also, if you stop taking this medicine too soon, your symptoms may return.

This medicine works best when there is a constant amount in the blood or urine. **To help keep this amount constant, do not miss any doses. Also, it is best to take each dose at evenly spaced times day and night.** For example, if you are to take 4 doses a day, each dose should be spaced about 6 hours apart. If this interferes with your sleep or other daily activities, or if you need help in planning the best times to take your medicine, check with your doctor, nurse, or pharmacist.

If you do miss a dose of this medicine, take it as soon as possible. This will help to keep a constant amount of medicine in the blood or urine. However, if it is almost time for your next dose and your dosing schedule is:

• 1 dose a day—Space the missed dose and the next dose 10 to 12 hours apart.

• 2 doses a day—Space the missed dose and the next dose 5 to 6 hours apart.

• 3 or more doses a day—Space the missed dose and the next dose 2 to 4 hours apart or double your next dose.

Then go back to your regular dosing schedule.

How to store this medicine:

• Store the liquid form of most cephalosporins in the refrigerator because heat will cause this medicine to break down. Follow the directions on the label. However, keep the medicine from freezing.

• **Keep out of the reach of children.**

• Do not keep outdated medicine or medicine no longer needed. Flush the contents of the container down the toilet, unless otherwise directed.

Precautions While Using This Medicine

If your symptoms do not improve within a few days or if they become worse, check with your doctor.

Diabetics—This medicine may cause false test results with some urine sugar tests. Check with your doctor before changing your diet or the dosage of your diabetes medicine.

If diarrhea occurs, do not take any diarrhea medicine without first checking with your doctor or pharmacist. These medicines may make your diarrhea worse or make it last longer.

For patients receiving cefamandole, cefoperazone, or moxalactam by injection:

• Drinking alcoholic beverages or taking other alcohol-containing preparations (for example, elixirs, cough syrups, tonics, or injections of alcohol) while receiving these medicines and for several days after stopping them may cause increased side effects such as abdominal or stomach cramps, nausea, vomiting, headache, fainting, fast or irregular heartbeat, difficult breathing, sweating, or redness of the face or skin. These effects usually start within 15 to 30 minutes after taking alcohol and may not go away for up to several hours. Therefore, **you should not drink alcoholic beverages or take other alcohol-containing preparations while you are receiving these medicines and for several days after stopping them.**

Side Effects of This Medicine

Along with its needed effects, a medicine may cause some unwanted effects. Although not all of these side effects appear very often, when they do occur they may require medical attention. **Stop taking this medicine and check with your doctor immediately if any of the following side effects occur:**

Less common or rare

Unusual bleeding or bruising (cefamandole, cefoperazone, or moxalactam only)

Rare

Abdominal or stomach cramps, pain, and bloating (severe)

Diarrhea (watery and severe) which may also be bloody

Fever

Nausea or vomiting

Unusual thirst

Unusual tiredness or weakness

Unusual weight loss

(the above side effects may also occur up to several weeks after you stop taking this medicine)

Convulsions (seizures)—moxalactam only

Other side effects may occur which usually do not require medical attention. These side effects may go away during treatment as your body adjusts to the medicine. However, check with your doctor if any of the following side effects continue or are bothersome:

More common (less common with some cephalosporins)

Diarrhea (mild)

Skin rash, itching, redness, or swelling

Sore mouth or tongue

Stomach cramps or upset (mild)

Less common or rare

Itching of the rectal or genital (sex organ) areas

Other side effects not listed above may also occur in some patients. If you notice any other effects, check with your doctor.

CHENODIOL (Systemic)

A commonly used brand name is Chenix.

Chenodiol (kee-noe-DYE-ole) is used in the treatment of gallstone disease. It is taken by mouth to dissolve the gallstones.

Chenodiol is used in patients who do not need to have their gallbladder removed or in those in whom surgery is best avoided because of other medical problems. However, chenodiol works only in those patients who have a working gallbladder and whose gallstones are made of cholesterol. Chenodiol works best when these stones are small and of the "floating" type.

Chenodiol is available only with your doctor's prescription.

Before Using This Medicine

Importance of diet—If you have gallstones, your doctor may prescribe chenodiol and a personal high-fiber diet for you. Some foods that are high in fiber are whole grain breads and cereals, bran, fruit, and green, leafy vegetables. It has been found that such a diet may help dissolve the stones faster and may keep new stones from forming.

It may also be important for you to go on a reducing diet. However, check with your doctor before going on any diet.

In order to decide on the best treatment for your medical problem, your doctor should be told:

—if you have ever had any unusual or allergic reaction to chenodiol.

—if you are pregnant or if you intend to become pregnant while taking this medicine. Chenodiol is not recommended during pregnancy since it has been shown to cause liver and kidney problems in animals when given in doses many times the human dose. Be sure you have discussed this with your doctor.

—if you are breast-feeding an infant. Although it is not known whether chenodiol passes into the breast milk and this medicine has not been shown to cause problems in humans, the chance always exists.

—if you have any of the following medical problems:

Biliary tract problems
Blood vessel disease
Bowel inflammation disease
Liver disease
Pancreas disease

—if you are now taking any of the following medicines or types of medicine:

Antacids (aluminum-containing)
Cholestyramine
Colestipol
Estrogens
Oral contraceptives (birth control pills)

Proper Use of This Medicine

Take chenodiol with food or milk for best results, unless otherwise directed by your doctor.

Take chenodiol for the full time of treatment, even if you begin to feel better. If you stop taking this medicine too soon the gallstones may not dissolve as fast or may not dissolve at all.

If you miss a dose of this medicine, take it as soon as possible. However, if it is almost time for your next dose, skip the missed dose and go back to your regular dosing schedule. Do not double doses.

How to store this medicine:

• Store away from heat and direct light.

• **Keep out of the reach of children.**

• Do not store in the bathroom medicine cabinet because the heat or moisture may cause the medicine to break down.

• Do not keep outdated medicine or medicine no longer needed. Flush the contents of the container down the toilet, unless otherwise directed.

Precautions While Using This Medicine

It is important that your doctor check your progress at regular visits. **Laboratory tests will have to be done every few months** while you are taking this medicine in order to make sure the gallstones are dissolving and your liver is working properly.

Check with your doctor immediately if severe abdominal or stomach pain, especially toward the upper right side, and severe nausea and vomiting occur. These symptoms may mean that you have other medical problems or that your gallstone condition needs your doctor's attention.

Side Effects of This Medicine

Along with its needed effects, a medicine may cause some unwanted effects. Although not all of these side effects appear very often, when they do occur they may require medical attention. Check with your doctor as soon as possible if the following side effect occurs:

Less common or rare
   Diarrhea (severe)

Other side effects may occur which usually do not require medical attention. These side effects may go away during treatment as your body adjusts to the medicine. However, check with your doctor if any of the following side effects continue or are bothersome:

More common
   Diarrhea (mild)
Less common or rare
   Constipation
   Frequent urge for bowel movement
   Gas or indigestion (usually disappears within 2 to 4 weeks from the beginning of treatment)

Loss of appetite
Nausea or vomiting
Stomach cramps or pain

Other side effects not listed above may also occur in some patients. If you notice any other effects, check with your doctor.

CHLORDIAZEPOXIDE AND AMITRIPTYLINE (Systemic)

A commonly used brand name is Limbitrol.

Chlordiazepoxide (klor-dye-az-e-POX-ide) and amitriptyline (a-mee-TRIP-ti-leen) combination is used to treat depression that occurs with anxiety or nervous tension.

This medicine is available only with your doctor's prescription.

For information about the precautions and side effects of the medicines in this combination, see:

Benzodiazepines (Systemic)
Antidepressants, Tricyclic (Systemic)

Combination products are designed for specific uses. These uses may not be the same as the uses of the individual ingredients. Therefore, some of the information provided in the individual listings may not be relevant to the combination product. If questions arise, check with your doctor, nurse, or pharmacist.

CHLORDIAZEPOXIDE AND CLIDINIUM (Systemic)

Some commonly used brand names are:

Chlordinium	Clipoxide
Clindex	Librax
Clinoxide	Lidox

Chlordiazepoxide (klor-dye-az-e-POX-ide) and clidinium (kli-DI-nee-um) is a combination of medicines used to relax the digestive system and to reduce stomach acid. It is used to treat stomach and intestinal problems such as ulcers and colitis.

This combination is available only with your doctor's prescription.

Before Using This Medicine

In order to decide on the best treatment for your medical problem, your doctor should be told:

—if you have ever had any unusual or allergic reaction to benzodiazepines such as alprazolam, chlordiazepoxide, clonazepam, clorazepate, diazepam, flurazepam, halazepam, lorazepam, oxazepam, prazepam, or temazepam.

—if you are on a low-salt, low-sugar, or any other special diet, or if you are allergic to any substance, such as sulfites or other preservatives or dyes. Most medicines contain more than their active ingredient. Your doctor or pharmacist can help you avoid products that may cause a problem.

—if you are pregnant or if you intend to become pregnant while using this medicine. Clidinium (contained in this combination) has not been shown to cause birth defects or other problems in humans. However, chlordiazepoxide (contained also in this combination) may cause birth defects if taken during the first 3 months of pregnancy. In addition, too much use of this medicine during pregnancy may cause the baby to become dependent on the medicine. This may lead to withdrawal side effects after birth.

—if you are breast-feeding an infant. Chlordiazepoxide (contained in this combination) may pass into the breast milk and cause unwanted effects, such as excessive drowsiness, in infants.

—if you have any of the following medical problems:
  Difficult urination
  Dry mouth (severe and continuing)
  Emphysema, asthma, bronchitis, or other chronic lung disease
  Enlarged prostate
  Glaucoma
  Hiatal hernia
  High blood pressure
  Intestinal blockage
  Kidney disease
  Liver disease
  Mental depression
  Myasthenia gravis
  Overactive thyroid
  Severe mental illness
  Severe ulcerative colitis

—if you are taking *any* other medicines including over-the-counter (OTC) or nonprescription medicines (for example, antacids or diarrhea medicine). Many medicines change the way clidinium affects your body. Also, the effect of other medicines may be reduced by clidinium.

—if you are now taking central nervous system (CNS) depressants such as:
  Anticonvulsants (seizure medicine)
  Antihistamines or medicine for hay fever, other allergies, or colds
  Barbiturates
  Muscle relaxants
  Narcotics
  Prescription pain medicine
  Sedatives, tranquilizers, or sleeping medicine

—if you are now taking tricyclic antidepressants such as:
  Amitriptyline
  Amoxapine
  Clomipramine
  Desipramine
  Doxepin
  Imipramine
  Nortriptyline
  Protriptyline
  Trimipramine

—if you are now taking or have taken within the past 2 weeks monoamine oxidase (MAO) inhibitors such as:

Furazolidone
Isocarboxazid
Pargyline
Phenelzine
Procarbazine
Tranylcypromine

Proper Use of This Medicine

Take this medicine about ½ to 1 hour before meals unless otherwise directed by your doctor.

Take this medicine only as directed by your doctor. Do not take more of it, do not take it more often, and do not take it for a longer period of time than your doctor ordered. If too much is taken, it may become habit-forming.

If you miss a dose of this medicine, take it as soon as possible. However, if it is almost time for your next dose, skip the missed dose and go back to your regular dosing schedule. Do not double doses.

How to store this medicine:

• Store away from heat and direct light.

• **Keep out of the reach of children.**

• Do not store in the bathroom medicine cabinet because the heat or moisture may cause the medicine to break down.

• Do not keep outdated medicine or medicine no longer needed. Flush the contents of the container down the toilet, unless otherwise directed.

Precautions While Using This Medicine

If you will be taking this medicine regularly for a long period of time your doctor should check your progress at regular visits.

Do not take this medicine within an hour of taking medicine for diarrhea. Taking them too close together will make this medicine less effective.

This medicine may cause some people to become dizzy, light-headed, drowsy, or less alert than they are normally. **Make sure you know how you react to this medicine before you drive, use machines, or do other jobs that require you to be alert.**

This medicine will add to the effects of alcohol and other CNS depressants (medicines that slow down the nervous system, possibly causing drowsiness). Some examples of CNS depressants are sedatives, tranquilizers, or sleeping medicine; prescription pain medicine or narcotics; barbiturates; medicine for seizures; muscle relaxants; or anesthetics, including some dental anesthetics. **Check with your doctor before taking any of the above while you are using this medicine and also for a few days after you stop taking it.**

This medicine will often make you sweat less, causing your body temperature to increase. **Use extra care not to become overheated during exercise or hot weather while you are taking this medicine as this could possibly result in heat stroke.**

Your mouth, nose, and throat may feel very dry while you are taking this medicine. To help relieve mouth dryness, chew sugarless gum or dissolve bits of ice in your mouth.

Check with your doctor if you develop intestinal problems such as constipation. This is especially important if you are taking other medicine while you are taking chlordiazepoxide and clidinium. If not corrected, serious complications may result.

If you will be taking this medicine in large doses or for a long period of time, do not stop taking it without first checking with your doctor. Your doctor may want you to reduce gradually the amount you are taking before stopping completely.

Side Effects of This Medicine

Along with its needed effects, a medicine may cause some unwanted effects. Although not all of these side effects appear very often, when they do occur they may require medical attention. Check with your doctor as soon as possible if any of the following side effects occur:

Less common or rare
    Constipation
    Eye pain
    Mental depression
    Skin rash or hives
    Sore throat and fever
    Trouble in sleeping
    Unusual excitement, nervousness, or
        irritability
    Unusually slow heartbeat, shortness of
        breath, or troubled breathing
    Yellowing of eyes or skin

Signs of overdose
    Confusion
    Difficult urination
    Drowsiness (severe)
    Dryness of mouth, nose, or throat (severe)
    Unusually fast heartbeat
    Unusual warmth, dryness, and flushing of
        skin

Other side effects may occur which usually do not require medical attention. These side effects may go away during treatment as your body adjusts to the medicine. However, check with your doctor if any of the following side effects continue or are bothersome:

More common
    Bloated feeling
    Dizziness
    Drowsiness
    Dry mouth
    Headache
    Reduced sweating

Less common
    Blurred vision
    Decreased sexual ability
    Nausea
    Unusual tiredness or weakness

After you stop using this medicine, your body may need time to adjust. The length of time this takes depends on the amount of medicine you were using and how long you used it. During this period of time check with your doctor if you notice any of the following side effects:
    Convulsions (seizures)
    Muscle cramps
    Nausea or vomiting
    Stomach cramps
    Trembling

Children and elderly patients are usually more sensitive to the effects of this medicine. Excitement, agitation, drowsiness, or confusion are more likely to occur in elderly patients.

Other side effects not listed above may also occur in some patients. If you notice any other effects, check with your doctor.

CHLORZOXAZONE AND ACETAMINOPHEN (Systemic)

Some commonly used brand names are:

Blanex	Mus-Lax
Chlorofon-F	Paracet Forte
Chlorzone Forte	Parafon Forte
Flexaphen	Polyflex
Flexin	Zoxaphen
Lobac	

Generic name product may also be available (tablets only).

Chlorzoxazone (klor-ZOX-a-zone) and acetaminophen (a-seat-a-MEE-noe-fen) combination medicine is taken by mouth to help relax certain muscles in your body and relieve the pain and discomfort caused by strains, sprains, or other injury to your muscles. However, this medicine does not take the place of rest, exercise or physical therapy, or other treatment that your doctor may recommend for your medical problem.

Chlorzoxazone acts in the central nervous system (CNS) to produce its muscle relaxant effects. Its actions in the CNS may also produce some of its side effects.

In the United States, this medicine is available only with your doctor's prescription. In Canada, this medicine is available without a prescripton.

For information about the precautions and side effects of the medicines in this combination, see:

Skeletal Muscle Relaxants (Systemic)
Acetaminophen (Systemic)

Combination products are designed for specific uses. These uses may not be the same as the uses of the individual ingredients. Therefore, some of the information provided in the individual listings may not be relevant to the combination product. If questions arise, check with your doctor, nurse, or pharmacist.

CIMETIDINE (Systemic)

A commonly used brand name is Tagamet.

Cimetidine (sye-MET-i-deen) is a medicine used to treat duodenal ulcers and prevent their return. It is also used to treat gastric ulcers and in some conditions in which the stomach produces too much acid, such as in Zollinger-Ellison disease. Cimetidine may also be used for other conditions as determined by your doctor.

Cimetidine works by decreasing the amount of acid produced by the stomach.

Cimetidine is available only with your doctor's prescription.

Before Using This Medicine

In order to decide on the best treatment for your medical problem, your doctor should be told:

—if you have ever had any unusual or allergic reaction to cimetidine or ranitidine.

—if you are pregnant or if you intend to become pregnant while using this medicine. Studies have not been done in humans. However, one study in rats suggested that cimetidine may affect male sexual development. More studies are needed to confirm this.

—if you are breast-feeding an infant. Although cimetidine has not been shown to cause problems in humans, the chance always exists since this medicine passes into the breast milk.

—if you have any of the following medical problems:

Kidney disease
Liver disease

—if you are now taking any other medicine, especially the following medicines or types of medicine:

Aminophylline
Antacids
Anticoagulants (blood thinners)
Chlordiazepoxide
Diazepam
Ketoconazole
Metoprolol
Metronidazole
Oxtriphylline
Phenytoin
Procainamide
Propranolol
Sucralfate
Theophylline

—if you are now taking tricyclic antidepressants, such as:

Amitriptyline
Amoxapine
Clomipramine
Desipramine
Doxepin

Imipramine
Nortriptyline
Protriptyline
Trimipramine

Proper Use of This Medicine

If you are taking several doses of cimetidine a day, take them with meals and at bedtime for best results, unless otherwise directed by your doctor. If you are taking a single daily dose, it is most often taken at bedtime.

It may take several days for cimetidine to begin to relieve stomach pain. Antacids may be taken with cimetidine, but not at the same time, to help relieve pain, unless your doctor has told you not to use them. However, one hour should pass between taking the antacid and the cimetidine. For example, if you are taking cimetidine with meals, then wait an hour after the meal before taking the antacid.

Take this medicine for the full time of treatment, even if you begin to feel better. Also, it is important that you keep your doctor's appointments for check-ups so that your doctor will be better able to tell you when to stop taking this medicine.

If you miss a dose of this medicine, take it as soon as possible. However, if it is almost time for your next dose, skip the missed dose and go back to your regular dosing schedule. Do not double doses.

How to store this medicine:

• Store away from heat and direct light.

• **Keep out of the reach of children.**

• Do not store in the bathroom medicine cabinet because the heat or moisture may cause the medicine to break down.

• Keep the oral solution form of this medicine from freezing.

• Do not keep outdated medicine or medicine no longer needed. Flush the contents of the container down the toilet, unless otherwise directed.

Precautions While Using This Medicine

Before you have any skin tests for allergies, tell the doctor in charge that you are taking this medicine. The results of the test may be affected by this medicine.

Remember that certain medicines, such as aspirin, and certain foods and drinks irritate the stomach and may make your problem worse.

Cigarette smoking tends to decrease the effect of cimetidine. This is more likely to affect the stomach's nighttime production of acid. While taking cimetidine, stop smoking completely, or at least do not smoke after taking the last dose of the day.

Follow your doctor's orders and check with him or her if your ulcer pain continues or gets worse.

Side Effects of This Medicine

Along with its needed effects, a medicine may cause some unwanted effects. Although not all of these side effects appear very often, when they do occur they may require medical attention. Check with your doctor as soon as possible if any of the following side effects occur:

Rare

    Confusion (especially in the elderly and/ or very ill, or with very large doses)
    Sore throat and fever
    Unusual bleeding or bruising
    Unusual tiredness or weakness

Other side effects may occur which usually do not require medical attention. These side effects may go away during treatment as your body adjusts to the medicine. However, check with your doctor if

any of the following side effects continue or are bothersome:

Less common or rare

Decreased sexual ability (especially in patients with Zollinger-Ellison disease who have received high doses for at least 1 year)
Diarrhea
Dizziness or headache
Muscle cramps or pain
Skin rash
Swelling of breasts or breast soreness in females and males

Dizziness and confusion are more likely to occur in elderly patients with kidney or liver disease, who are usually more sensitive to the effects of cimetidine.

Other side effects not listed above may also occur in some patients. If you notice any other effects, check with your doctor.

CLONIDINE (Systemic)

Some commonly used brand names are Catapres and Catapres-TTS.

Clonidine (KLOE-ni-deen) belongs to the general class of medicines called antihypertensives. It is used to treat high blood pressure.

High blood pressure adds to the workload of the heart and arteries. If it continues for a long time, they may not function properly. This can damage the blood vessels of the brain, heart, and kidneys, resulting in a stroke, heart attack, or kidney failure. These problems may be avoided if blood pressure is controlled.

Clonidine works by controlling nerve impulses along certain nerve pathways. As a result, it relaxes blood vessels so that blood passes through them more easily. This helps to lower blood pressure.

Clonidine may also be used for other conditions as determined by your doctor.

Clonidine is available only with your doctor's prescription.

Before Using This Medicine

In order to decide on the best treatment for your medical problem, your doctor should be told:

—if you have ever had any unusual or allergic reaction to clonidine.

—if you are on a low-salt, low-sugar, or any other special diet, or if you are allergic to any substance, such as sulfites or other preservatives or dyes. Most medicines contain more than their active ingredient. Your doctor or pharmacist can help you avoid products that may cause a problem.

—if you are pregnant or if you intend to become pregnant while using this medicine. Studies have not been done in humans. Although clonidine has not been shown to cause birth defects in animals, it has been shown to cause toxic or harmful effects in the animal fetus, even at doses of only one-third the maximum human dose.

—if you are breast-feeding an infant. Although clonidine has not been shown to cause problems in humans, the chance always exists since this medicine passes into breast milk.

—if you have any of the following medical problems:

Heart or blood vessel disease
Kidney disease
Mental depression (history of)
Raynaud's syndrome

—if you are now taking any of the following medicines or types of medicine:

Acebutolol
Antidepressants, tricyclic
Appetite suppressants
Atenolol
Fenfluramine

Inflammation medicines, especially indomethacin
Labetalol
Diuretics (water pills)
Metoprolol
Nadolol
Other antihypertensives (high blood pressure medicine)
Oxprenolol
Pindolol
Propranolol
Sotalol
Timolol

—if you are now taking central nervous system (CNS) depressants such as:

Anticonvulsants (seizure medicine)
Antihistamines or medicine for hay fever, other allergies, or colds
Barbiturates
Muscle relaxants
Narcotics
Prescription pain medicine
Sedatives, tranquilizers, or sleeping medicine

Proper Use of This Medicine

Importance of diet—When prescribing medicine for your condition, your doctor will probably try to control your condition by prescribing a personal diet for you. Such a diet may be low in sodium (salt). Most people eat much more sodium than they need and too much sodium in the diet may increase blood pressure. Some foods that contain large amounts of sodium include canned soup, pickles, ketchup, green and ripe olives, relish, frankfurters, soy sauce, and carbonated beverages. Your doctor may want you to limit the amounts of these and other high-sodium foods in your diet. Medicine is usually more effective when such a diet is properly followed.

Also, it may be very important for you to go on a reducing diet. However, check with your doctor before going on any diet.

Many patients who have high blood pressure will not notice any signs of the problem. In fact, many may feel normal. It is very important that you take your medicine exactly as directed and that you keep your doctor's appointments even if you feel well.

Remember that this medicine will not cure your high blood pressure but it does help control it. Therefore, you must continue to use it as directed if you expect to lower your blood pressure and keep it down. **You may have to take medicine for the rest of your life.** If high blood pressure is not treated, it can cause serious problems such as heart failure, blood vessel disease, stroke, or kidney disease.

For patients using the transdermal (stick-on patch) system:

• **Use this medicine exactly as directed by your doctor.** It will work only if applied correctly. **This medicine usually comes with patient instructions. Read them carefully before using.**

• Do not try to trim or cut the adhesive patch to adjust the dosage. Check with your doctor if you think the medicine is not working as it should.

• Apply the patch to a clean, dry skin area on your upper arm or chest with little or no hair and free of scars, cuts, or irritation.

• The system should stay in place even during showering, bathing, or swimming. If the patch becomes loose, cover it with the extra adhesive overlay. Apply a new patch if the first one becomes too loose or falls off.

• Each dose is best applied to a different area of skin to prevent skin problems or other irritation.

In order to help remember to use your medicine, try to get into the habit of using it at regular times. If you are taking the tablets, take them at the same time each day. If you are using the transdermal system, try to use it at the same time of day each week.

If you do miss a dose of this medicine, take it or use it as soon as possible. Then go back to your regular dosing schedule. **If you miss more than one dose of the tablets in a row or if you miss changing the transdermal patch for more than one day, check with your doctor right away.** If your body goes without this medicine for too long, your blood pressure may go up to a dangerously high level and some unpleasant effects may occur.

How to store this medicine:
- Store away from heat and direct light.
- **Keep out of the reach of children.**
- Do not store in the bathroom medicine cabinet because the heat or moisture may cause the medicine to break down.
- Do not keep outdated medicine or medicine no longer needed. Flush the tablets down the toilet, unless otherwise directed.

Precautions While Using This Medicine

It is important that your doctor check your progress at regular visits in order to make sure that this medicine is working properly.

Check with your doctor before you stop using this medicine. Your doctor may want you to reduce gradually the amount you are using before stopping completely.

Make sure that you have enough clonidine on hand to last through weekends, holidays, or vacations. You should not miss any doses. You may want to ask your doctor for another prescription for clonidine to carry in your wallet or purse. You could then have it filled if you run out when you are away from home.

Clonidine will add to the effects of alcohol and other CNS depressants (medicines that slow down the nervous system, possibly causing drowsiness). Some examples of CNS depressants are antihistamines or medicine for hay fever, other allergies, or colds; sedatives, tranquilizers, or sleeping medicine; prescription pain medicine or narcotics; barbiturates; medicine for seizures; muscle relaxants; or anesthetics, including some dental anesthetics. **Check with your doctor before taking any of the above while you are using this medicine.**

Clonidine may cause some people to become drowsy or less alert than they are normally. This is more likely to happen when you begin to take it or when you increase the amount of medicine you are taking. **Make sure you know how you react to this medicine before you drive, use machines, or do other jobs that require you to be alert.**

Before having any kind of surgery (including dental surgery) or emergency treatment, **tell the physician or dentist in charge that you are using this medicine.**

Dizziness, lightheadedness, or fainting may occur, especially when you get up from a lying or sitting position. Getting up slowly may help but if the problem continues or gets worse, check with your doctor.

The dizziness, lightheadedness, or fainting is also more likely to occur if you drink alcohol, stand for long periods of time, exercise, or if the weather is hot. **While you are taking clonidine, be careful in the amount of alcohol you drink. Also, use extra care during exercise or hot weather or if you must stand for long periods of time.**

Your mouth, nose, and throat may feel very dry while you are taking this medicine. To help relieve mouth dryness, chew sugarless gum or dissolve bits of ice in your mouth.

Do not take other medicines unless they have been discussed with your doctor. This especially includes over-the-counter (nonprescription) medicines for appetite control, asthma, colds, cough, hay fever, or sinus problems, since they may tend to increase your blood pressure.

Side Effects of This Medicine

Along with its needed effects, a medicine may cause some unwanted effects. Although not all of these side effects appear very often, when they do occur they may require medical attention. **Check with your doctor immediately** if any of the following side effects occur:

Signs of overdose
    Difficulty in breathing
    Dizziness (extreme) or faintness
    Unusually slow heartbeat
    Unusual tiredness or weakness

Check with your doctor as soon as possible if any of the following side effects occur:

More common—with transdermal system only
    Itching or redness of skin

Less common
    Darkening of skin—with transdermal
        system only
    Swelling of feet and lower legs

Rare
    Mental depression
    Paleness or cold feeling in fingertips and
        toes
    Vivid dreams or nightmares

Other side effects may occur which usually do not require medical attention. These side effects may go away during treatment as your body adjusts to the medicine. However, check with your doctor if any of the following side effects continue or are bothersome:

More common
    Dizziness
    Drowsiness
    Dry mouth

Less common
    Constipation
    Decreased sexual ability
    Difficulty in sleeping
    Dizziness, lightheadedness, or
        fainting, especially when getting up
        from a lying or sitting position
    Loss of appetite
    Nausea or vomiting
    Painful salivary glands

After you have been using this medicine for a while, it may cause unpleasant or even harmful effects if you stop taking it too suddenly. After you stop taking this medicine, **check with your doctor immediately** if any of the following occur:
    Anxiety or tenseness
    Chest pain
    Difficulty in sleeping
    Flushing or redness of face
    Headache
    Increased salivation
    Nausea
    Nervousness
    Rapid or irregular heartbeat
    Restlessness
    Shaking or trembling of hands and
        fingers
    Stomach cramps
    Sweating
    Vomiting

Dizziness or faintness may be more likely to occur in the elderly, who are more sensitive to the effects of clonidine.

Other side effects not listed above may also occur in some patients. If you notice any other effects, check with your doctor.

CLONIDINE AND CHLORTHALIDONE (Systemic)

A commonly used brand name is Combipres.

Clonidine (KLOE-ni-deen) and chlorthalidone (klor-THAL-i-done) combinations are used in the treatment of high blood pressure. High blood pressure adds to the workload of the heart and arteries. If it continues for a long time, they may not function properly. This can damage the blood vessels of the brain, heart, and kidneys resulting in a stroke, heart attack, or kidney failure. These problems may be avoided if blood pressure is controlled.

Clonidine works by controlling nerve impulses along certain body nerve pathways. As a result, it relaxes blood vessels so that blood passes through them more easily. The chlorthalidone in this combination helps reduce the amount of water in the body by increasing the flow of urine.

Clonidine and chlorthalidone combination is available only with your doctor's prescription.

For information about the precautions and side effects of the medicines in this combination, see:

Clonidine (Systemic)
Diuretics, Thiazide (Systemic)

Combination products are designed for specific uses. These uses may not be the same as the uses of the individual ingredients. Therefore, some of the information provided in the individual listings may not be relevant to the combination product. If questions arise, check with your doctor, nurse, or pharmacist.

COUGH/COLD COMBINATIONS— ANTIHISTAMINES AND ANTITUSSIVES (Systemic)

This information applies to the following medicines:

Bromodiphenhydramine (broe-moe-dye-fen-HYE-dra-meen) and Codeine (KOE-deen)
Chlorpheniramine (klor-fen-EER-a-meen) and Codeine
Doxylamine (dox-ILL-a-meen) and Dextromethorphan (dex-troe-meth-OR-fan)
Phenyltoloxamine (fen-ill-tole-OX-a-meen) and Hydrocodone (hye-droe-KOE-done)
Promethazine (proe-METH-a-zeen) and Codeine
Promethazine and Dextromethorphan

Some commonly used brand names are:	Generic names:
Ambay Cough Ambenyl Cough	Bromodiphenhydramine and Codeine
Penntuss*	Chlorpheniramine and Codeine
Vicks Formula 44 Cough Mixture	Doxylamine and Dextromethorphan
Tussionex	Phenyltoloxamine and Hydrocodone
Phenergan with Codeine	Promethazine and Codeine
Phenergan with Dextromethorphan	Promethazine and Dextromethorphan

*Not available in the United States.

Antihistamine and antitussive combinations are used to relieve the cough due to colds or influenza. They are not to be used for chronic cough that occurs with smoking, asthma, or emphysema, or when there is an unusually large amount of mucus or phlegm (pronounced flem) with the cough.

Antihistamines are used to relieve or prevent the symptoms of hay fever and other types of allergy. They work by preventing the effects of a substance called histamine, which is produced by the body. However, in these combination medicines, the antihistamine is used to increase the effects of the antitussive.

To help relieve coughing these combinations contain either a narcotic (codeine or hydrocodone) or non-narcotic (dextromethorphan) antitussive. These antitussives act directly on the cough center in the brain. Narcotics may become habit-forming, causing mental or physical dependence, if used for a long time. Physical dependence may lead to withdrawal side effects when you stop taking the medicine.

Some of these combinations are available only with your doctor's prescription. Others are available without a prescription; however, your doctor or pharmacist may have special instructions on the proper dose of the medicine for your medical condition.

Before Using This Medicine

Before you use this medicine, check with your doctor, nurse, or pharmacist:

—if you have ever had any unusual or allergic reaction to antihistamines, codeine, dextromethorphan, or hydrocodone.

—if you are on a low-salt, low-sugar, or any other special diet, or if you are allergic to any substance, such as sulfites or other preservatives or dyes. Most medicines contain more than their active ingredient, and many liquid medicines contain alcohol. Your doctor or pharmacist can help you avoid products that may cause a problem.

—if you are pregnant or if you intend to become pregnant while taking this medicine. Although most antihistamines and dextromethorphan have not been shown to cause problems in humans, the chance always exists.

Promethazine (contained in some of these combination medicines) has been shown to cause jaundice and muscle tremors in a few newborn infants whose mothers received phenothiazines such as promethazine during pregnancy. To avoid these effects, medicines that contain promethazine should be stopped 1 or 2 weeks before the expected delivery date.

Although studies on birth defects with narcotic antitussives, such as codeine and hydrocodone (contained in some of these combination medicines), have not been done in humans, these medicines have not been reported to cause birth defects in humans. However, hydrocodone has been shown to cause birth defects in animals when given in very large doses. Codeine has not been shown to cause birth defects in animal studies, but it caused other unwanted effects. Also, regular use of narcotics during pregnancy may cause the baby to become dependent on the medicine. This may lead to withdrawal side effects after birth. In addition, narcotics may cause breathing problems in the newborn infant if taken just before delivery.

—if you are breast-feeding an infant. Small amounts of antihistamines and codeine pass into the breast milk. Use is not recommended since the chances of this medicine causing side effects, such as unusual excitement or irritability, in the infant are greater. Also, since antihistamines tend to decrease the secretions of the body, it is possible that the flow of breast milk may be reduced in some patients.

—if you have any of the following medical problems:

Emphysema, asthma, or chronic lung
  disease (especially in children)
Enlarged prostate
Glaucoma
Liver disease
Urinary tract blockage or problems with
  urination

—if you are taking a medicine containing codeine or hydrocodone and also have any of the following medical problems:

Brain disease or injury
Colitis
Convulsions or seizures (history of)
Gallbladder disease or gallstones
Heart or blood vessel disease
Kidney disease
Underactive thyroid

—if you are now taking any of the following medicines or types of medicine:

Amantadine
Antimuscarinics (medicine for abdominal or stomach spasms or cramps)
Aspirin or other salicylates
Cisplatin
Paromomycin
Procainamide
Quinidine
Vancomycin

—if you are now taking central nervous system (CNS) depressants such as:

Anticonvulsants (seizure medicine)
Barbiturates
Muscle relaxants
Other antihistamines or medicine for hay fever, other allergies, or colds
Other narcotics
Prescription pain medicine
Sedatives, tranquilizers, or sleeping medicine

—if you are now taking tricyclic antidepressants (medicine for depression) such as:

Amitriptyline
Amoxapine
Desipramine
Doxepin
Imipramine
Nortriptyline
Protriptyline
Trimipramine

—if you are now taking or have taken within the past 2 weeks monoamine oxidase (MAO) inhibitors such as:

Furazolidone
Isocarboxazid
Pargyline
Phenelzine
Procarbazine
Tranylcypromine

Proper Use of This Medicine

Take this medicine with food or a glass of water or milk to reduce stomach irritation, if necessary.

To help loosen mucus or phlegm in the lungs, **drink a glass of water after each dose of this medicine,** unless otherwise directed by your doctor.

Take this medicine only as directed. Do not take more of it, and do not take it more often than recommended on the label, unless otherwise directed by your doctor. To do so may increase the chance of side effects.

If you must take this medicine regularly and you miss a dose, take it as soon as possible. However, if it is almost time for your next dose, skip the missed dose and go back to your regular dosing schedule. Do not double doses.

How to store this medicine:

• Store away from heat and direct light.

• **Keep this medicine out of the reach of children** since overdose is very dangerous in young children.

• Do not store in the bathroom medicine cabinet because the heat or moisture may cause the medicine to break down.

• Keep from freezing. Do not refrigerate the syrup.

• Do not keep outdated medicine or medicine no longer needed. Flush the contents of the container down the toilet, unless otherwise directed.

Precautions While Using This Medicine

If your cough has not improved after 7 days or if you have a high fever, skin rash, continuing headache, or sore throat with the cough, check with your doctor. These signs may mean that you have other medical problems.

Tell the doctor in charge that you are taking this medicine before you have any skin tests for allergies. The results of the test may be affected by the antihistamine in this medicine.

This medicine will add to the effects of alcohol and other CNS depressants (medicines that slow down the nervous system, possibly causing drowsiness). Some examples of CNS depressants are antihistamines or medicine for hay fever, other allergies, or colds; sedatives, tranquilizers, or sleeping medicine; prescription pain medicine or narcotics; barbiturates; medicine for seizures; muscle relaxants; or anesthetics, including some dental anesthetics. **Check with your doctor before taking any of the above while you are using this medicine.**

This medicine may cause some people to become drowsy or less alert than they are normally. **Make sure you know how you react to this medicine before you drive, use machines, or do other jobs that require you to be alert.**

When taking antihistamines (contained in this combination medicine) on a regular basis, make sure your doctor knows if you are taking large amounts of aspirin (as in arthritis or rheumatism) at the same time. Effects of too much aspirin, such as ringing in the ears, may be covered up by this medicine.

For patients taking codeine- or hydrocodone-containing medicine:

• Before having any kind of surgery (including dental surgery) or emergency treatment, tell the physician or dentist in charge that you are taking this medicine.

• Dizziness, lightheadedness, or fainting may be especially likely to occur when you get up suddenly from a lying or sitting position. Getting up slowly may help lessen this problem.

• Nausea or vomiting may occur after taking a narcotic antitussive. This effect may go away if you lie down for a while. However, if nausea or vomiting continues, check with your doctor.

• **If you think you or someone else in your home may have taken an overdose of this medicine, get emergency help at once.** Taking an overdose of this medicine or taking alcohol or CNS depressants with this medicine may lead to unconsciousness or death. Signs of overdose include confusion, convulsions or seizures, severe nervousness or restlessness, severe dizziness, severe drowsiness, unusually slow or troubled breathing, and severe weakness.

Side Effects of This Medicine

Along with its needed effects, a medicine may cause some unwanted effects. Although serious side effects occur rarely when this medicine is taken as recommended, they may be more likely to occur if:

—too much medicine is taken.
—it is taken in large doses.
—it is taken for a long period of time.

Get emergency help immediately if any of the following signs of overdose occur:

> Clumsiness or unsteadiness
> Cold, clammy skin
> Confusion
> Convulsions (seizures)
> Drowsiness or dizziness (severe)
> Dryness of mouth, nose, or throat
> Flushing or redness of face
> Muscle spasms (especially of neck and back)
> Nervousness or restlessness
> Shortness of breath or troubled breathing
> Shuffling walk
> Tic-like (jerky) movements of head and face
> Trembling and shaking of hands
> Weakness (severe)

Other side effects may occur which usually do not require medical attention. These

side effects may go away during treatment as your body adjusts to the medicine. However, check with your doctor if any of the following side effects continue or are bothersome:

More common
　Drowsiness

Less common or rare
　Constipation
　Difficult or painful urination
　Dizziness or lightheadedness
　Dryness of mouth, nose, or throat
　False sense of well-being
　Nausea or vomiting
　Nightmares
　Skin rash
　Unusual excitement, nervousness, restlessness, or irritability

Although not all of the side effects listed above have been reported for all of these medicines, they have been reported for at least one of them. However, since there are some similarities among these combination medicines, most of the above side effects may occur with any of these medicines.

Use of this medicine is not recommended in premature or newborn infants. Serious side effects, such as convulsions (seizures) and unusually fast or irregular heartbeats, are more likely to occur in children and would be of greater risk to these infants.

Children and elderly patients are usually more sensitive to the effects of this medicine. Confusion, convulsions, difficult and painful urination, dizziness, drowsiness, or dryness of mouth may be more likely to occur in elderly patients. Nightmares or unusual excitement, nervousness, restlessness, or irritability may be more likely also to occur in children and in elderly patients. Also, breathing problems may be more likely to occur in very young children and elderly patients, or those patients who are very ill, and are

taking combinations containing codeine or hydrocodone.

Other side effects not listed above may also occur in some patients. If you notice any other effects, check with your doctor.

COUGH/COLD COMBINATIONS— ANTIHISTAMINES, ANTITUSSIVES, AND ANALGESICS (Systemic)

This information applies to the following medicines:

Chlorpheniramine (klor-fen-EER-a-meen), Codeine (KOE-deen), and Aspirin

Chlorpheniramine, Dextromethorphan (dextroe-meth-OR-fan), and Acetaminophen (a-seat-a-MEE-noe-fen)

Some commonly used brand names are:	Generic names:
Coricidin with Codeine*	Chlorpheniramine, Codeine, and Aspirin
Remcol-C	Chlorpheniramine, Dextromethorphan, and Acetaminophen

*Not available in the United States.

Antihistamine, antitussive, and analgesic combinations are used to relieve cough and aches and pain due to colds, influenza or hay fever. They are not to be used for the chronic cough that occurs with smoking, asthma, or emphysema or when there is an unusually large amount of mucus or phlegm (pronounced flem) with the cough.

Antihistamines are used to relieve or prevent the symptoms of hay fever and other types of allergy. They work by preventing the effects of a substance called histamine, which is produced by the body. However, in these combination medicines, antihistamines help mainly to produce a drying effect in the nose and chest.

To relieve coughing these combinations contain a narcotic (codeine) or a non-narcotic (dextromethorphan) antitussive. These antitussives act directly on the cough center in the brain. Narcotics may become habit-forming, causing mental or physical dependence, if used for a long time. Physical dependence may lead to withdrawal side effects when you stop taking the medicine.

Analgesics, such as acetaminophen and aspirin, are used in these combination medicines mainly to help relieve the aches and pain that may occur with the common cold.

There have been reports suggesting that use of aspirin in children with fever due to a viral infection (especially flu or chicken pox) may cause a serious illness called Reye's syndrome. Do not give medicines containing aspirin or other salicylates to a child or a teenager with symptoms of flu or chicken pox unless you have first discussed this with your child's doctor.

Some of these combinations are available only with your doctor's prescription. Others are available without a prescription; however, your doctor or pharmacist may have special instructions on the proper dose of the medicine for your medical condition.

For information about the precautions and side effects of the medicines in this combination, see:

Cough/Cold Combinations—
   Antihistamines and Antitussives
   (Systemic)
Acetaminophen (Systemic) or
   Salicylates (Systemic)

Combination products are designed for specific uses. These uses may not be the same as the uses of the individual ingredients. Therefore, some of the information provided in the individual listings may not be relevant to the combination product. If questions arise, check with your doctor, nurse, or pharmacist.

COUGH/COLD COMBINATIONS— ANTIHISTAMINES, ANTITUSSIVES, AND EXPECTORANTS (Systemic)

This information applies to the following medicines:

Bromodiphenhydramine (broe-moe-dye-fen-HYE-dra-meen), Diphenhydramine (dye-fen-HYE-dra-meen), Codeine (KOE-deen), Ammonium Chloride (a-MOE-nee-um KLOR-ide), and Potassium Guaiacolsulfonate (poe-TAS-ee-um gwye-a-kol-SUL-fon-ate)

Chlorpheniramine (klor-fen-EER-a-meen), Codeine, Carbetapentane, Guaifenesin (gwye-FEN-e-sin), Sodium Citrate (SOE-dee-um SI-trate), and Citric (SI-trik) Acid

Phenindamine (fen-IN-da-meen), Hydrocodone (hye-droe-KOE-done), and Guaifenesin

Pheniramine (fen-EER-a-meen), Pyrilamine (peer-ILL-a-meen), Hydrocodone, and Potassium Citrate

Pyrilamine, Codeine, and Terpin Hydrate (TER-pin HYE-drate)

Pyrilamine, Dextromethorphan (dex-troe-meth-OR-fan), and Ammonium Chloride

Some commonly used brand names are:	Generic names
Ambophen Expectorant A-Nil Expectorant	Bromodiphen-hydramine, Diphenhydramine, Codeine, Ammonium Chloride, and Potassium Guaiacol-sulfonate
Tussar SF Tussar-2 Cough	Chlorpheniramine, Codeine, Carbetapentane, Guaifenesin, Sodium Citrate, and Citric Acid
P-V-Tussin	Phenindamine, Hydrocodone, and Guaifenesin

Citra Forte	Pheniramine, Pyrilamine, Hydrocodone, and Potassium Citrate
Tricodene #1 Tricodene #2	Pyrilamine, Codeine, and Terpin Hydrate
Endotussin-NN	Pyrilamine, Dextromethorphan, and Ammonium Chloride

Antihistamine, antitussive, and expectorant combinations are used to relieve the cough due to colds, influenza, or hay fever. They are not to be used for the chronic cough that occurs with smoking, asthma, or emphysema or when there is an unusually large amount of mucus or phlegm (pronounced flem) with the cough.

Antihistamines are used to relieve or prevent the symptoms of hay fever and other types of allergy. They work by preventing the effects of a substance called histamine, which is produced by the body. However, in these combination medicines, antihistamines help mainly to produce a drying effect in the nose and chest.

To help relieve coughing these combinations contain either a narcotic (codeine or hydrocodone) or a non-narcotic (dextromethorphan) antitussive. These antitussives act directly on the cough center in the brain. Narcotics may become habit-forming, causing mental or physical dependence, if used for a long time. Physical dependence may lead to withdrawal side effects when you stop taking the medicine.

Guaifenesin works by loosening the mucus or phlegm in the lungs. Other expectorants (for example, ammonium chloride) may have a similar effect.

Some of these combinations are available only with your doctor's prescription. Others are available without a prescription; however, your doctor or pharmacist may have special instructions on the proper dose of the medicine for your medical condition.

For information about the precautions and side effects of the medicines in this combination, see:

Cough/Cold Combinations—
Antihistamines and Antitussives
(Systemic)
Guaifenesin (Systemic) or Terpin
Hydrate (Systemic)

Combination products are designed for specific uses. These uses may not be the same as the uses of the individual ingredients. Therefore, some of the information provided in the individual listings may not be relevant to the combination product. If questions arise, check with your doctor, nurse, or pharmacist.

COUGH/COLD COMBINATIONS— ANTIHISTAMINES, DECONGESTANTS, AND ANTITUSSIVES (Systemic)

Note: For quick reference the following antihistamine, decongestant, and antitussive combinations are numbered to match the corresponding brand names.

This information applies to the following medicines:

1. Brompheniramine (brome-fen-EER-a-meen), Phenylephrine (fen-ill-EF-rin), Phenylpropanolamine (fen-ill-proe-pa-NOLE-a-meen), and Codeine (KOE-deen)
2. Brompheniramine, Phenylephrine, Phenylpropanolamine, and Dextromethorphan (dex-troe-meth-OR-fan)
3. Brompheniramine, Phenylpropanolamine, and Codeine
4. Carbinoxamine, Pseudoephedrine (soo-doe-e-FED-rin), and Dextromethorphan
5. Chlorpheniramine (klor-fen-EER-a-meen), Ephedrine (e-FED-rin), Phenylephrine, and Carbetapentane

6. Chlorpheniramine, Phenylephrine, and Hydrocodone (hye-droe-KOE-done)
7. Chlorpheniramine, Phenylephrine, Phenylpropanolamine, and Codeine
8. Chlorpheniramine, Phenylephrine, Phenylpropanolamine, and Dextromethorphan
9. Chlorpheniramine, Phenylephrine, Phenylpropanolamine, and Drocode
10. Chlorpheniramine, Phenylephrine, and Dextromethorphan
11. Chlorpheniramine, Phenylpropanolamine, and Dextromethorphan
12. Chlorpheniramine, Pseudoephedrine, and Codeine
13. Chlorpheniramine, Pseudoephedrine, and Dextromethorphan
14. Chlorpheniramine, Pseudoephedrine, and Hydrocodone
15. Diphenylpyraline (dye-fen-il-PEER-a-leen), Phenylephrine, and Codeine
16. Diphenylpyraline, Phenylephrine, and Dextromethorphan
17. Diphenylpyraline, Phenylephrine, and Hydrocodone
18. Doxylamine, Phenylpropanolamine, and Dextromethorphan
19. Pheniramine, Pyrilamine (peer-ILL-a-meen), Phenylephrine, Phenylpropanolamine, and Hydrocodone
20. Pheniramine, Pyrilamine, Phenylpropanolamine, and Dextromethorphan
21. Pheniramine, Pyrilamine, Phenylpropanolamine, and Hydrocodone
22. Promethazine, Phenylephrine, and Codeine
23. Pyrilamine, Phenylephrine, and Codeine
24. Pyrilamine, Phenylephrine, and Dextromethorphan
25. Pyrilamine, Phenylephrine, and Hydrocodone
26. Triprolidine (trye-PROE-li-deen), Pseudoephedrine, and Codeine
27. Triprolidine, Pseudoephedrine, and Dextromethorphan
28. Triprolidine, Pseudoephedrine, and Noscapine

Some commonly used brand names are:

Actifed with Codeine Cough[26]	Biphetane DC Cough[3]
Actifed DM*[27]	Carbodec DM Drops[4]
Actifed-Plus*[28]	Cheracol Plus Liquid[11]
Alamine-C Liquid[12]	CoActifed*[26]
Bayaminicol[11]	Codehist DH[12]
Baydec DM Drops[4]	Codimal DH[25]
Bayhistine DH[12]	Codimal DM[24]
	Codimal PH[23]

Colrex Cough[10]	Phenergan VC with Codeine[22]
Cophene-S[9]	Poly-Histine-CS[3]
Cremacoat 4 Throat Coating Cough Medicine[18]	Promist HD Liquid[14]
Dimetane-DC Cough[3]	Pseudo-Car DM[4]
Dimetapp with Codeine*[1]	Pseudodine C Cough[26]
Dimetapp-DM*[2]	Rhinosyn-DM[13]
Dondril[10]	Rondec-DM[4]
Efficol Cough Whip (Cough Suppressant/ Decongestant/ Antihistamine)[11]	Ru-Tuss with Hydrocodone Liquid[19]
Histalet DM[13]	Ryna-C Liquid[12]
Kleer[10]	Rynatuss[5]
Nasahist Liquid[10]	Rynatuss Pediatric[5]
Novahistex C*[15]	Spantuss[10]
Novahistex DH*[17]	Thenylate S.F.[10]
Novahistex DM*[16]	T-Koff[7]
Novahistine Cough & Cold Formula Liquid[13]	Torfan DM*[4]
	Triaminicol DM*[20]
	Tricodene Forte[11]
Novahistine DH*[17]	Trimedine Liquid[10]
Novahistine DH Liquid[12]	Trind DM Liquid[11]
Ornade-DM*[11]	Tusquelin[8]
PediaCare 3 Children's Cold Relief[4]	Tussafed[4]
	Tussaminic DH Forte*[21]
	Tussaminic DH Pediatric*[21]
	Tussanil DH[6]
	Tussar DM Cough[10]

*Not available in the United States.

Antihistamine, decongestant, and antitussive combinations are used to relieve the cough and nasal congestion due to colds, influenza, or hay fever. They are not to be used for the chronic cough that occurs with smoking, asthma, or emphysema or when there is an unusually large amount of mucus or phlegm (pronounced flem) with the cough.

Antihistamines are used to relieve or prevent the symptoms of hay fever and other types of allergy. They work by preventing the effects of a substance called histamine, which is produced by the body. However, in these medicines antihistamines help mainly to produce a drying effect in the nose and chest.

Decongestants, such as phenylpropanolamine (also known as PPA), produce a narrowing of blood vessels. This leads to clearing of nasal congestion, but it may also increase blood pressure in patients who have high blood pressure.

To help relieve coughing these combinations contain either a narcotic (codeine, drocode, or hydrocodone) or a non-narcotic (carbetapentane, dextromethorphan, or noscapine) antitussive. These antitussives act directly on the cough center in the brain. Narcotics may become habit-forming, causing mental or physical dependence, if used for a long time. Physical dependence may lead to withdrawal side effects when you stop taking the medicine.

Some of these combinations are available only with your doctor's prescription. Others are available without a prescription; however, your doctor or pharmacist may have special instructions on the proper dose of the medicine for your medical condition.

Before Using This Medicine

Before you use this medicine, check with your doctor, nurse, or pharmacist:

—if you have ever had any unusual or allergic reaction to antihistamines, carbetapentane, codeine, dextromethorphan, drocode, hydrocodone, noscapine, or to amphetamine, dextroamphetamine, ephedrine, epinephrine, isoproterenol, metaproterenol, methamphetamine, norepinephrine, phenylephrine, pseudoephedrine, PPA, or terbutaline.

—if you are on a low-salt, low-sugar, or any other special diet, or if you are allergic to any substance, such as sulfites or other preservatives or dyes. Most medicines contain more than their active ingredient, and many liquid medicines contain alcohol. Your doctor or pharmacist can help you avoid products that may cause a problem.

—if you are pregnant or if you intend to become pregnant while taking this medicine. Although antihistamines and dextromethorphan have not been shown to cause problems in humans, the chance always exists.

Studies on birth defects have not been done in either animals or humans with decongestants such as ephedrine, phenylephrine, or phenylpropanolamine. Studies on birth defects have not been done in humans with the decongestant pseudoephedrine; however, in animal studies pseudoephedrine did not cause birth defects but did cause a reduction in average weight, length, and rate of bone formation in the animal fetus.

Although studies on birth defects with narcotic antitussives, such as codeine, drocode, and hydrocodone, have not been done in humans, these medicines have not been reported to cause birth defects in humans. However, hydrocodone has been shown to cause birth defects in animals when given in very large doses. Codeine has not been shown to cause birth defects in animal studies, but it caused other unwanted effects. Also, regular use of narcotics during pregnancy may cause the baby to become dependent on the medicine. This may lead to withdrawal side effects after birth. In addition, narcotics may cause breathing problems in the newborn infant if taken just before delivery.

—if you are breast-feeding an infant. Small amounts of antihistamines, some decongestants, and codeine pass into the breast milk. Use is not recommended since the chances of this medicine causing side effects, such as unusual excitement or irritability, in the infant are greater. Also, since antihistamines tend to decrease the secretions of the body, it is possible that the flow of breast milk may be reduced in some patients.

—if you have any of the following medical problems:

Diabetes mellitus (sugar diabetes)
Emphysema, asthma, or chronic lung disease (especially in children)
Enlarged prostate
Glaucoma
Heart or blood vessel disease
High blood pressure
Liver disease
Overactive thyroid
Urinary tract blockage or problems with urination

—if you are taking a combination medicine containing codeine, drocode, or hydrocodone and also have any of the following medical problems:

Brain disease or injury
Colitis
Convulsions or seizures (history of)
Gallbladder disease or gallstones
Kidney disease
Underactive thyroid

—if you are now taking any of the following medicines or types of medicine:

Acebutolol
Amantadine
Amphetamines
Antimuscarinics (medicine for abdominal or stomach spasms or cramps)
Aspirin or other salicylates
Atenolol
Caffeine
Cisplatin
Diet aids, phenylpropanolamine-containing (medicines used for appetite control)
Digitalis glycosides (heart medicine)
Guanethidine
Labetalol
Medicine for asthma or other breathing problems
Methyldopa
Metoprolol
Nadolol
Paromomycin
Pindolol
Procainamide
Propranolol
Quinidine
Reserpine
Timolol
Vancomycin

—if you are now taking any central nervous system (CNS) depressants such as:

Anticonvulsants (seizure medicine)
Barbiturates
Muscle relaxants
Narcotics
Other antihistamines or medicine for hay fever, other allergies, or colds
Prescription pain medicine
Sedatives, tranquilizers, or sleeping medicine

—if you are now taking tricyclic antidepressants such as:

Amitriptyline
Amoxapine
Desipramine
Doxepin
Imipramine
Nortriptyline
Protriptyline
Trimipramine

—if you are now taking or have taken within the past 2 weeks monoamine oxidase (MAO) inhibitors such as:

Furazolidone
Isocarboxazid
Pargyline
Phenelzine
Procarbazine
Tranylcypromine

Proper Use of This Medicine

Take this medicine with food or a glass of water or milk to lessen stomach irritation, if necessary.

To help loosen mucus or phlegm in the lungs, **drink a glass of water after each dose of this medicine,** unless otherwise directed by your doctor.

Take this medicine only as directed. Do not take more of it and do not take it more often than recommended on the label, unless otherwise directed by your doctor. To do so may increase the chance of side effects.

For patients taking the extended-release tablet form of this medicine:

• Swallow it whole.

• Do not crush, break, or chew before swallowing.

If you must take this medicine regularly and you miss a dose, take it as soon as possible. However, if it is almost time for your next dose, skip the missed dose and go back to your regular dosing schedule. Do not double doses.

How to store this medicine:

• Store away from heat and direct light.

• **Keep this medicine out of the reach of children** since overdose is very dangerous in young children.

• Do not store in the bathroom medicine cabinet because the heat or moisture may cause the medicine to break down.

• Keep the medicine from freezing. Do not refrigerate the syrup.

• Do not keep outdated medicine or medicine no longer needed. Flush the contents of the container down the toilet, unless otherwise directed.

Precautions While Using This Medicine

If your cough has not improved after 7 days or if you have a high fever, skin rash, continuing headache, or sore throat with the cough, check with your doctor. These signs may mean that you have other medical problems.

Tell the doctor in charge that you are taking this medicine before you have any skin tests for allergies. The results of the test may be affected by the antihistamine in this medicine.

This medicine will add to the effects of alcohol and other CNS depressants (medicines that slow down the nervous system, possibly causing drowsiness). Some examples of CNS depressants are antihistamines or medicine for hay fever, other allergies, or colds; sedatives, tranquilizers, or sleeping medicine; prescription pain medicine or narcotics; barbiturates; medicine for seizures; muscle relaxants; or anesthetics, including some dental anesthetics. **Check with your doctor before taking any of the above while you are taking this medicine.**

This medicine may cause some people to become drowsy, dizzy, or less alert than they are normally. **Make sure you know how you react to this medicine before you drive, use machines, or do other jobs that require you to be alert.**

This medicine may add to the central nervous system (CNS) stimulant and other effects of phenylpropanolamine (PPA)-containing diet aids. **Do not use medicines for diet or appetite control while taking this medicine unless you have checked with your doctor.**

This medicine may cause some people to be nervous or restless or to have trouble in sleeping. If you have trouble in sleeping, **take the last dose of this medicine for each day a few hours before bedtime.** If you have any questions about this, check with your doctor.

When taking antihistamines (contained in this combination medicine) on a regular basis, make sure your doctor knows if you are taking large amounts of aspirin at the same time (as in arthritis or rheumatism). Effects of too much aspirin, such as ringing in the ears, may be covered up by the antihistamine.

Before having any kind of surgery (including dental surgery) or emergency treatment, tell the physician or dentist in charge that you are taking this medicine.

For patients taking codeine-, drocode-, or hydrocodone-containing medicine:

• Dizziness, lightheadedness, or fainting may be especially likely to occur when you get up suddenly from a lying or sitting position. Getting up slowly may help lessen this problem.

• Nausea or vomiting may occur after taking a narcotic antitussive (contained in this combination medicine). This effect may go away if you lie down for a while. However, if nausea or vomiting continues, check with your doctor.

• **If you think you or someone else in your home may have taken an overdose of this medicine, get emergency help at once.** Taking an overdose of this medicine or taking alcohol or CNS depressants with this medicine may lead to unconsciousness or death. Signs of overdose include confusion, convulsions or seizures, severe nervousness or restlessness, severe dizziness, severe drowsiness, unusually slow or troubled breathing, and severe weakness.

Side Effects of This Medicine

Along with its needed effects, a medicine may cause some unwanted effects. Although serious side effects occur rarely when this medicine is taken as recommended, they may be more likely to occur if:

—too much medicine is taken.
—it is taken in large doses.
—it is taken for a long period of time.

Get emergency help immediately if any of the following signs of overdose occur:

Clumsiness or unsteadiness
Cold, clammy skin
Confusion (severe)
Convulsions (seizures)
Drowsiness or dizziness (severe)
Dryness of mouth, nose, or throat (severe)
Flushing or redness of face
Hallucinations (seeing, hearing, or feeling things that are not there)
Headache (continuing)
Nervousness or restlessness (severe)
Shortness of breath or troubled breathing
Unusually slow or fast heartbeat
Weakness (severe)

Other side effects may occur which usually do not require medical attention. These side effects may go away during treatment as your body adjusts to the medicine. However, check with your doctor or pharmacist if any of the following side effects continue or are bothersome:

More common

Drowsiness

Less common

Constipation
Difficult or painful urination
Dizziness or lightheadedness
Dryness of mouth, nose, or throat
False sense of well-being
Nausea or vomiting
Nightmares
Skin rash
Trouble in sleeping
Unusual excitement, nervousness, restlessness, or irritability

Although not all of the side effects listed above have been reported for all of these medicines, they have been reported for at least one of them. However, since there are some similarities among these combination medicines, most of the above side effects may occur with any of these medicines.

Use of this medicine is not recommended in premature or newborn infants. Serious side effects, such as convulsions (seizures) and unusually fast or irregular heartbeats, are more likely to occur in children and would be of greater risk to these infants.

Children and elderly patients are usually more sensitive to the effects of this medicine. Confusion, convulsions, difficult and painful urination, dizziness, drowsiness, or dryness of mouth may be more likely to occur in elderly patients. Nightmares or unusual excitement, nervousness, restlessness, or irritability may be more likely also to occur in children and in elderly patients. Also, breathing problems may be more likely to occur in very young children and elderly patients, or those patients who are very ill, and are taking codeine-, drocode-, or hydrocodone-containing medicine.

Other side effects not listed above may also occur in some patients. If you notice any other effects, check with your doctor.

COUGH/COLD COMBINATIONS— ANTIHISTAMINES, DECONGESTANTS, ANTITUSSIVES, AND ANALGESICS (Systemic)

Note: For quick reference the following antihistamine, decongestant, antitussive, and analgesic combinations are numbered to match the corresponding brand names.

This information applies to the following medicines:

1. Chlorpheniramine (klor-fen-EER-a-meen), Phenindamine (fen-IN-da-meen), Phenylephrine (fen-ill-EF-rin), Dextromethorphan (dex-troe-meth-OR-fan), Acetaminophen (a-seat-a-MEE-noe-fen), Salicylamide (sal-i-SILL-a-mide), Caffeine, and Ascorbic (a-SKOR-bik) Acid
2. Chlorpheniramine, Pheniramine, Pyrilamine, Phenylephrine, Hydrocodone, Salicylamide, Caffeine, and Ascorbic Acid
3. Chlorpheniramine, Phenylephrine, Codeine (KOE-deen), and Acetaminophen
4. Chlorpheniramine, Phenylephrine, Dextromethorphan, Acetaminophen, and Salicylamide
5. Chlorpheniramine, Phenylephrine, Hydrocodone (hye-droe-KOE-done), Acetaminophen, and Caffeine
6. Chlorpheniramine, Phenylpropanolamine (fen-ill-proe-pa-NOLE-a-meen), Dextromethorphan, and Acetaminophen
7. Chlorpheniramine, Phenylpropanolamine, Dextromethorphan, Acetaminophen, and Caffeine
8. Chlorpheniramine, Pseudoephedrine (soo-doe-e-FED-rin), Dextromethorphan, and Acetaminophen
9. Doxylamine (dox-ILL-a-meen), Pseudoephedrine, Dextromethorphan, and Acetaminophen
10. Pheniramine, Pyrilamine (peer-ILL-a-meen), Phenylpropanolamine, Codeine, Acetaminophen, and Caffeine
11. Pyrilamine, Phenylephrine, Codeine, and Sodium Salicylate
12. Pyrilamine, Phenylephrine, Dextromethorphan, and Acetaminophen
13. Pyrilamine, Phenylpropanolamine, Dextromethorphan, and Sodium Salicylate

Some commonly used brand names are:

Citra Forte[2]	Contac Severe Cold
Co-Apap[8]	Formula Night
Colrex Compound[3]	Strength[9]
Comtrex Multi-	CoTylenol Cold
Symptom	Medication[8]
Cold Reliever[6]	Dristan Ultra Colds
Contac Severe Cold	Formula[8]
Formula[8]	Hycomine Compound[5]

Improved Sino-Tuss[4]
Kolephrin with Codeine Liquid[11]
Kolephrin/DM[7]
Kolephrin NN Liquid[13]
NyQuil Nighttime Colds Medicine[9]

Nytime Cold Medicine Liquid[9]
Omnicol[1]
Robitussin Night Relief Colds Formula Liquid[12]
Triaminicin with Codeine*[10]

---

*Not available in the United States.

Antihistamine, decongestant, antitussive, and analgesic combinations are used to relieve cough, nasal congestion, and aches and pain due to colds, influenza, or hay fever. They are not to be used for the chronic cough that occurs with smoking, asthma, or emphysema or when there is an unusually large amount of mucus or phlegm (pronounced flem) with the cough.

Antihistamines are used to relieve or prevent the symptoms of hay fever and other types of allergy. They work by preventing the effects of a substance called histamine, which is produced by the body. However, in these combination medicines, antihistamines help mainly to produce a drying effect in the nose and chest.

Decongestants, such as phenylpropanolamine (also known as PPA), produce a narrowing of blood vessels. This leads to clearing of nasal congestion, but it may also cause an increase in blood pressure in patients who have high blood pressure.

To help relieve coughing these combinations contain either a narcotic (codeine or hydrocodone) or a non-narcotic (dextromethorphan) antitussive. These antitussives act directly on the cough center in the brain. Narcotics may become habit-forming, causing mental or physical dependence, if used for a long time. Physical dependence may lead to withdrawal side effects when you stop taking the medicine.

Analgesics, such as acetaminophen and salicylates, are used in these combination medicines mainly to help relieve the aches and pain that may occur with the common cold.

A few reports have suggested that acetaminophen and salicylates may work together to cause kidney damage or cancer of the kidney or urinary bladder. This may occur if large amounts of both medicines are taken together for a long period of time. However, taking usual amounts of these combinations medicines for short periods of time has not been shown to cause these unwanted effects.

There have been reports suggesting that use of aspirin in children with fever due to a viral infection (especially flu or chicken pox) may cause a serious illness called Reye's syndrome. Do not give medicines containing aspirin or other salicylates to a child or a teenager with symptoms of flu or chicken pox unless you have first discussed this with your child's doctor.

Some of these combinations are available only with your doctor's prescription. Others are available without a prescription; however, your doctor or pharmacist may have special instructions on the proper dose of the medicine for your medical condition.

For information about the precautions and side effects of the medicines in this combination, see:

Cough/Cold Combinations—
    Antihistamines, Decongestants, and
    Antitussives (Systemic)
Acetaminophen (Systemic) or
    Salicylates (Systemic)

Combination products are designed for specific uses. These uses may not be the same as the uses of the individual ingredients. Therefore, some of the information provided in the individual listings may not be relevant to the combination product. If questions arise, check with your doctor, nurse, or pharmacist.

COUGH/COLD COMBINATIONS— ANTIHISTAMINES, DECONGESTANTS, ANTITUSSIVES, AND EXPECTORANTS (Systemic)

Note: For quick reference the following antihistamine, decongestant, antitussive, and expectorant combinations are numbered to match the corresponding brand names.

This information applies to the following medicines:

1. Brompheniramine (brome-fen-EER-a-meen), Phenylephrine (fen-ill-EF-rin), Phenylpropanolamine (fen-ill-proe-pa-NOLE-a-meen), Codeine (KOE-deen), and Guaifenesin (gwye-FEN-e-sin)
2. Brompheniramine, Phenylephrine, Phenylpropanolamine, Hydrocodone (hye-droe-KOE-done), and Guaifenesin
3. Chlorpheniramine (klor-fen-EER-a-meen), Phenindamine (fen-IN-da-meen), Pyrilamine (peer-ILL-a-meen), Phenylephrine, Hydrocodone, and Ammonium Chloride
4. Chlorpheniramine, Phenyltoloxamine (fen-ill-tole-OX-a-meen), Ephedrine (e-FED-rin), Codeine, and Guaiacol Carbonate
5. Chlorpheniramine, Ephedrine, Phenylephrine, Dextromethorphan (dex-troe-meth-OR-fan), Ammonium Chloride, and Ipecac
6. Chlorpheniramine, Ephedrine, Codeine, and Ammonium Chloride
7. Chlorpheniramine, Phenylephrine, Codeine, and Ammonium Chloride
8. Chlorpheniramine, Phenylephrine, Codeine, Ammonium Chloride, Potassium Guaiacolsulfonate, and Sodium Citrate
9. Chlorpheniramine, Phenylephrine, Codeine, and Potassium Iodide
10. Chlorpheniramine, Phenylephrine, Dextromethorphan, and Guaifenesin
11. Chlorpheniramine, Phenylephrine, Phenylpropanolamine, Carbetapentane, and Potassium Guaiacolsulfonate
12. Chlorpheniramine, Phenylephrine, Dextromethorphan, Guaifenesin, and Ammonium Chloride
13. Chlorpheniramine, Phenylpropanolamine, Dextromethorphan, and Ammonium Chloride
14. Chlorpheniramine, Phenylpropanolamine, Dextromethorphan, Ammonium Chloride, Terpin Hydrate (TER-pin HYE-drate), and Sodium Citrate
15. Diphenylpyraline (dye-fen-il-PEER-a-leen), Phenylephrine, Hydrocodone, and Guaifenesin
16. Phenindamine (fen-IN-da-meen), Phenylephrine, Dextromethorphan, Potassium Guaiacolsulfonate, Sodium Citrate, Citric Acid, and Ipecac
17. Pheniramine (fen-EER-a-meen), Pyrilamine, Phenylpropanolamine, Dextromethorphan, and Ammonium Chloride
18. Pheniramine, Pyrilamine, Phenylpropanolamine, Dextromethorphan, and Guaifenesin
19. Pheniramine, Pyrilamine, Phenylpropanolamine, Hydrocodone, and Guaifenesin
20. Pyrilamine, Phenylephrine, Hydrocodone, and Ammonium Chloride
21. Triprolidine (trye-PROE-li-deen), Pseudoephedrine (soo-doe-e-FED-rin), Codeine, and Guaifenesin

Some commonly used brand names:

Cerose-DM Expectorant[16]	Novahistex Expectorant*[15]
CoActifed Expectorant*[20]	Novahistine Expectorant*[15]
Cophene-X[11]	Omni-Tuss*[4]
Cophene-XP[11]	Pediacof Cough[9]
Dimetane Expectorant-C*[1]	Prominicol Cough[17]
Dimetane Expectorant-DC*[2]	P-V- Tussin[3]
Donatussin[10]	Quelidrine Cough[5]
Dristan Cough Formula[10]	Ru-Tuss Expectorant[7]
Efricon Expectorant Liquid[8]	Triaminic Expectorant DH[19]
Father John's Medicine Plus[12]	Triaminic-DM Expectorant*[18]
Histadyl E.C.[6]	Tricodene NN Cough and Cold Medication[14]
Hycomine*[20]	
Hycomine-S Pediatric*[20]	
Kophane[13]	

---

*Not available in the United States.

Antihistamine, decongestant, antitussive, and expectorant combinations are used to relieve the cough and nasal congestion due to colds, influenza, or hay fever. They are not to be used for the chronic cough that occurs with smoking, asthma, or emphysema or when there is an unusually large amount of mucus or phlegm (pronounced flem) with the cough.

Antihistamines are used to relieve or prevent the symptoms of hay fever and other types of allergy. They work by preventing the effects of a substance called histamine, which is produced by the body. However, in these combination medicines, antihistamines help mainly to produce a drying effect in the nose and chest.

Decongestants, such as phenylpropanolamine (also known as PPA), produce a narrowing of blood vessels. This leads to clearing of nasal congestion, but it may also increase blood pressure in patients who have high blood pressure.

To help relieve coughing these combinations contain either a narcotic (codeine or hydrocodone) or a non-narcotic (carbetapentane or dextromethorphan) antitussive. These antitussives act directly on the cough center in the brain. Narcotics may become habit-forming, causing mental or physical dependence, if used for a long time. Physical dependence may lead to withdrawal side effects when you stop taking the medicine.

Guaifenesin works by loosening the mucus or phlegm in the lungs. Other expectorants (for example, ammonium chloride) may have a similar effect.

Some of these combinations are available only with your doctor's prescription. Others are available without a prescription; however, your doctor or pharmacist may have special instructions on the proper dose of the medicine for your medical condition.

Before Using This Medicine

Before you use this medicine, check with your doctor, nurse, or pharmacist:

—if you have ever had any unusual or allergic reaction to antihistamines, carbetapentane, codeine, dextromethorphan, guaifenesin, hydrocodone, terpin hydrate, or to amphetamine, dextroamphetamine, ephedrine, epinephrine, isoproterenol, metaproterenol, methamphetamine, norepinephrine, phenylephrine, pseudoephedrine, PPA, or terbutaline.

—if you are on a low-salt, low-sugar, or any other special diet, or if you are allergic to any substance, such as sulfites or other preservatives or dyes. Most medicines contain more than their active ingredient, and many liquid medicines contain alcohol. Your doctor or pharmacist can help you avoid products that may cause a problem.

—if you are pregnant or if you intend to become pregnant while taking this medicine. Although antihistamines, dextromethorphan, and expectorants like guaifenesin have not been shown to cause problems in humans, the chance always exists.

Studies on birth defects have not been done in either animals or humans with decongestants such as ephedrine, phenylephrine, or phenylpropanolamine. Studies on birth defects have not been done in humans with the decongestant pseudoephedrine; however, in animal studies, pseudoephedrine did not cause birth defects but did cause a reduction in average weight, length, and rate of bone formation in the animal fetus.

Although studies on birth defects with narcotic antitussives, such as codeine and hydrocodone, have not been done in humans, these medicines have not been reported to cause birth defects in humans. However, hydrocodone has been shown to cause birth defects in animals when given in very large doses. Codeine has not been shown to cause birth defects in animal studies, but it caused other unwanted effects. Also, regular use of narcotics during pregnancy may cause the baby to become dependent on the medicine. This may lead to withdrawal side effects after birth. In addition, narcotics may cause breathing problems in the newborn infant if taken just before delivery.

Potassium iodide (contained in one of these combination medicines) is not recommended during pregnancy. Iodides have caused enlargement of the thyroid gland in the fetus and breathing problems in newborn infants whose mothers took iodides in large doses for a long period of time.

Some of these combination medicines contain a large amount of alcohol. Too much use of alcohol during pregnancy may cause birth defects.

—if you are breast-feeding an infant. Small amounts of antihistamines, some decongestants, and codeine pass into the breast milk. Also, iodides such as potassium iodide (contained in one of these combination medicines) pass into the breast milk and may cause unwanted effects, such as underactive thyroid in the infant. Use is not recommended since the chances of this medicine causing side effects, such as unusual excitement or irritability, in the infant are greater. Also, since antihistamines tend to decrease the secretions of the body, it is possible that the flow of breast milk may be reduced in some patients.

—if you have any of the following medical problems:

Diabetes mellitus (sugar diabetes)
Emphysema, asthma, or chronic lung disease (especially in children)
Enlarged prostate
Glaucoma

Heart or blood vessel disease
High blood pressure
Liver disease
Overactive thyroid
Urinary tract blockage or difficult urination

—if you are taking a combination medicine containing codeine or hydrocodone and have any of the following medical problems:

Brain disease or injury
Colitis
Convulsions or seizures (history of)
Gallbladder disease or gallstones
Kidney disease
Underactive thyroid

—if you are now taking any of the following medicines or types of medicine:

Acebutolol
Amantadine
Amphetamines
Antimuscarinics (medicine for abdominal or stomach spasms or cramps)
Aspirin or other salicylates
Atenolol
Caffeine
Cisplatin
Diet aids, phenylpropanolamine-containing (medicines used for appetite control)
Digitalis glycosides (heart medicine)
Guanethidine
Labetalol
Medicine for asthma or other breathing problems
Methyldopa
Metoprolol
Nadolol
Paromomycin
Pindolol
Procainamide
Propranolol
Quinidine
Reserpine
Timolol
Vancomycin

—if you are now taking any central nervous system (CNS) depressants such as:

Anticonvulsants (seizure medicine)
Barbiturates
Muscle relaxants
Narcotics

Other antihistamines or medicine for hay
fever, other allergies, or colds
Prescription pain medicine
Sedatives, tranquilizers, or sleeping
medicine

—if you are now taking tricyclic antidepressants such as:

Amitriptyline
Amoxapine
Desipramine
Doxepin
Imipramine
Nortriptyline
Protriptyline
Trimipramine

—if you are now taking or have taken
within the past 2 weeks monoamine oxidase (MAO) inhibitors such as:

Furazolidone
Isocarboxazid
Pargyline
Phenelzine
Procarbazine
Tranylcypromine

Proper Use of This Medicine

Take this medicine with food or a glass of
water or milk to lessen stomach irritation, if necessary.

To help loosen mucus or phlegm in the
lungs, **drink a glass of water after each
dose of this medicine,** unless otherwise
directed by your doctor.

Take this medicine only as directed. Do not
take more of it and do not take it more
often than recommended on the label,
unless otherwise directed by your doctor. To do so may increase the chance of
side effects.

If you must take this medicine regularly
and you miss a dose, take it as soon as
possible. However, if it is almost time for
your next dose, skip the missed dose and
go back to your regular dosing schedule.
Do not double doses.

How to store this medicine:

• Store away from heat and direct light.

• **Keep this medicine out of the reach of
children** since overdose is very dangerous in young children.

• Do not store in the bathroom medicine
cabinet because the heat or moisture
may cause the medicine to break down.

• Keep the medicine from freezing. Do
not refrigerate the syrup.

• Do not keep outdated medicine or medicine no longer needed. Flush the contents of the container down the toilet,
unless otherwise directed.

Precautions While Using This Medicine

If your cough has not improved after 7 days
or if you have a high fever, skin rash,
continuing headache, or sore throat with
the cough, check with your doctor.
These signs may mean that you have
other medical problems.

Tell the doctor in charge that you are taking
this medicine before you have any skin
tests for allergies. The results of the test
may be affected by the antihistamine in
this medicine.

This medicine will add to the effects of alcohol and other CNS depressants (medicines that slow down the nervous system, possibly causing drowsiness). Some
examples of CNS depressants are antihistamines or medicine for hay fever,
other allergies, or colds; sedatives, tranquilizers, or sleeping medicine; prescription pain medicine or narcotics; barbiturates; medicine for seizures; muscle
relaxants; or anesthetics, including
some dental anesthetics. **Check with
your doctor before taking any of the
above while you are taking this medicine.**

This medicine may cause some people to
become drowsy, dizzy, or less alert than
they are normally. **Make sure you know**

how you react to this medicine before you drive, use machines, or do other jobs that require you to be alert.

This medicine may add to the central nervous system (CNS) stimulant and other effects of phenylpropanolamine (PPA)-containing diet aids. **Do not use medicines for diet or appetite control while taking this medicine unless you have checked with your doctor.**

This medicine may cause some people to be nervous or restless or to have trouble in sleeping. If you have trouble in sleeping, **take the last dose of this medicine for each day a few hours before bedtime.** If you have any questions about this, check with your doctor.

Before having any kind of surgery (including dental surgery) or emergency treatment, tell the physician or dentist in charge that you are taking this medicine.

When taking antihistamines (contained in this combination medicine) on a regular basis, make sure your doctor knows if you are taking large amounts of aspirin at the same time (as in arthritis or rheumatism). Effects of too much aspirin, such as ringing in the ears, may be covered up by the antihistamine.

For patients taking codeine- or hydrocodone-containing medicine:

• Dizziness, lightheadedness, or fainting may be especially likely to occur when you get up suddenly from a lying or sitting position. Getting up slowly may help lessen this problem.

• Nausea or vomiting may occur after taking a narcotic antitussive. This effect may go away if you lie down for a while. However, if nausea or vomiting continues, check with your doctor.

• If you think you or someone else in your home may have taken an overdose of this medicine, get emergency help at once. Taking an overdose of this medicine or taking alcohol or CNS depressants with this medicine may lead to unconsciousness or death. Signs of overdose include confusion, convulsions or seizures, severe nervousness or restlessness, severe dizziness, severe drowsiness, unusually slow or troubled breathing, and severe weakness.

For patients taking potassium iodide–containing medicine:

• Make sure your doctor knows if you are planning to have any future thyroid tests. The results of the thyroid test may be affected by the potassium iodide contained in one of these combination medicines.

Side Effects of This Medicine

Along with its needed effects, a medicine may cause some unwanted effects. Although serious effects occur rarely when this medicine is taken as recommended, they may be more likely to occur if:

—too much medicine is taken.
—it is taken in large doses.
—it is taken for a long period of time.

Get emergency help immediately if any of the following signs of overdose occur:

Clumsiness or unsteadiness
Cold, clammy skin
Confusion
Convulsions (seizures)
Drowsiness or dizziness (severe)
Dryness of mouth, nose, or throat (severe)
Flushing or redness of face
Hallucinations (seeing, hearing, or feeling things that are not there)
Headache (continuing and severe)
Nervousness or restlessness (severe)
Shortness of breath or troubled breathing
Unusually slow or fast heartbeat
Weakness (severe)

Other side effects may occur which usually do not require medical attention. These

side effects may go away during treatment as your body adjusts to the medicine. However, check with your doctor or pharmacist if any of the following side effects continue or are bothersome:

More common

Drowsiness

Less common

Constipation
Difficult or painful urination
Dizziness or lightheadedness
Dryness of mouth, nose, or throat
Nausea or vomiting
Nightmares
Skin rash
Trouble in sleeping
Unusual excitement, nervousness, restlessness, or irritability

Although not all of the side effects listed above have been reported for all of these medicines, they have been reported for at least one of them. However, since there are some similarities among these combination medicines, most of the above side effects may occur with any of these medicines.

Use of this medicine is not recommended in premature or newborn infants. Serious side effects, such as convulsions (seizures) and unusually fast or irregular heartbeats, are more likely to occur in children and would be of greater risk to these infants.

Children and elderly patients are usually more sensitive to the effects of this medicine. Confusion, convulsions, difficult and painful urination, dizziness, drowsiness, or dryness of mouth may be more likely to occur in elderly patients. Nightmares or unusual excitement, nervousness, restlessness, or irritability may be more likely also to occur in children and in elderly patients. Also, breathing problems may be more likely to occur in very young children and elderly patients, or those patients who are very ill, and are

taking combinatons containing codeine or hydrocodone.

Other side effects not listed above may also occur in some patients. If you notice any other effects, check with your doctor.

COUGH/COLD COMBINATIONS— ANTIHISTAMINES, DECONGESTANTS, ANTITUSSIVES, EXPECTORANTS, AND ANALGESICS (Systemic)

This information applies to the following medicines:

Chlorpheniramine (klor-fen-EER-a-meen), Phenylephrine (fen-ill-EF-rin), Phenylpropanolamine (fen-ill-proe-pa-NOLE-a-meen), Dextromethorphan (dex-troe-meth-OR-fan), Guaifenesin (gwye-FEN-e-sin), and Acetaminophen (a-seat-a-MEE-noe-fen)

Chlorpheniramine, Phenylephrine, Dextromethorphan, Guaifenesin, and Acetaminophen

Chlorpheniramine, Phenylpropanolamine, Codeine (KOE-deen), Guaifenesin, and Acetaminophen

Chlorpheniramine, Phenylpropanolamine, Hydrocodone (hye-droe-KOE-done), Guaifenesin, and Salicylamide (sal-i-SILL-a-mide)

Chlorpheniramine, Pseudoephedrine (soo-doe-e-FED-rin), Dextromethorphan, Guaifenesin, and Aspirin

Pheniramine (fen-EER-a-meen), Pyrilamine (peer-ILL-a-meen), Phenylpropanolamine, Dextromethorphan, Terpin Hydrate (TER-pin HYE-drate), and Acetaminophen

Pheniramine, Phenylephrine, Codeine, Sodium Citrate (SOE-dee-um SI-trate), Sodium Salicylate (sa-LI-sill-ate), and Caffeine

Some commonly used brand names are:	Generic names:
Anatuss	Chlorpheniramine, Phenylephrine, Phenylpropanolamine, Dextromethorphan, Guaifenesin, and Acetaminophen
Phenilar Cough and Cold	Chlorpheniramine, Phenylephrine, Dextromethorphan, Guaifenesin, and Acetaminophen
Anatuss with Codeine	Chlorpheniramine, Phenylpropanolamine, Codeine, Guaifenesin, and Acetaminophen
Tussanil DH	Chlorpheniramine, Phenylpropanolamine, Hydrocodone, Guaifenesin, and Salicylamide
Viro-Med	Chlorpheniramine, Pseudoephedrine, Dextromethorphan, Guaifenesin, and Aspirin
Chexit Tussagesic	Pheniramine, Pyrilamine, Phenylpropanolamine, Dextromethorphan, Terpin Hydrate, and Acetaminophen
Tussirex with Codeine Liquid	Pheniramine, Phenylephrine, Codeine, Sodium Citrate, Sodium Salicylate, and Caffeine

Antihistamine, decongestant, antitussive, expectorant, and analgesic combinations are used to relieve cough, nasal congestion, and aches and pain due to colds, influenza, or hay fever. They are not to be used for the chronic cough that occurs with smoking, asthma, or emphysema or when there is an unusually large amount of mucus or phlegm (pronounced flem) with the cough.

Antihistamines are used to relieve or prevent the symptoms of hay fever and other types of allergy. They work by preventing the effects of a substance called histamine, which is produced by the body. However, in these combination medicines, antihistamines help mainly to produce a drying effect in the nose and chest.

The decongestants, such as phenylpropanolamine (also known as PPA), produce a narrowing of blood vessels. This leads to clearing of nasal congestion, but it may also increase blood pressure in patients who have high blood pressure.

To help relieve coughing these combinations contain either a narcotic (codeine or hydrocodone) or a non-narcotic (dextromethorphan) antitussive. These antitussives act directly on the cough center in the brain. Narcotics may become habit-forming, causing mental or physical dependence, if used for a long time. Physical dependence may lead to withdrawal side effects when you stop taking the medicine.

Guaifenesin works by loosening the mucus or phlegm in the lungs. Other expectorants (for example, sodium citrate) may have a similar effect.

Analgesics, such as acetaminophen, aspirin, and other salicylates (such as salicylamide and sodium salicylate), are used in these combination medicines mainly to help relieve the aches and pain that may occur with the common cold.

There have been reports suggesting that use of aspirin in children with fever due to a viral infection (especially flu or chicken pox) may cause a serious illness called Reye's syndrome. Do not give medicines containing aspirin or other salicylates to a child or a teenager with symptoms of flu or chicken pox unless you have first discussed this with your child's doctor.

Some of these combinations are available only with your doctor's prescription. Others are available without a prescription; however, your doctor or pharmacist may have special instructions on the proper dose of the medicine for your medical condition.

For information about the precautions and side effects of the medicines in this combination, see:

Cough/Cold Combinations—
    Antihistamines, Decongestants, and
    Antitussives (Systemic)
Guaifenesin (Systemic) or Terpin
    Hydrate (Systemic)
Acetaminophen (Systemic) or
    Salicylates (Systemic)

Combination products are designed for specific uses. These uses may not be the same as the uses of the individual ingredients. Therefore, some of the information provided in the individual listings may not be relevant to the combination product. If questions arise, check with your doctor, nurse, or pharmacist.

Phenylpropanolamine (fen-ill-proe-pa-NOLE-a-meen), and Guaifenesin (gwye-FEN-e-sin)
2. Carbinoxamine (kar-bi-NOX-a-meen), Pseudoephedrine (soo-doe-e-FED-rin), and Guaifenesin
3. Chlorpheniramine (klor-fen-EER-a-meen), Ephedrine (e-FED-rin), and Guaifenesin
4. Chlorpheniramine, Phenylephrine, and Guaifenesin
5. Chlorpheniramine, Phenylpropanolamine, and Guaifenesin
6. Chlorpheniramine, Phenylpropanolamine, Guaifenesin, Sodium Citrate (SOE-dee-um SI-trate), and Citric (SI-trik) Acid
7. Chlorpheniramine, Pseudoephedrine, and Guaifenesin
8. Dexchlorpheniramine (dex-klor-fen-EER-a-meen), Pseudoephedrine, and Guaifenesin
9. Pheniramine (fen-EER-a-meen), Pyrilamine (peer-ILL-a-meen), Phenylpropanolamine, and Guaifenesin

Some commonly used brand names are:

Brexin[2]	Lanatuss
Bronkotuss	Expectorant[6]
Expectorant[3]	Ornade
Dimetane	Expectorant[*5]
Expectorant[*1]	Polaramine
Donatussin Drops[4]	Expectorant[2]
Fedahist Expectorant[7]	Triaminic
Guistrey Fortis[4]	Expectorant[9]
	Trinex[7]

COUGH/COLD COMBINATIONS— ANTIHISTAMINES, DECONGESTANTS, AND EXPECTORANTS (Systemic)

Note: For quick reference the following antihistamine, decongestant, and expectorant combinations are numbered to match the corresponding brand names.

This information applies to the following medicines:

1. Brompheniramine (brome-fen-EER-a-meen), Phenylephrine (fen-ill-EF-rin),

Antihistamine, decongestant, and expectorant combinations are used to relieve cough and nasal congestion due to colds, influenza, or hay fever. They are not to be used for the chronic cough that occurs with smoking, asthma, or emphysema or when there is an unusually large amount of mucus or phlegm (pronounced flem) with the cough.

Antihistamines are used to relieve or prevent the symptoms of hay fever and other types of allergy. They work by preventing the effects of a substance called histamine, which is produced by the body. However, in these medicines antihistamines help mainly to produce a drying effect in the nose and chest.

Decongestants, such as phenylpropanolamine (also known as PPA), produce a narrowing of blood vessels. This leads to clearing of nasal congestion, but it may also increase blood pressure in patients who have high blood pressure.

Guaifenesin works by loosening the mucus or phlegm in the lungs. Other expectorants (for example, sodium citrate and citric acid) may have a similar effect.

Some of these combinations are available only with your doctor's prescription. Others are available without a prescription; however, your doctor or pharmacist may have special instructions on the proper dose of the medicine for your medical condition.

For information about the precautions and side effects of the medicines in this combination, see:

Antihistamines and Decongestants
    (Systemic)
Guaifenesin (Systemic)

Combination products are designed for specific uses. These uses may not be the same as the uses of the individual ingredients. Therefore, some of the information provided in the individual listings may not be relevant to the combination product. If questions arise, check with your doctor, nurse, or pharmacist.

COUGH/COLD COMBINATIONS— ANTITUSSIVES AND ANTIMUSCARINICS (Systemic)

This information applies to the following medicines:

Hydrocodone (hye-droe-KOE-done) and Homatropine (hoe-MA-troe-peen)†

Some commonly used brand names are Baycodan, Hycodan, and Hydropane.

---

† Generic name product may also be available.

Antitussive and antimuscarinic combinations are used to relieve coughs due to colds, influenza, or hay fever. They are not to be used for chronic cough that occurs with smoking, asthma, or emphysema or when there is an unusually large amount of mucus or phlegm (pronounced flem) with the cough.

The narcotic antitussive, hydrocodone, acts directly on the cough center of the brain. Narcotics may become habit-forming, causing mental or physical dependence, if used for a long time. Physical dependence may lead to withdrawal side effects when you stop taking the medicine.

The homatropine in this medicine belongs to the group of medicines called antimuscarinics. In this medicine, it may help produce a drying effect in the nose and chest.

This combination medicine is available only with your doctor's prescription.

Before Using This Medicine

In order to decide on the best treatment for your medical problem, your doctor should be told:

—if you have ever had an unusual reaction to hydrocodone, homatropine, or to any of the belladonna alkaloids, such as atropine, belladonna, hyoscyamine, and scopolamine.

—if you are on a low-salt, low-sugar, or any other special diet, or if you are allergic to any substance, such as sulfites or other preservatives or dyes. Most medicines contain more than their active ingredient, and many liquid medicines contain alcohol. Your doctor or pharmacist can help you avoid products that may cause a problem.

—if you are pregnant or if you intend to become pregnant while using this medicine. Although studies on birth defects with hydrocodone have not been done in humans, it has not been reported to cause birth defects in humans. However, studies in animals have shown that hydrocodone causes birth defects when given in very large doses.

Too much use of narcotics during pregnancy may cause the fetus to become dependent on the medicine. This may lead to withdrawal side effects in the newborn baby. Also, if taken just before or during delivery, hydrocodone may cause breathing problems in the newborn baby.

Although homatropine has not been shown to cause birth defects or other problems in humans, the chance always exists.

—if you are breast-feeding an infant. Although hydrocodone and homatropine have not been shown to cause problems in humans, the chance always exists. It is not known whether hydrocodone or homatropine pass into the breast milk.

—if you have any of the following medical problems:
    Brain disease or injury
    Colitis
    Convulsions or seizures (history of)
    Down's syndrome (mongolism)
    Emphysema, asthma, or chronic lung disease
    Enlarged prostate, urinary tract blockage, or problems with urination
    Gallbladder disease or gallstones
    Glaucoma
    Intestinal blockage or other intestinal problems
    Kidney disease
    Liver disease
    Spastic paralysis (in children)
    Underactive or overactive thyroid

—if you are now taking other antimuscarinics (medicine for stomach spasms or cramps) or any of the following eye medicines used for glaucoma:
    Demecarium
    Echothiophate
    Isoflurophate

—if you are now using central nervous system (CNS) depressants such as:
    Anticonvulsants (seizure medicine)
    Antihistamines or medicine for hay fever, other allergies, or colds
    Barbiturates
    Muscle relaxants
    Other narcotics
    Prescription pain medicine
    Sedatives, tranquilizers, or sleeping medicine
    Tricyclic antidepressants (medicine for depression)

—if you are now taking or have taken within the past 2 weeks monoamine oxidase (MAO) inhibitors such as:
    Furazolidone
    Isocarboxazid
    Pargyline
    Phenelzine
    Procarbazine
    Tranylcypromine

Proper Use of This Medicine

Take this medicine only as directed by your doctor. Do not take more of it, do not take it more often, and do not take it for a longer period of time than your doctor ordered. If too much hydrocodone is taken, it may become habit-forming (causing mental or physical dependence) or lead to medical problems because of an overdose.

To help loosen mucus or phlegm in the lungs, **drink a glass of water after each dose of this medicine,** unless otherwise directed by your doctor.

If you must take this medicine regularly and you miss a dose, take it as soon as possible. However, if it is almost time for your next dose, skip the missed dose and go back to your regular dosing schedule.

Do not double doses. Or, you may take the missed dose as soon as you remember and take the rest of the doses for the day at least 4 hours apart, unless otherwise directed by your doctor.

How to store this medicine:

• Store away from heat and direct light.

• **Keep this medicine out of the reach of children** since overdose is very dangerous in young children.

• Do not store in the bathroom medicine cabinet because the heat or moisture may cause the medicine to break down.

• Keep the medicine from freezing. Do not refrigerate the syrup.

• Do not keep outdated medicine or medicine no longer needed. Flush the contents of the container down the toilet, unless otherwise directed.

Precautions While Using This Medicine

If your cough has not improved after 7 days or if you have a high fever, skin rash, continuing headache, or sore throat with the cough, check with your doctor. These signs may mean that you have other medical problems.

This medicine will add to the effects of alcohol and other CNS depressants (medicines that slow down the nervous system, possibly causing drowsiness). Some examples of CNS depressants are antihistamines or medicine for hay fever, other allergies, or colds; sedatives, tranquilizers, or sleeping medicine; prescription pain medicine or other narcotics; barbiturates; medicine for seizures; muscle relaxants; or anesthetics, including some dental anesthetics. **Check with your doctor before taking any of the above while you are using this medicine.**

This medicine may cause some people to become drowsy, dizzy, or lightheaded, or to feel a false sense of well-being. **Make sure you know how you react to this medicine before you drive, use machines, or do other jobs that require you to be alert and clearheaded.**

Dizziness, lightheadedness, or fainting may be especially likely to occur when you get up suddenly from a lying or sitting position. Getting up slowly may help lessen this problem.

Nausea or vomiting may occur, especially after the first couple of doses. This effect may go away if you lie down for a while. However, if nausea or vomiting continues, check with your doctor.

The homatropine in this medicine may make you sweat less, causing your body temperature to increase. **Use extra care not to become overheated during exercise or hot weather while you are taking this medicine,** since overheating may result in heat stroke.

Before having any kind of surgery (including dental surgery) or emergency treatment, tell the physician or dentist in charge that you are taking this medicine.

If you think you or someone else in your home may have taken an overdose of this medicine, get emergency help at once. Taking an overdose of this medicine or taking alcohol or CNS depressants with this medicine may lead to unconsciousness or death. Signs of overdose include confusion, convulsions or seizures, severe nervousness or restlessness, severe dizziness, severe drowsiness, unusually slow or troubled breathing, and severe weakness.

Side Effects of This Medicine

Along with its needed effects, a medicine may cause some unwanted effects. Although serious side effects occur rarely when this medicine is taken as recommended, they may be more likely to occur if:

—too much medicine is taken.
—it is taken in large doses.
—it is taken for a long period of time.

Get emergency help immediately if any of the following signs of overdose occur:

Blurred or double vision or other changes in vision
Cold, clammy skin
Confusion
Convulsions or seizures
Dizziness (severe)
Drowsiness (severe)
Fever
Nervousness or restlessness (severe)
Pinpoint pupils of eyes
Shortness of breath or troubled breathing
Unusually slow or fast heartbeat
Unusually slow or troubled breathing
Unusual warmth, dryness, and flushing of skin
Weakness (severe)

Other side effects may occur which usually do not require medical attention. These side effects may go away during treatment as your body adjusts to the medicine. However, check with your doctor if any of the following side effects continue or are bothersome:

More common

Constipation
Dizziness or lightheadedness
Drowsiness
Dryness of mouth, nose, throat, or skin
Nausea or vomiting

In infants and children, especially those with spastic paralysis or brain damage, this medicine may be more likely to cause severe side effects. Fever or unusual warmth, dryness, and flushing of skin are more likely to occur in children. Also, when it is given to children during hot weather, a rapid increase in body temperature may occur.

Breathing problems, excitement, agitation, drowsiness, or confusion are more likely to occur in children and the elderly, who are usually more sensitive to the effects of this medicine.

Other side effects not listed above may also occur in some patients. If you notice any other effects, check with your doctor.

COUGH/COLD COMBINATIONS— ANTITUSSIVES AND EXPECTORANTS (Systemic)

Note: For quick reference the following antitussive and expectorant combinations are numbered to match the corresponding brand names.

This information applies to the following medicines:

1. Codeine (KOE-deen) and Calcium Iodide (KAL-see-um EYE-oh-dyed)
2. Codeine and Guaifenesin (gwye-FEN-e-sin)
3. Codeine and Iodinated Glycerol (EYE-oh-di-nay-ted GLI-ser-ole)
4. Codeine, Potassium Guaiacolsulfonate (poe-TASS-ee-um gwye-a-kole-SUL-foe-nate), Sodium Citrate (SOE-dee-um SI-trate), Citric (SI-trik)Acid, and Ipecac (IP-e-kak)
5. Codeine and Terpin Hydrate (TER-pin HYE-drate)†
6. Dextromethorphan (dex-troe-meth-OR-fan) and Ammonium Chloride (a-MOE-nee-um KLOR-ide)
7. Dextromethorphan, Ammonium Chloride, and Ipecac Alkaloids
8. Dextromethorphan and Guaifenesin
9. Dextromethorphan, Guaifenesin, Ammonium Chloride, and Sodium Citrate
10. Dextromethorphan and Iodinated Glycerol
11. Dextromethorphan and Terpin Hydrate†
12. Hydrocodone (hye-droe-KOE-done) and Guaifenesin

13. Hydrocodone and Potassium Guaiacolsulfonate
14. Hydromorphone (hye-droe-MOR-fone) and Guaifenesin
15. Noscapine (NOSS-ka-peen) and Guaifenesin

Some commonly used brand names are:

2/G-DM Cough[8]	Kwelcof Liquid[12]
Actol Expectorant[15]	Nortussin with
Adatuss D.C.	Codeine[2]
Expectorant[12]	Novahistine
Anti-Tuss DM	Cough
Expectorant[8]	Formula Liquid[8]
Baytussin AC[2]	Pedi-Tot Pediatric
Baytussin DM[8]	Cough[9]
Calcidrine[1]	Peedee Dose
Cetro-Cirose[4]	Cough
Cheracol[2]	Suppressant
Cheracol D Cough[8]	Liquid[8]
Codiclear DH[13]	Pertussin Original[8]
Codistan No.1[8]	Prunicodeine[5]
Dilaudid Cough[14]	Queltuss[8]
Efficol Cough Whip	Rhinosyn-DMX
(Cough Suppres-	Expectorant[8]
sant/Expectorant)[8]	Robitussin A-C[2]
Endotussin-NN	Robitussin-DM[8]
Pediatric[6]	Robitussin-DM
Entuss Expectorant[12] [13]	Cough Calmers[8]
Glycotuss-dM[8]	Silexin Cough[8]
Glydeine Cough[2]	SK-Terpin Hydrate
Glydm Cough[8]	and Codeine[5]†
Guiamid D.M. Liquid[8]	Terphan[11]
Guiatuss A.C.[2]	Terpin-Dex[11]
Guiatuss-DM[8]	Tolu-Sed Cough[2]
Guiatussin with	Tolu-Sed DM
Codeine Liquid[2]	Cough[8]
Halotussin with	Trocal[8]
Codeine Liquid[2]	Tussi-Organidin
Halotussin-DM	DM Liquid[10]
Expectorant[8]	Tussi-Organidin
Hycotuss Expectorant[12]	Liquid[3]
Iophen-C[3]	Unproco[8]
Ipsatol DM	Vicks Children's
Cough[7]	Cough[8]
Kolephrin GG/	
DM[8]	

---

*Not available in the United States.
†Generic name product may also be available.

Antitussive and expectorant combinations are used to relieve coughs due to colds, influenza, or hay fever. They are not to be used for the chronic cough that occurs with smoking, asthma, or emphysema or when there is an unusually large amount of mucus or phlegm (pronounced flem) with the cough.

To help relieve coughing these combinations contain either a narcotic (codeine, hydrocodone, or hydromorphone) or a nonnarcotic (dextromethorphan or noscapine) antitussive. These antitussives act directly on the cough center in the brain. Narcotics may become habit-forming, causing mental or physical dependence, if used for a long time. Physical dependence may lead to withdrawal side effects when you stop taking the medicine.

Guaifenesin works by loosening the mucus or phlegm in the lungs. Other expectorants (for example, ammonium chloride) may have a similar effect.

Some of these combinations are available only with your doctor's prescription. Others are available without a prescription; however, your doctor or pharmacist may have special instructions on the proper dose of the medicine for your medical condition.

Before Using This Medicine

Before you use this medicine, check with your doctor, nurse, or pharmacist:

—if you have ever had any unusual or allergic reaction to codeine, dextromethorphan, guaifenesin, hydrocodone, hydromorphone, noscapine, or terpin hydrate, or to medicines that contain iodine such as calcium iodide or iodinated glycerol.

—if you are on a low-salt, low-sugar, or any other special diet, or if you are allergic to any substance, such as sulfites or other preservatives or dyes. Most medicines contain more than their active ingredient, and many liquid medicines contain alcohol. Your doctor or pharmacist can help you avoid products that may cause a problem.

—if you are pregnant or if you intend to become pregnant while taking this medicine. Dextromethorphan and guaifenesin have not been shown to cause problems in humans; however, the chance always exists.

Although studies on birth defects with narcotic antitussives, such as codeine, hydrocodone, and hydromorphone, have not been done in humans, these medicines have not been reported to cause birth defects in humans. However, hydrocodone and hydromorphone have been shown to cause birth defects in animals when given in very large doses. Codeine has not been shown to cause birth defects in animal studies, but it caused other unwanted effects. Also, regular use of narcotics during pregnancy may cause the baby to become dependent on the medicine. This may lead to withdrawal side effects after birth. In addition, if taken just before delivery, narcotics may cause breathing problems in the newborn infant.

Calcium iodide and iodinated glycerol (contained in some of these combination medicines) are not recommended during pregnancy. Iodides have caused enlargement of the thyroid gland in the fetus and resulted in breathing problems in newborn infants whose mothers took iodides in large doses for a long period of time.

Some of these combination medicines contain a large amount of alcohol. Too much use of alcohol during pregnancy may cause birth defects.

—if you are breast-feeding an infant. Iodides, such as calcium iodide and iodinated glycerol (contained in some of these combination medicines) pass into the breast milk and may cause unwanted effects, such as underactive thyroid in the infant. Also, the alcohol and codeine (contained in some of these combination medicines) pass into the breast milk. Although the amount of alcohol

and codeine in recommended doses of this medicine does not usually cause problems, the chance always exists.

—if you have any of the following medical problems:
> Emphysema, asthma, or chronic lung disease (especially in children)
> Liver disease

—if you are taking a combination medicine containing codeine, hydrocodone, or hydromorphone and have any of the following medical problems:
> Brain disease or injury
> Colitis
> Convulsions or seizures (history of)
> Enlarged prostate or problems with urination
> Gallbladder disease or gallstones
> Heart disease
> Kidney disease
> Underactive thyroid

—if you are taking a combination medicine containing calcium iodide or iodinated glycerol and have any of the following medical problems:
> Acne (in teenagers)
> Cystic fibrosis (in children)
> Thyroid disease (or history of)

—if you are taking a combination medicine containing codeine, hydrocodone, or hydromorphone and also take antimuscarinics (medicine for stomach spasms or cramps).

—if you are taking a combination medicine containing codeine, hydrocodone, or hydromorphone and also take any central nervous system (CNS) depressants such as:
> Anticonvulsants (seizure medicine)
> Antihistamines or medicine for hay fever, other allergies, or colds
> Barbiturates
> Muscle relaxants
> Narcotics
> Prescription pain medicine
> Sedatives, tranquilizers, or sleeping medicine

—if you are taking a combination medicine containing codeine, hydrocodone, or hydromorphone and also take tricyclic antidepressants such as:

Amitriptyline
Amoxapine
Desipramine
Doxepin
Imipramine
Nortriptyline
Protriptyline
Trimipramine

—if you are taking any of these combination medicines and are also taking or have taken within the past 2 weeks monoamine oxidase (MAO) inhibitors such as:

Furazolidone
Isocarboxazid
Pargyline
Phenelzine
Procarbazine
Tranylcypromine

Proper Use of This Medicine

To help loosen mucus or phlegm in the lungs, **drink a glass of water after each dose of this medicine,** unless otherwise directed by your doctor.

Take this medicine only as directed. Do not take more of it and do not take it more often than recommended on the label, unless otherwise directed by your doctor. To do so may increase the chance of side effects.

If you must take this medicine regularly and you miss a dose, take it as soon as possible. However, if it is almost time for your next dose, skip the missed dose and go back to your regular dosing schedule. Do not double doses.

How to store this medicine:

• Store away from heat and direct light.

• **Keep this medicine out of the reach of children** since overdose is very dangerous in young children.

• Do not store in the bathroom medicine cabinet because the heat or moisture may cause the medicine to break down.

• Keep the medicine from freezing. Do not refrigerate the syrup.

• Do not keep outdated medicine or medicine no longer needed. Flush the contents of the container down the toilet, unless otherwise directed.

Precautions While Using This Medicine

If your cough has not improved after 7 days or if you have a high fever, skin rash, continuing headache, or sore throat with the cough, check with your doctor. These signs may mean that you have other medical problems.

For patients taking codeine-, hydrocodone-, or hydromorphone-containing medicine:

• This medicine will add to the effects of alcohol and other CNS depressants (medicines that slow down the nervous system, possibly causing drowsiness). Some examples of CNS depressants are antihistamines or medicine for hay fever, other allergies, or colds; sedatives, tranquilizers, or sleeping medicine; prescription pain medicine or narcotics; barbiturates; medicine for seizures; muscle relaxants; or anesthetics, including some dental anesthetics. **Check with your doctor before taking any of the above while you are taking this medicine.**

• This medicine may cause some people to become drowsy, dizzy, or less alert than they are normally. **Make sure you know how you react to this medicine before you drive, use machines, or do other jobs that require you to be alert.**

• Before having any kind of surgery (including dental surgery) or emergency treatment, tell the physician or dentist in charge that you are taking this medicine.

• Dizziness, lightheadedness, or fainting may be especially likely to occur when you get up suddenly from a lying or sitting position. Getting up slowly may help lessen this problem.

• Nausea or vomiting may occur after taking a narcotic antitussive. This effect may go away if you lie down for a while. However, if nausea or vomiting continues, check with your doctor.

• **If you think you or someone else in your home may have taken an overdose of this medicine, get emergency help at once.** Taking an overdose of this medicine or taking alcohol or CNS depressants with this medicine may lead to unconsciousness or death. Signs of overdose include confusion, convulsions or seizures, severe nervousness or restlessness, severe dizziness, severe drowsiness, unusually slow or troubled breathing, and severe weakness.

For patients taking calcium iodide– or iodinated glycerol–containing medicine:

• Make sure your doctor knows if you are planning to have any future thyroid tests. The results of the thyroid test may be affected by the iodine in this medicine.

Side Effects of This Medicine

Along with its needed effects, a medicine may cause some unwanted effects. Although serious side effects occur rarely when this medicine is taken as recommended, they may be more likely to occur if:

—too much medicine is taken.
—it is taken in large doses.
—it is taken for a long period of time.

Get emergency help immediately if you are taking codeine-, hydrocodone-, or hydromorphone-containing medicine and any of the following signs of overdose occur:

　　Cold, clammy skin
　　Confusion (severe)
　　Convulsions (seizures)
　　Drowsiness or dizziness (severe)
　　Nervousness or restlessness (severe)
　　Shortness of breath or troubled breathing
　　Weakness (severe)

Also, check with your doctor as soon as possible if you are taking iodine-containing medicine and any of the following side effects occur:

　　Headache (continuing)
　　Loss of appetite
　　Metallic taste
　　Skin rash, hives, or redness
　　Sore throat
　　Swelling of face, lips, or eyelids
　　Unusual increase in salivation

Other side effects may occur which usually do not require medical attention. These side effects may go away during treatment as your body adjusts to the medicine. However, check with your doctor or pharmacist if any of the following side effects continue or are bothersome:

More common
　　Drowsiness

Less common
　　Constipation
　　Dizziness or lightheadedness
　　Nausea or vomiting

Although not all of the side effects listed above have been reported for all of these medicines, they have been reported for at least one of them. However, since there are some similarities among these combination medicines, most of the above side effects may occur with any of these medicines.

Very young children and elderly patients may be more sensitive to the effects of codeine, hydrocodone, or hydromorphone (contained in some of these combination medicines). Breathing problems may be more likely to occur in very young children and elderly patients, or those patients who are very ill and are taking codeine-, hydrocodone-, or hydromorphone-containing medicine.

Other side effects not listed above may also occur in some patients. If you notice any other effects, check with your doctor.

COUGH/COLD COMBINATIONS— DECONGESTANTS AND ANTITUSSIVES (Systemic)

Note: For quick reference the following decongestant and antitussive combinations are numbered to match the corresponding brand names.

This information applies to the following medicines:

1. Phenylephrine (fen-ill-EF-rin) and Noscapine (NOSS-ka-peen)
2. Phenylephrine, Phenylpropanolamine (fen-ill-proe-pa-NOLE-a-meen), and Codeine (KOE-deen)
3. Phenylpropanolamine and Caramiphen (kar-AM-i-fen)
4. Phenylpropanolamine and Dextromethorphan (dex-troe-meth-OR-fan)
5. Phenylpropanolamine and Hydrocodone (hye-droe-KOE-done)
6. Pseudoephedrine (soo-doe-e-FED-rin) and Codeine
7. Pseudoephedrine and Dextromethorphan
8. Pseudoephedrine and Hydrocodone

Some commonly used brand names are:

Am-Tuss Expectorant[2]	Hydro-
Baycomine[5]	Propanolamine[5]
BayCotussend Liquid[6]	Nucofed[6]
Bayer Cough Syrup for	Ornacol[4]
Children[4]	Rescaps-D S.R.[3]
Codamine[5]	Romilar III
Conar[1]	Decongestant
Contac Cough[7]	Cough[4]
De-Tuss[6]	Sudafed DM*[7]
Detussin Liquid[6]	Syracol Liquid[4]
Efficol Cough Whip	Triaminic-DM
(Cough Suppres-	Cough Formula[4]
sant/Decongestant)[4]	Tricodene
Entuss-D[6]	Pediatric[4]
Halls Mentho-Lyptus	Tuss-Ade[3]
Decongestant Cough	Tuss Allergine
Formula[4]	Modified T.D.[3]
Hold (Children's	Tussend[6]
Formula)[4]	Tussend Liquid[6]
Hycodan-D*[5]	Tussogest[3]
Hycomine[5]	Tuss-Ornade
Hydrophen[5]	Spansules[3]

*Not available in the United States.

Decongestant and antitussive combinations are used to relieve cough and nasal congestion due to colds, influenza, or hay fever. They are not to be used for the chronic cough that occurs with smoking, asthma, or emphysema or when there is an unusually large amount of mucus or phlegm (pronounced flem) with the cough.

Decongestants, such as phenylephrine, phenylpropanolamine (also known as PPA), and pseudoephedrine, produce a narrowing of blood vessels. This leads to clearing of nasal congestion, but it may also increase blood pressure in patients who have high blood pressure.

To help relieve coughing these combinations contain either a narcotic (codeine or hydrocodone) or non-narcotic (caramiphen, dextromethorphan, or noscapine) antitussive. These antitussives act directly on the cough center in the brain. Narcotics may become habit-forming, causing mental or physical dependence, if used for a long time. Physical dependence may lead to withdrawal side effects when you stop taking the medicine.

Some of these combinations are available only with your doctor's prescription. Others are available without a prescription; however, your doctor or pharmacist may have special instructions on the proper dose of the medicine for your medical condition.

Before Using This Medicine

Before you use this medicine, check with your doctor, nurse, or pharmacist:

—if you have ever had any unusual or allergic reaction to caramiphen, codeine, dextromethorphan, hydrocodone, or noscapine, or to amphetamine, dextroamphetamine, ephedrine, epinephrine, isoproterenol, metaproterenol, methamphetamine, norepinephrine, phenylephrine, pseudoephedrine, PPA, or terbutaline.

—if you are on a low-salt, low-sugar, or any other special diet, or if you are allergic to any substance, such as sulfites or other preservatives or dyes. Most medicines contain more than their active ingredient, and many liquid medicines contain alcohol. Your doctor or pharmacist can help you avoid products that may cause a problem.

—if you are pregnant or if you intend to become pregnant while taking this medicine. Although dextromethorphan has not been shown to cause problems in humans, the chance always exists.

Studies on birth defects have not been done in either animals or humans with decongestants such as phenylephrine or phenylpropanolamine. Studies on birth defects have not been done in humans with the decongestant pseudoephedrine; however, in animal studies pseudoephedrine did not cause birth defects but did cause a reduction in average weight, length, and rate of bone formation in the animal fetus.

Although studies on birth defects with narcotic antitussives, such as codeine and hydrocodone, have not been done in humans, these medicines have not been reported to cause birth defects in humans. However, when given in very large doses, hydrocodone has been shown to cause birth defects in animals. Codeine has not been shown to cause birth defects in animal studies, but it caused other unwanted effects. Also, regular use of narcotics during pregnancy may cause the baby to become dependent on the medicine. This may lead to withdrawal side effects after birth. In addition, if taken just before delivery, narcotics may cause breathing problems in the newborn infant.

Some of these combination medicines contain a large amount of alcohol. Too much use of alcohol during pregnancy may cause birth defects.

—if you are breast-feeding an infant. Although this medicine has not been shown to cause problems in humans, the chance always exists since alcohol and small amounts of some decongestants and some antitussives pass into the breast milk.

—if you have any of the following medical problems:

>   Diabetes mellitus (sugar diabetes)
>   Emphysema, asthma, or chronic lung disease (especially in children)
>   Heart or blood vessel disease
>   High blood pressure
>   Liver disease
>   Overactive thyroid

—if you are taking a combination medicine containing codeine or hydrocodone and have any of the following medical problems:

>   Brain disease or injury
>   Colitis
>   Convulsions or seizures (history of)
>   Gallbladder disease or gallstones
>   Kidney disease
>   Liver disease
>   Underactive thyroid

—if you are now taking any of the following medicines or types of medicine:

>   Acebutolol
>   Amphetamines
>   Atenolol
>   Caffeine
>   Diet aids, phenylpropanolamine-containing (medicines used for appetite control)
>   Digitalis glycosides (heart medicine)
>   Guanethidine
>   Labetalol
>   Medicine for asthma or other breathing problems
>   Metoprolol
>   Nadolol
>   Pindolol
>   Propranolol
>   Reserpine
>   Timolol

—if you are taking a combination medicine containing caramiphen, codeine, or hydrocodone and also take any central nervous system (CNS) depressants such as:

>   Anticonvulsants (seizure medicine)
>   Antihistamines or medicine for hay fever, other allergies, or colds
>   Barbiturates

Muscle relaxants
Narcotics
Prescription pain medicine
Sedatives, tranquilizers, or sleeping
    medicine

—if you are taking a combination medicine containing codeine or hydrocodone and also take antimuscarinics (medicine for stomach spasms or cramps).

—if you are now taking tricyclic antidepressants such as:

Amitriptyline
Amoxapine
Desipramine
Doxepin
Imipramine
Nortriptyline
Protriptyline
Trimipramine

—if you are now taking or have taken within the past 2 weeks monoamine oxidase (MAO) inhibitors such as:

Furazolidone
Isocarboxazid
Pargyline
Phenelzine
Procarbazine
Tranylcypromine

Proper Use of This Medicine

To help loosen mucus or phlegm in the lungs, **drink a glass of water after each dose of this medicine,** unless otherwise directed by your doctor.

Take this medicine only as directed. Do not take more of it and do not take it more often than recommended on the label, unless otherwise directed by your doctor. To do so may increase the chance of side effects.

For patients taking the extended-release capsule form of this medicine:

• Swallow it whole.

• Do not crush, break, or chew before swallowing.

• If the capsule is too large to swallow, you may mix the contents of the capsule

with applesauce, jelly, honey, or syrup and swallow without chewing.

If you must take this medicine regularly and you miss a dose, take it as soon as possible. However, if it is almost time for your next dose, skip the missed dose and go back to your regular dosing schedule. Do not double doses.

How to store this medicine:

• Store away from heat and direct light.

• **Keep this medicine out of the reach of children** since overdose is very dangerous in young children.

• Do not store in the bathroom medicine cabinet because the heat or moisture may cause the medicine to break down.

• Keep the medicine from freezing. Do not refrigerate the syrup.

• Do not keep outdated medicine or medicine no longer needed. Flush the contents of the container down the toilet, unless otherwise directed.

Precautions While Using This Medicine

If your cough has not improved after 7 days or if you have a high fever, skin rash, continuing headache, or sore throat with the cough, check with your doctor. These signs may mean that you have other medical problems.

This medicine may add to the central nervous system (CNS) stimulant and other effects of phenylpropanolamine (PPA)-containing diet aids. **Do not use medicines for diet or appetite control while taking this medicine unless you have checked with your doctor.**

This medicine may cause some people to be nervous or restless or to have trouble in sleeping. If you have trouble in sleeping, **take the last dose of this medicine for each day a few hours before bedtime.** If you have any questions about this, check with your doctor.

Before having any kind of surgery (including dental surgery) or emergency treatment, tell the physician or dentist in charge that you are taking this medicine.

For patients taking caramiphen-, codeine-, or hydrocodone-containing medicine:

• This medicine will add to the effects of alcohol and other CNS depressants (medicines that slow down the nervous system, possibly causing drowsiness). Some examples of CNS depressants are antihistamines or medicine for hay fever, other allergies, or colds; sedatives, tranquilizers, or sleeping medicine; prescription pain medicine or narcotics; barbiturates; medicine for seizures; muscle relaxants; or anesthetics, including some dental anesthetics. **Check with your doctor before taking any of the above while you are taking this medicine.**

• This medicine may cause some people to become drowsy, dizzy, or less alert than they are normally. **Make sure you know how you react to this medicine before you drive, use machines, or do other jobs that require you to be alert.**

For patients taking codeine- or hydrocodone-containing medicine:

• Dizziness, lightheadedness, or fainting may be especially likely to occur when you get up suddenly from a lying or sitting position. Getting up slowly may help lessen this problem.

• Nausea or vomiting may occur after taking a narcotic antitussive. This effect may go away if you lie down for a while. However, if nausea or vomiting continues, check with your doctor.

• **If you think you or someone else in your home may have taken an overdose of this medicine, get emergency help at once.** Taking an overdose of this medicine or taking alcohol or CNS depressants with this medicine may lead to unconsciousness or death. Signs of overdose include

confusion, convulsions or seizures, severe nervousness or restlessness, severe dizziness, severe drowsiness, unusually slow or troubled breathing, and severe weakness.

Side Effects of This Medicine

Along with its needed effects, a medicine may cause some unwanted effects. Although serious side effects occur rarely when this medicine is taken as recommended, they may be more likely to occur if:

—too much medicine is taken.
—it is taken in large doses.
—it is taken for a long period of time.

Get emergency help immediately if you are taking codeine- or hydrocodone-containing medicine and any of the following signs of overdose occur:

Cold, clammy skin
Confusion (severe)
Convulsions (seizures)
Drowsiness or dizziness (severe)
Nervousness or restlessness (severe)
Shortness of breath or troubled breathing
Weakness (severe)

Also, check with your doctor as soon as possible if any of the following side effects occur:

Headache (continuing and severe)
Nausea or vomiting (severe)
Unusually fast, pounding, or irregular heartbeat

Other side effects may occur which usually do not require medical attention. These side effects may go away during treatment as your body adjusts to the medicine. However, check with your doctor or pharmacist if any of the following side effects continue or are bothersome:

More common
Drowsiness
Less common
Constipation
Difficult or painful urination
Dizziness or lightheadedness

Dryness of nose or mouth
False sense of well-being
Nausea or vomiting
Nervousness or restlessness
Trouble in sleeping

Although not all of the side effects listed above have been reported for all of these medicines, they have been reported for at least one of them. However, since there are similarities among these combination medicines, most of the above side effects may occur with any of these medicines.

Very young children and elderly patients are usually more sensitive to the effects of this medicine. Breathing problems may be more likely to occur in very young children and elderly patients, or those patients who are very ill, and are taking medicine containing codeine or hydrocodone.

Use of caramiphen and phenylpropanolamine combination medicine is not recommended in infants less than 6 months of age or under 15 pounds of weight, since side effects, such as unusual excitement and irritability, are more likely to occur in very young children.

Other side effects not listed above may also occur in some patients. If you notice any other effects, check with your doctor.

COUGH/COLD COMBINATIONS—DECONGESTANTS, ANTITUSSIVES, AND ANALGESICS (Systemic)

This information applies to the following medicines:

Phenylpropanolamine (fen-ill-proe-pa-NOLE-a-meen), Dextromethorphan (dex-troe-meth-OR-fan), and Acetaminophen (a-seat-a-MEE-noe-fen)
Pseudoephedrine (soo-doe-e-FED-rin), Dextromethorphan, and Acetaminophen

Some commonly used brand names are:	Generic names:
Contac Jr. Children's Cold Medicine Saleto-CF	Phenylpropanolamine, Dextromethorphan, and Acetaminophen
Viro-Med Liquid	Pseudoephedrine, Dextromethorphan, and Acetaminophen

Decongestant, antitussive, and analgesic combinations are used to relieve cough, nasal congestion, and aches and pain due to colds, influenza, or hay fever. They are not to be used for the chronic cough that occurs with smoking, asthma, or emphysema or when there is an unusually large amount of mucus or phlegm (pronounced flem) with the cough.

Decongestants, such as phenylpropanolamine (also known as PPA) and pseudoephedrine, produce a narrowing of blood vessels. This leads to clearing of nasal congestion, but it may also increase blood pressure in patients who have high blood pressure.

The antitussive dextromethorphan is used to relieve coughing. It acts directly on the cough center in the brain.

The analgesic acetaminophen helps relieve the aches and pain that may occur with the common cold.

These medicines are available without a prescription; however, your doctor or pharmacist may have special instructions on the proper dose of the medicine for your medical condition.

For information about the precautions and side effects of the medicines in this combination, see:

Cough/Cold Combinations—
Decongestants and Antitussives
(Systemic)
Acetaminophen (Systemic)

Combination products are designed for specific uses. These uses may not be the same as the uses of the individual ingredients. Therefore, some of the information provided in the individual listings may not be relevant to the combination product. If questions arise, check with your doctor, nurse, or pharmacist.

COUGH/COLD COMBINATIONS— DECONGESTANTS, ANTITUSSIVES, AND EXPECTORANTS (Systemic)

This information applies to the following medicines:

Phenylephrine (fen-ill-EF-rin), Hydrocodone (hye-droe-KOE-done), and Guaifenesin (gwye-FEN-e-sin)
Phenylephrine, Noscapine (NOSS-ka-peen), and Guaifenesin
Phenylpropanolamine, Codeine (KOE-deen), and Guaifenesin
Phenylpropanolamine (fen-ill-proe-pa-NOLE-a-meen), Dextromethorphan (dex-troe-meth-OR-fan), and Guaifenesin
Pseudoephedrine (soo-doe-e-FED-rin), Codeine, and Guaifenesin
Pseudoephedrine, Dextromethorphan, and Guaifenesin
Pseudoephedrine, Hydrocodone, and Guaifenesin

Some commonly used brand names are: Generic names:

Donatussin DC	Phenylephrine, Hydrocodone, and Guaifenesin
Conar Expectorant	Phenylephrine, Noscapine, and Guaifenesin
Conex with Codeine Naldecon-CX Triaminic Expectorant with Codeine	Phenylpropanolamine, Codeine, and Guaifenesin
Coricidin Cough Cremacoat 3 Throat Coating Cough Medicine Kiddy Koff Naldecon-DX Robitussin-CF	Phenylpropanolamine, Dextromethorphan, and Guaifenesin
Alamine Expectorant Bayhistine Expectorant C-Tussin Expectorant Deproist Expectorant with Codeine Isoclor Expectorant Novahistine Expectorant Nucofed Expectorant Phenhist Expectorant Robitussin-DAC Ryna-CX Liquid	Pseudoephedrine, Codeine, and Guaifenesin
Ambenyl-D Decongestant Cough Formula Dimacol Dorcol Children's Cough Noratuss II Liquid Novahistine DMX Rhinosyn-X Sudafed Cough Trizone DM* Vicks Formula 44D Decongestant Cough Mixture	Pseudoephedrine, Dextromethorphan, and Guaifenesin
Detussin Expectorant Entuss-D Pseudo-Hist Expectorant SRC Expectorant Tussend Expectorant	Pseudoephedrine, Hydrocodone, and Guaifenesin

*Not available in the United States.

Decongestant, antitussive, and expectorant combinations are used to relieve cough and nasal congestion due to colds, influenza, or hay fever. They are not to be used for the chronic cough that occurs with smoking, asthma, or emphysema or when there is an unusually large amount of mucus or phlegm (pronounced flem) with the cough.

Decongestants, such as phenylephrine, phenylpropanolamine (also known as PPA), and pseudoephedrine, produce a narrowing of blood vessels. This leads to clearing of nasal congestion, but it may also increase blood pressure in patients who have high blood pressure.

To help relieve coughing these combinations contain either a narcotic (codeine or hydrocodone) or a non-narcotic (dextromethorphan or noscapine) antitussive. These antitussives act directly on the cough center in the brain. Narcotics may become habit-forming, causing mental or physical dependence, if used for a long time. Physical dependence may lead to withdrawal side effects when you stop taking the medicine.

Guaifenesin, an expectorant, works by loosening the mucus or phlegm in the lungs.

Some of these combinations are available only with your doctor's prescription. Others are available without a prescription; however, your doctor or pharmacist may have special instructions on the proper dose of the medicine for your medical condition.

For information about the precautions and side effects of the medicines in this combination, see:

Cough/Cold Combinations—
Decongestants and Antitussives
(Systemic)
Guaifenesin (Systemic)

Combination products are designed for specific uses. These uses may not be the same as the uses of the individual ingredients. Therefore, some of the information provided in the individual listings may not be relevant to the combination product. If questions arise, check with your doctor, nurse, or pharmacist.

COUGH/COLD COMBINATIONS— DECONGESTANTS, ANTITUSSIVES, EXPECTORANTS, AND ANALGESICS (Systemic)

This information applies to the following medicines:

Phenylephrine (fen-ill-EF-rin), Dextromethorphan (dex-troe-meth-OR-fan), Guaifenesin (gwye-FEN-e-sin), and Acetaminophen (a-seat-a-MEEN-noe-fen)

Phenylephrine, Noscapine (NOSS-ka-peen), Guaifenesin, and Acetaminophen

Pseudoephedrine (soo-doe-e-FED-rin), Dextromethorphan, Guaifenesin, and Acetaminophen

Some commonly used brand names are:	Generic names:
Coryban-D Cough	Phenylephrine, Dextromethorphan, Guaifenesin, and Acetaminophen
Conar-A	Phenylephrine, Noscapine, Guaifenesin, and Acetaminophen
Day Care Vicks Formula 44M Multi-symptom Cough Mixture	Pseudoephedrine, Dextromethorphan, Guaifenesin, and Acetaminophen

Decongestant, antitussive, expectorant, and analgesic combinations are used to relieve cough, nasal congestion, and aches and pain due to colds, influenza, or hay fever. They are not to be used for the chronic cough that occurs with smoking, asthma, or emphysema or when there is an unusually large amount of mucus or phlegm (pronounced flem) with the cough.

The decongestants phenylephrine and pseudoephedrine produce a narrowing of blood vessels. This leads to clearing of nasal congestion, but it may also increase blood pressure in patients who have high blood pressure.

To help relieve coughing these combinations contain dextromethorphan or noscapine. These antitussives act directly on the cough center in the brain.

Guaifenesin, an expectorant, works by loosening the mucus or phlegm in the lungs.

The analgesic acetaminophen relieves the aches and pain that may occur with the common cold.

These medicines are available without a prescription; however, your doctor or pharmacist may have special instructions on the proper dose of the medicine for your medical condition.

For information about the precautions and side effects of the medicines in this combination, see:

Cough/Cold Combinations—
    Decongestants and Antitussives
    (Systemic)
Guaifenesin (Systemic)
Acetaminophen (Systemic)

Combination products are designed for specific uses. These uses may not be the same as the uses of the individual ingredients. Therefore, some of the information provided in the individual listings may not be relevant to the combination product. If questions arise, check with your doctor, nurse, or pharmacist.

COUGH/COLD COMBINATIONS— DECONGESTANTS AND EXPECTORANTS (Systemic)

This information applies to the following medicines:

Ephedrine (e-FED-rin) and Guaifenesin (gwye-FEN-e-sin)

Ephedrine and Potassium Iodide (poe-TAS-ee-um EYE-oh-dyed)

Phenylephrine (fen-ill-EF-rin), Phenylpropanolamine (fen-ill-proe-pa-NOLE-a-meen), and Guaifenesin

Phenylpropanolamine and Guaifenesin

Pseudoephedrine (soo-doe-e-FED-rin) and Guaifenesin

Some commonly used brand names are:	Generic names:
Broncholate	Ephedrine and Guaifenesin
KIE	Ephedrine and Potassium Iodide
Entex Entex Liquid Respinol-G Respinol LA Rymed Rymed Liquid Rymed-TR	Phenylephrine, Phenylpropanolamine, and Guaifenesin
Bayaminic Expectorant Codimal Expectorant Conex Dura-Vent Entex LA Head & Chest Naldecon-EX Poly-Histine Expectorant Plain Prominic Expectorant Triaminic Expectorant Triphenyl Expectorant	Phenylpropanolamine and Guaifenesin

Congess	
Guaifed	
Histalet X	
Promist	
Promist LA	
Pseudo-Bid	
Respaire-120 SR	Pseudoephedrine
Robitussin-PE	and Guaifenesin
Sinufed Timecelles	
Sudafed Expectorant*	
Sueda-G	
T-Moist	
Zephrex	

*Not available in the United States.

Decongestant and expectorant combinations are used to relieve cough and nasal congestion due to colds, influenza, or hay fever. They are not to be used for the chronic cough that occurs with smoking, asthma, or emphysema or when there is an unusually large amount of mucus or phlegm (pronounced flem) with the cough.

The decongestants, such as ephedrine, phenylephrine, phenylpropanolamine (also known as PPA), and pseudoephedrine, produce a narrowing of blood vessels. This leads to clearing of nasal congestion, but it may also increase blood pressure in patients who have high blood pressure.

Guaifenesin works by loosening the mucus or phlegm in the lungs. Other expectorants, such as potassium iodide, may have a similar effect.

Some of these combinations are available only with your doctor's prescription. Others are available without a prescription; however, your doctor or pharmacist may have special instructions on the proper dose of the medicine for your medical condition.

Before Using This Medicine

Before you use this medicine, check with your doctor, nurse, or pharmacist:

—if you have ever had any unusual or allergic reaction to guaifenesin, potassium iodide or iodine, or to amphetamine, dextroamphetamine, ephedrine, epinephrine, isoproterenol, metaproterenol, methamphetamine, norepinephrine, phenylephrine, pseudoephedrine, PPA, or terbutaline.

—if you are pregnant or if you intend to become pregnant while taking this medicine. Although the expectorant guaifenesin has not been shown to cause problems in humans, the chance always exists. However, the expectorant potassium iodide, contained in one of these combination medicines, is not recommended during pregnancy. Iodides have caused enlargement of the thyroid gland in the fetus and resulted in breathing problems in newborn infants whose mothers took iodides in large doses for a long period of time.

Studies on birth defects have not been done in either animals or humans with the decongestants ephedrine, phenylephrine, or phenylpropanolamine. Studies on birth defects have not been done in humans with the decongestant pseudoephedrine; however, in animal studies pseudoephedrine did not cause birth defects but did cause a reduction in average weight, length, and rate of bone formation in the animal fetus.

—if you are breast-feeding an infant. Iodides, such as potassium iodide (contained in one of these combinations) pass into the breast milk and may cause unwanted effects, such as underactive thyroid in the infant. Also, small amounts of some decongestants pass into the breast milk.

—if you have any of the following medical problems:

    Acne (in teenagers) (for potassium iodide–containing only)

    Cystic fibrosis (in children) (for potassium iodide–containing only)

    Diabetes mellitus (sugar diabetes)

    Enlarged prostate

    Heart or blood vessel disease

    High blood pressure

    Thyroid disease (or history of)

—if you are now taking any of the following medicines or types of medicine:

    Acebutolol

    Amphetamines

    Antihypertensives

    Antithyroid medicine (for potassium iodide–containing only)

    Atenolol

    Caffeine

    Diet aids, phenylpropanolamine-containing (medicines used for appetite control)

    Digitalis glycosides (heart medicine)

    Guanethidine

    Labetalol

    Lithium (for potassium iodide–containing only)

    Medicine for asthma or other breathing problems

    Metoprolol

    Methyldopa

    Nadolol

    Pindolol

    Propranolol

    Reserpine

    Timolol

—if you are now taking tricyclic antidepressants (medicine for depression) such as:

    Amitriptyline

    Amoxapine

    Desipramine

    Doxepin

    Imipramine

    Nortriptyline

    Protriptyline

    Trimipramine

—if you are now taking or have taken within the past 2 weeks monoamine oxidase (MAO) inhibitors such as:

    Furazolidone

    Isocarboxazid

    Pargyline

    Phenelzine

    Procarbazine

    Tranylcypromine

Proper Use of This Medicine

To help loosen mucus or phlegm in the lungs, **drink a glass of water after each dose of this medicine,** unless otherwise directed by your doctor.

Take this medicine only as directed. Do not take more of it and do not take it more often than recommended on the label, unless otherwise directed by your doctor. To do so may increase the chance of side effects.

For patients taking the extended-release capsule or tablet form of this medicine:

• Swallow it whole.

• Do not crush, break, or chew before swallowing.

• If the capsule is too large to swallow, you may mix the contents of the capsule with applesauce, jelly, honey, or syrup and swallow without chewing.

If you must take this medicine regularly and you miss a dose, take it as soon as possible. However, if it is almost time for your next dose, skip the missed dose and go back to your regular dosing schedule. Do not double doses.

How to store this medicine:

- Store away from heat and direct light.

- **Keep this medicine out of the reach of children** since overdose is very dangerous in young children.

- Do not store in the bathroom medicine cabinet because the heat or moisture may cause the medicine to break down.

- Keep the medicine from freezing. Do not refrigerate the syrup.

- Do not keep outdated medicine or medicine no longer needed. Flush the contents of the container down the toilet, unless otherwise directed.

Precautions While Using This Medicine

If your cough has not improved after 7 days or if you have a high fever, skin rash, continuing headache, or sore throat with the cough, check with your doctor. These signs may mean that you have other medical problems.

The decongestant in this medicine may add to the central nervous system (CNS) stimulant and other effects of phenylpropanolamine (PPA)-containing diet aids. **Do not use medicines for diet or appetite control while taking this medicine unless you have checked with your doctor.**

This medicine may cause some people to be nervous or restless or to have trouble in sleeping. If you have trouble in sleeping, **take the last dose of this medicine for each day a few hours before bedtime.** If you have any questions about this, check with your doctor.

Before having any kind of surgery (including dental surgery) or emergency treatment, tell the physician or dentist in charge that you are taking this medicine.

Side Effects of This Medicine

Along with its needed effects, a medicine may cause some unwanted effects. Although serious side effects occur rarely when this medicine is taken as recommended, they may be more likely to occur if:

—too much medicine is taken.
—it is taken in large doses.
—it is taken for a long period of time.

Check with your doctor as soon as possible if the following signs of overdose occur:

Headache (continuing and severe)
Nausea or vomiting (severe)
Nervousness or restlessness (severe)
Shortness of breath or troubled breathing (severe or continuing)
Unusually fast, pounding, or irregular heartbeat

Other side effects may occur which usually do not require medical attention. These side effects may go away during treatment as your body adjusts to the medicine. However, check with your doctor or pharmacist if any of the following side effects continue or are bothersome:

Less common

Difficult or painful urination
Dizziness
Dryness of nose or mouth
Trouble in sleeping
Unusual excitement, nervousness, restlessness, or irritability

Although not all of the side effects listed above have been reported for all of these medicines, they have been reported for at least one of them. However, since these combination medicines are very similar, any of the above side effects may occur with any of these medicines.

The above side effects are more likely to occur in children and elderly patients, who are usually more sensitive to the effects of this medicine.

Other side effects not listed above may also occur in some patients. If you notice any other effects, check with your doctor.

CROMOLYN (Inhalation)

Some commonly used brand names or other names are Intal and Sodium Cromoglycate.

Cromolyn (KROE-moe-lin) is taken by oral inhalation to prevent asthma attacks. It is also used before and during exposure to substances that cause allergic reactions to prevent bronchospasm (wheezing or difficulty in breathing). In addition, this medicine is used to prevent bronchospasm caused by exercise.

Cromolyn inhalation works by acting on certain cells in the body, called mast cells, to prevent them from releasing substances which cause the asthma or bronchospasm attack.

Cromolyn will not help an asthma attack that has already started. If this medicine is used during a severe attack, it may cause irritation and make the attack worse.

This medicine is available only with your doctor's prescription.

Before Using This Medicine

In order to decide on the best treatment for your medical problem, your doctor should be told:

—if you have ever had any unusual or allergic reaction to cromolyn.

—if you are using the capsule form of cromolyn for inhalation and you have ever had any unusual or allergic reaction to lactose, milk, or milk products.

—if you are pregnant or if you intend to become pregnant while using this medicine. Studies have not been done in humans. However, studies in animals have shown that cromolyn causes a decrease in the weight of the fetus and increases the chance of death of the animal fetus when given by injection in very large amounts.

—if you are breast-feeding an infant. Although it is not known whether cromolyn passes into the breast milk and this medicine has not been shown to cause problems in humans, the chance always exists.

—if you have either of the following medical problems:
    Kidney disease
    Liver disease

Proper Use of This Medicine

Cromolyn inhalation is used to prevent asthma or bronchospasm (wheezing or difficulty in breathing) attacks. It will not relieve an attack that has already started. If this medicine is used during a severe attack, it may cause irritation and make the attack worse.

Use cromolyn inhalation only as directed. Do not use more of it and do not use it more often than your doctor ordered. To do so may increase the chance of side effects.

For patients using cromolyn inhalation regularly (for example, every day):

• **In order for cromolyn to work properly, it must be inhaled every day in regularly spaced doses as ordered by your doctor.** Up to 4 weeks may pass before you feel the full effects of the medicine.

• If you miss a dose of this medicine, take it as soon as possible. Then take any remaining doses for that day at regularly spaced intervals. Do not double doses.

For patients using the capsule form of cromolyn for inhalation:

• This medicine is used with a special inhaler and usually comes with patient directions. Read the directions carefully before using.

• **Do not swallow the capsules because the medicine will not work if you swallow it.**

For patients using the solution form of cromolyn for inhalation:

• Use this medicine only in a power-operated nebulizer with an adequate flow rate and equipped with a face mask or mouthpiece. Make sure you understand exactly how to use it. Hand-operated nebulizers are not suitable for using this medicine. If you have any questions about this, check with your doctor.

How to store this medicine:

• Store away from heat and direct light.

• **Keep out of the reach of children.**

• Do not store in the bathroom medicine cabinet because the heat or moisture may cause the medicine to break down.

• Keep the liquid form of this medicine from freezing.

• Do not keep outdated medicine or medicine no longer needed. Flush the contents of the container down the toilet, unless otherwise directed.

Precautions While Using This Medicine

If your symptoms do not improve or if your condition gets worse, check with your doctor.

If you are also taking an adrenocorticoid (cortisone-like medicine, such as cortisone or prednisone) for your asthma along with this medicine, do not stop taking the adrenocorticoid even if your asthma seems better, unless told to do so by your doctor.

If you are also using a bronchodilator inhaler to help you breathe better, use the bronchodilator first. Then wait 20 to 30 minutes before using cromolyn, unless otherwise directed by your doctor. This will help to increase the absorption of cromolyn and to reduce the possibility of side effects. If your bronchodilator does not seem to be working or if you have any questions, check with your doctor.

Dryness of the mouth, throat irritation, and hoarseness may occur after using this medicine. Gargling and rinsing the mouth after each dose may help prevent these effects.

Side Effects of This Medicine

Along with its needed effects, a medicine may cause some unwanted effects. Although not all of these side effects appear very often, when they do occur they may require medical attention. Check with your doctor as soon as possible if any of the following side effects occur:

Less common
> Difficult or painful urination
> Dizziness
> Frequent urge to urinate
> Headache (severe or continuing)
> Increased wheezing
> Joint pain or swelling
> Muscle pain or weakness
> Nausea or vomiting
> Skin rash, hives, or itching
> Swelling of the lips and eyes
> Tightness in chest
> Troubled breathing
> Trouble in swallowing

Rare
> Chest pain
> Chills
> Difficulty in breathing (severe)
> Unusual sweating
> Wheezing (severe)

Other side effects may occur which usually do not require medical attention. These side effects may go away during treatment as your body adjusts to the medicine. However, check with your doctor if any of the following side effects continue or are bothersome:

More common
> Cough
> Hoarseness

Less common
    Dryness of the mouth
    Sneezing
    Stuffy nose
    Throat irritation
    Watering of the eyes

Other side effects not listed above may also occur in some patients. If you notice any other effects, check with your doctor.

CYCLOBENZAPRINE
(Systemic)
A commonly used brand name is Flexeril.

Cyclobenzaprine (sye-kloe-BEN-za-preen) is a medicine that is used to help relax certain muscles in your body. It is used to relieve the pain and discomfort caused by strains, sprains, or other injury to your muscles. However, this medicine does not take the place of rest, exercise or physical therapy, or other treatment that your doctor may recommend for your medical problem. Cyclobenzaprine acts on the central nervous system (CNS) to produce its muscle relaxant effects. Its actions on the CNS may also cause some of this medicine's side effects.

Cyclobenzaprine is available only with your doctor's prescription.

Before Using This Medicine

In order to decide on the best treatment for your medical problem, your doctor should be told:

—if you have ever had any unusual or allergic reaction to cyclobenzaprine.

—if you are on a low-salt, low-sugar, or any other special diet, or if you are allergic to any substance, such as sulfites or other preservatives. Most medicines contain more than their active ingredient. Your doctor or pharmacist can help you avoid products that may cause a problem.

—if you are pregnant or if you intend to become pregnant while using this medicine. Studies on birth defects with cyclobenzaprine have not been done in humans. However, cyclobenzaprine has not been shown to cause birth defects or other problems in animal studies.

—if you are breast-feeding an infant. Although cyclobenzaprine has not been shown to cause problems, the chance always exists. It is not known whether cyclobenzaprine passes into the breast milk.

—if you have any of the following medical problems:
    Glaucoma
    Heart or blood vessel disease
    Overactive thyroid
    Problems with urination

—if you are now taking other central nervous system (CNS) depressants such as:
    Anticonvulsants (seizure medicine)
    Antihistamines or medicine for hay fever, other allergies, or colds
    Barbiturates
    Narcotics
    Other muscle relaxants
    Prescription pain medicine
    Sedatives, tranquilizers, or sleeping medicine
    Tricyclic antidepressants (medicine for depression)

—if you are now taking any of the following medicines or types of medicine:
    Antimuscarinics (prescription medicine for stomach cramps or spasms)
    Benztropine
    Biperidin
    Ethopropazine
    Guanadrel
    Guanethidine
    Procyclidine
    Trihexyphenidyl

—if you are now taking or have taken within the past 2 weeks monoamine oxidase (MAO) inhibitors such as:

    Furazolidone
    Isocarboxazid
    Pargyline
    Phenelzine
    Procarbazine
    Tranylcypromine

Proper Use of This Medicine

Take this medicine only as directed by your doctor. Do not take more of it and do not take it more often than your doctor ordered. To do so may increase the chance of serious side effects.

If you miss a dose of this medicine and remember within an hour or so of the missed dose, take it right away. Then go back to your regular dosing schedule. But if you do not remember until later, skip the missed dose and go back to your regular dosing schedule. Do not double doses.

How to store this medicine:

• Store away from heat and direct light.

• **Keep out of the reach of children.**

• Do not store in the bathroom medicine cabinet because the heat or moisture may cause the medicine to break down.

• Do not keep outdated medicine or medicine no longer needed. Flush the contents of the container down the toilet, unless otherwise directed.

Precautions While Using This Medicine

This medicine will add to the effects of alcohol and other CNS depressants (medicines that slow down the nervous system, possibly causing drowsiness). Some examples of CNS depressants are antihistamines or medicine for hay fever, other allergies, or colds; sedatives, tranquilizers, or sleeping medicine; prescription pain medicine or narcotics; barbiturates; medicine for seizures; tricyclic antidepressants (medicine for depression); other muscle relaxants; or anesthetics, including some dental anesthetics. **Check with your doctor before taking any of the above while you are using this medicine.**

This medicine may cause some people to have blurred vision or to become drowsy, dizzy, or less alert than they are normally. **Make sure you know how you react to this medicine before you drive, use machines, or do other jobs that require you to be alert and see well.**

Dryness of the mouth may occur while you are taking this medicine. Sucking on sugarless hard candy or ice chips or chewing sugarless gum may help relieve the dry mouth.

Side Effects of This Medicine

Along with its needed effects, a medicine may cause some unwanted effects. Although not all of these side effects appear very often, when they do occur they may require medical attention. **Check with your doctor immediately** if any of the following side effects occur:

Rare
    Swelling of face, lips, or tongue

Signs of overdose
    Convulsions (seizures)
    Drowsiness, severe
    Fainting
    Hallucinations (seeing, hearing, or feeling things that are not there)
    Increase or decrease in body temperature
    Troubled breathing
    Unexplained muscle stiffness
    Unusually fast or irregular heartbeat
    Unusual nervousness or restlessness, severe
    Vomiting

Also, check with your doctor as soon as possible if any of the following side effects occur:

Rare

Clumsiness or unsteadiness
Confusion
Mental depression
Problems in urinating
Ringing or buzzing sound in the ears
Skin rash, hives, or itching

Other side effects may occur which usually do not require medical attention. These side effects may go away during treatment as your body adjusts to the medicine. However, check with your doctor if any of the following side effects continue or are bothersome:

More common

Dizziness or lightheadedness
Drowsiness
Dry mouth

Less common or rare

Bad taste in the mouth
Blurred vision
Constipation
Headache
Indigestion
Nausea
Numbness, tingling, pain, or weakness in hands or feet
Problems in speaking
Trembling
Trouble in sleeping
Unusual muscle weakness
Unusual pounding heartbeat
Unusual tiredness

Other side effects not listed above may also occur in some patients. If you notice any other effects, check with your doctor.

DEXTROMETHORPHAN
(Systemic)

Some commonly used brand names are:

Balminil D.M.*	Mediquell
Benylin DM Cough	Neo-DM*
Broncho-Grippol-DM*	Pertussin 8 Hour
Congespirin Cough	Cough Formula
Syrup	PediaCare 1
Cremacoat 1	Robidex*
Delsym	Romilar CF
Demo-Cineol*	Romilar Children's
DM Cough	Cough
DM Syrup*	Sedatuss*
Extend-12	St. Joseph for
Hold	Children
Koffex*	Sucrets Cough
	Control

---

*Not available in the United States.

Dextromethorphan (dex-troe-meth-OR-fan) is taken by mouth to relieve coughs due to colds or influenza (flu). It is not to be used for chronic cough that occurs with smoking, asthma, or emphysema or when there is an unusually large amount of mucus or phlegm with the cough.

Dextromethorphan relieves cough by acting directly on the cough center in the brain.

This medicine is available without a prescription; however, your doctor may have special instructions on the proper use of this medicine for your medical condition.

Before Using This Medicine

Before you use dextromethorphan, check with your doctor or pharmacist:

—if you have ever had any unusual or allergic reaction to dextromethorphan.

—if you are on a low-salt, low-sugar, or any other special diet, or if you are allergic to any substance, such as sulfites or other preservatives or dyes. Most medicines contain more than their active ingredient, and many liquid medicines contain alcohol. Your doctor or pharmacist can help you avoid products that may cause a problem.

—if you are pregnant or if you intend to become pregnant while taking this medicine. Although dextromethorphan has not been shown to cause problems in humans, the chance always exists.

—if you are breast-feeding an infant. Although dextromethorphan has not been shown to cause problems in humans, the chance always exists.

—if you have either of the following medical problems:

Asthma
Liver disease

—if you are now taking any of these medicines for high blood pressure:

Clonidine
Guanabenz
Methyldopa
Metyrosine

—if you are now taking any central nervous system (CNS) depressants, such as:

Anticonvulsants (seizure medicine)
Antihistamines or medicine for hay fever, other allergies, or colds
Barbiturates
Muscle relaxants
Narcotics
Prescription pain medicine
Sedatives, tranquilizers, or sleeping medicine

—if you are now taking tricyclic antidepressants, such as:

Amitriptyline
Amoxapine
Clomipramine
Desipramine
Doxepin
Imipramine
Nortriptyline
Protriptyline
Trimipramine

—if you are now taking or have taken within the past 2 weeks monoamine oxidase (MAO) inhibitors, such as:

Furazolidone
Isocarboxazid
Pargyline
Phenelzine
Procarbazine
Tranylcypromine

Proper Use of This Medicine

If you must take this medicine regularly and you miss a dose, take it as soon as possible. However, if it is almost time for your next dose, skip the missed dose and go back to your regular dosing schedule. Do not double doses.

How to store this medicine:

• Store away from heat and direct light.

• **Keep out of the reach of children.**

• Do not store in the bathroom medicine cabinet because the heat or moisture may cause the medicine to break down.

• Keep the syrup from freezing.

• Do not keep outdated medicine or medicine no longer needed. Flush the contents of the container down the toilet, unless otherwise directed.

Precautions While Using This Medicine

If your cough has not improved after 7 days or if you have a high fever, skin rash, or continuing headache with the cough, check with your doctor. These signs may mean that you have other medical problems.

Side Effects of This Medicine

Along with its needed effects, a medicine may cause some unwanted effects. Although not all of these side effects appear very often, when they do occur they may require medical attention. Check with your doctor as soon as possible if any of the following side effects occur:

Signs of overdose
Confusion
Unusual excitement, nervousness, restlessness, or irritability (severe)

Other side effects may occur which usually do not require medical attention. These side effects may go away during treatment as your body adjusts to the medicine. However, check with your doctor or pharmacist if any of the following side effects continue or are bothersome:

Less common or rare
Dizziness
Drowsiness
Nausea or vomiting
Stomach pain

Other side effects not listed above may also occur in some patients. If you notice any other effects, check with your doctor.

DICYCLOMINE (Systemic)

Some commonly used brand names are:

Antispas	Dibent
A-Spas	Dicen
Baycyclomine	Dilomine
Bentyl	Di-Spaz
Bentylol*	Neoquess
Byclomine	Nospaz
Cyclocen	Or-Tyl
	Spasmoject

Generic name product may also be available.

---

*Not available in the United States

Dicyclomine (dye-SYE-kloe-meen) belongs to the general family of medicines called antispasmodics. It helps to decrease cramping or spasms of the intestines.

Dicyclomine is available only with your doctor's prescription.

Before Using This Medicine

In order to decide on the best treatment for your medical problem, your doctor should be told:

—if you have ever had any unusual or allergic reaction to dicyclomine.

—if you are on a low-salt, low-sugar, or any other special diet, or if you are allergic to any substance, such as sulfites or other preservatives or dyes. Most medicines contain more than their active ingredient. Your doctor or pharmacist can help you avoid products that may cause a problem.

—if you are pregnant or if you intend to become pregnant while using this medicine. Although dicyclomine has not been shown to cause problems in humans, the chance always exists.

—if you are breast-feeding an infant. Although dicyclomine has not been shown to cause problems in humans, the chance always exists. Also, since· this medicine tends to decrease the secretions of the body, it is possible that the flow of breast milk may be reduced in some patients.

—if you have any of the following medical problems:
Bleeding (severe)
Colitis, ulcerative (severe)
Difficult urination
Enlarged prostate
Glaucoma (or predisposition to)
Heart disease
Hiatal hernia
Intestinal blockage or other intestinal problems
Kidney disease
Liver disease
Myasthenia gravis
Overactive thyroid
Urinary tract blockage

—if you are now taking any of the following medicines or types of medicine:
Amantadine
Antacids
Antidiarrhea medicine

Antimuscarinics, other (medicines for
abdominal or stomach spasms
or cramps)
Clonidine
Digoxin (heart medicine)
Guanabenz
Haloperidol
Medicine for Parkinson's disease
Medicine for myasthenia gravis
Methyldopa
Metoclopramide
Metyrosine
Nomifensine
Pimozide
Potassium chloride

—if you are now taking central nervous
system (CNS) depressants, such as:

Anticonvulsants (seizure medicine)
Antihistamines or medicine for hay fever,
other allergies, or colds
Narcotics
Prescription pain medicine
Sedatives, tranquilizers, or sleeping
medicine

—if you are now taking tricyclic antidepressants, such as:

Amitriptyline
Amoxapine
Clomipramine
Desipramine
Doxepin
Imipramine
Nortriptyline
Protriptyline
Trimipramine

—if you are now taking or have taken
within the past 2 weeks monoamine oxidase (MAO) inhibitors, such as:

Furazolidone
Isocarboxazid
Pargyline
Phenelzine
Procarbazine
Tranylcypromine

Proper Use of This Medicine

If this medicine upsets your stomach, take
it with food or milk, unless otherwise
directed by your doctor.

**Take this medicine exactly as directed by
your doctor.** Do not take more or less of
it, do not take it more often, and do not
take it for a longer period of time than
your doctor ordered. To do so may increase the chance of side effects.

If you miss a dose of this medicine, take it
as soon as possible. However, if it is almost time for your next dose, skip the
missed dose and go back to your regular
dosing schedule. Do not double doses.

How to store this medicine:

• Store away from heat and direct light.

• **Keep out of the reach of children.**

• Do not store in the bathroom medicine
cabinet because the heat or moisture
may cause the medicine to break down.

• Keep the syrup form of this medicine
from freezing.

• Do not keep outdated medicine or medicine no longer needed. Flush the contents of the container down the toilet,
unless otherwise directed.

Precautions While Using This Medicine

Do not take this medicine within 1 hour of
taking antacids or medicine for diarrhea. Taking them too close together will
make this medicine less effective.

This medicine will add to the effects of alcohol and other CNS depressants (medicines that slow down the nervous system, possibly causing drowsiness). Some
examples of CNS depressants are antihistamines or medicine for hay fever,
other allergies, or colds; sedatives, tranquilizers, or sleeping medicine; prescription pain medicine or narcotics; barbiturates; medicine for seizures; muscle
relaxants; or anesthetics, including
some dental anesthetics. **Check with
your doctor before taking any of the
above while you are using this medicine.**

This medicine may cause some people to have blurred vision or to become drowsy or less alert than they are normally. **Make sure you know how you react to this medicine before you drive, use machines, or do other jobs that require you to be alert.**

Check with your doctor if you develop intestinal problems such as constipation. This is especially important if you are taking other medicine while taking dicyclomine.

Although this side effect does not occur often, this medicine may make you sweat less, causing your body temperature to increase. Use extra care not to become overheated during exercise or hot weather while you are taking this medicine, as overheating could possibly result in heat stroke. Also, hot baths or saunas may make you feel dizzy or faint while you are taking this medicine.

Side Effects of This Medicine

In some very young infants this medicine has caused respiratory or breathing problems. These side effects were probably caused by not swallowing this medicine properly. Before giving dicyclomine to children, be sure you have discussed the use of it with your doctor.

Along with its needed effects, a medicine may cause some unwanted effects. Although not all of these side effects appear very often, when they do occur they may require medical attention. Check with your doctor as soon as possible if any of the following side effects occur:

More common
    Constipation (especially in the elderly)
Less common
    Difficult urination
Rare
    Skin rash

Other side effects may occur which usually do not require medical attention. These side effects may go away during treatment as your body adjusts to the medicine. However, check with your doctor if any of the following side effects continue or are bothersome:

More common
    Bloated feeling
    Dizziness
    Headache
Less common
    Blurred vision
    Confusion (especially in the elderly)
    Decreased sexual ability
    Drowsiness
    Nausea and vomiting
    Nervousness
Rare
    Decreased sweating
    Dry mouth
    Rapid pulse

Confusion, excitement, and constipation are more likely to occur in the elderly, who are usually more sensitive to the effects of dicyclomine.

Other side effects not listed above may also occur in some patients. If you notice any other effects, check with your doctor.

DIGITALIS MEDICINES
(Systemic)

This information applies to the following medicines:

Deslanoside (des-LAN-oh-side)
Digitalis (di-ji-TAL-iss)
Digitoxin (di-ji-TOX-in)
Digoxin (di-JOX-in)

Some commonly used brand names and other names are:	Generic names:
Cedilanid-D	Deslanoside
	Digitalis†
Crystodigin Purodigin	Digitoxin†
Lanoxin Lanoxicaps	Digoxin†

†Generic name product may also be available.

Digitalis medicines are taken by mouth or given by injection to improve the strength and efficiency of the heart, or to control the rate and rhythm of the heartbeat. This leads to better blood circulation and reduced swelling of hands and ankles in patients having such a problem.

Although digitalis has been prescribed to help some patients lose weight, it should **never** be used this way. When used improperly, digitalis can cause serious problems.

Digitalis medicines are available only with your doctor's prescription.

Before Using This Medicine

In order to decide on the best treatment for your medical problem, your doctor should be told:

—if you have ever had any unusual or allergic reaction to digitalis medicine.

—if you are on a low-salt, low-sugar, or any other special diet, or if you are allergic to any substance, such as sulfites or other preservatives or dyes. Most medicines contain more than their active ingredient, and many liquid medicines contain alcohol. Your doctor or pharmacist can help you avoid products that may cause a problem.

—if you are pregnant or if you intend to become pregnant while taking this medicine. Although digitalis medicines have not been shown to cause birth defects or other problems in humans, the chance always exists. These medicines pass from the mother to the fetus.

—if you are breast-feeding an infant. Although digitalis medicines have not been shown to cause problems in humans, since small amounts pass into the breast milk the chance always exists.

—if you have any of the following medical problems:
   Kidney disease
   Liver disease
   Lung disease (severe)

—if you have recently had a heart attack.

—if you have ever had rheumatic fever.

—if you are now taking any other medicine, especially the following medicines or types of medicine:
   Acetazolamide
   Antacids
   Antihypertensives (high blood pressure medicines)
   Antimuscarinics (medicine for abdominal or stomach spasms or cramps)
   Asthma or hay fever medicine
   Beta-blockers such as:
      Acebutolol
      Atenolol
      Labetalol
      Metoprolol
      Nadolol
      Oxprenolol
      Pindolol
      Propranolol
      Sotalol
      Timolol
   Cholestyramine
   Cold medicine
   Colestipol
   Decongestants
   Diarrhea medicine
   Dichlorphenamide
   Diuretics (water pills)
   Indomethacin
   Laxatives
   Medicine for appetite or diet control
   Methazolamide
   Metoclopramide
   Neomycin

Sinus congestion medicine
Sodium phosphates
Sulfasalazine

—if your diet contains large amounts of fiber, such as bran.

—if you are now taking or have taken within the past 2 weeks any of the following medicines or types of medicine:

Adrenocorticoids (cortisone-like medicine), especially prednisone
Any digitalis medicines or other heart medicines, especially quinidine
Barbiturates (does not apply to digoxin)
Diltiazem
Nifedipine
Oxyphenbutazone (does not apply to digoxin)
Phenylbutazone (does not apply to digoxin)
Primidone (does not apply to digoxin)
Potassium supplements
Rifampin (does not apply to digoxin)
Thyroid medicine
Verapamil

Proper Use of This Medicine

To help you remember to take your dose of medicine, try to take it at the same time every day.

Ask your doctor about checking your pulse rate. Then, while you are taking this medicine, check your pulse regularly. If it is much slower, or faster, than your usual rate (or less than 60 beats per minute), or if it changes in rhythm or force, check with your doctor. Such changes may mean that side effects are developing.

For patients taking the liquid form of digoxin:

• This medicine is to be taken by mouth even though it may come in a dropper bottle. The amount you should take is to be measured only with the specially marked dropper.

To keep your heart working properly, **take this medicine exactly as directed even though you may feel well.** Do not take more medicine than ordered and do not miss any doses.

If you do miss a dose of this medicine, do not take the missed dose at all and do not double the next one. Instead, go back to your regular dosing schedule. If you have any questions about this or if you miss doses for 2 or more days, check with your doctor.

How to store this medicine:

• Store away from heat and direct light.

• **Keep out of the reach of children.**

• Do not store in the bathroom medicine cabinet because the heat or moisture may cause the medicine to break down.

• Keep the oral liquid form of this medicine from freezing.

• Do not keep outdated medicine or medicine no longer needed. Flush the contents of the container down the toilet, unless otherwise directed.

Precautions While Using This Medicine

It is important that your doctor check your progress at regular visits in order to make sure the medicine is working properly. This will allow any needed changes in directions for taking it.

Do not stop taking this medicine without first checking with your doctor. Stopping suddenly may cause a serious change in heart function.

Keep this medicine out of the reach of children. Digitalis medicines are an important cause of accidental poisoning in children.

Watch for signs of overdose (too much medicine) while you are taking digitalis medicine. Follow directions carefully. The amount needed to help most people is very close to the amount that could cause serious problems from overdose. Some early warning signs of overdose are loss of appetite, nausea, vomiting, diarrhea, or extremely slow heartbeat. In infants and small children, the earliest signs of overdose are changes in the rate and rhythm of the heartbeat. They may not show the other signs as soon as adults.

Before having any kind of surgery (including dental surgery) or emergency treatment, tell the physician or dentist in charge that you are using this medicine.

Your doctor may want you to carry a medical identification card or bracelet stating that you are taking this medicine.

Do not take any other medicine unless ordered by your doctor. Many over-the-counter (OTC) or nonprescription medicines contain ingredients which interfere with digitalis medicines or which may make your condition worse. They include antacids; laxatives; asthma remedies; cold, cough, or sinus preparations; medicine for diarrhea; and reducing or diet medicines.

For patients taking the tablet or capsule forms of this medicine:

• This medicine may look like other tablets or capsules you now take. It is very important that you do not get the medicines mixed up since this may have serious results. Ask your pharmacist for ways to avoid mix-ups with medicines that look alike.

Side Effects of This Medicine

Along with its needed effects, a medicine may cause some unwanted effects. Although not all of these side effects appear very often, when they do occur they may require medical attention. Check with your doctor as soon as possible if any of the following side effects or signs of overdose occur:

Rare
  Skin rash or hives
Possible signs of overdose (in the order in which they may occur)
  Loss of appetite
  Nausea or vomiting
  Lower stomach pain
  Diarrhea
  Unusual tiredness or weakness (extreme)
  Unusually fast, slow, or uneven heartbeat
  Blurred vision or "yellow vision" (yellow halo seen around objects)
  Drowsiness
  Mental depression or confusion
  Headache

Note: Overdose symptoms in infants and small children may occur at first only as changes in the heartbeat rate or rhythm, while in adults and older children the first symptoms may be mostly stomach upset, stomach pain, loss of appetite, or unusually slow heartbeat.

The above signs of overdose may be more likely to occur in the elderly, who are usually more sensitive to the effects of digitalis medicines.

Other side effects not listed above may also occur in some patients. If you notice any other effects, check with your doctor.

DIPHENOXYLATE AND ATROPINE (Systemic)

Some commonly used brand names are:

Diphenatol	Lomotil
Enoxa	Lonox
Latropine	Lo-Trol
Lofene	Low-Quel
Lomanate	Nor-Mil
	SK-Diphenoxylate

Generic name product may also be available.

Diphenoxylate (dye-fen-OX-i-late) and atropine (A-troe-peen) is a combination medicine used along with other measures to treat severe diarrhea. Diphenoxylate helps stop diarrhea by slowing down the movements of the intestines. The atropine is included to prevent possible abuse, since diphenoxylate is chemically related to some narcotics.

This medicine is available only with your doctor's prescription.

Before Using This Medicine

In order to decide on the best treatment for your medical problem, your doctor should be told:

—if you have ever had any unusual or allergic reaction to diphenoxylate or atropine.

—if you are on a low-salt, low-sugar, or any other special diet, or if you are allergic to any substance, such as sulfites or other preservatives or dyes. Most medicines contain more than their active ingredient, and many liquid medicines contain alcohol. Your doctor or pharmacist can help you avoid products that may cause a problem.

—if you are pregnant or if you intend to become pregnant while taking this medicine. In animal studies this medicine given in larger doses than the usual human dose has not been shown to cause birth defects. However, some studies in animals have shown that this medicine may retard growth and lessen the chance of conceiving or becoming pregnant.

—if you are breast-feeding an infant. Although this medicine has not been shown to cause problems in humans, the chance always exists since both diphenoxylate and atropine pass into the breast milk.

—if you have any of the following medical problems:
Colitis (severe)
Difficult urination
Down's syndrome (mongolism) in children
Emphysema, asthma, bronchitis, or other chronic lung disease
Enlarged prostate
Gallbladder disease or gallstones
Glaucoma
Heart disease
Hiatal hernia
High blood pressure
Kidney disease
Liver disease
Myasthenia gravis
Overactive or underactive thyroid
Urinary tract blockage

—if you are now taking any of the following medicines or types of medicine:
Amantadine
Antimuscarinics, other (medicine for abdominal or stomach spasms or cramps)
Cephalosporins (a type of antibiotic)
Clonidine
Clindamycin
Guanabenz
Haloperidol
Lincomycins
Methyldopa
Metyrosine
Penicillins
Procainamide

—if you are now taking other central nervous system (CNS) depressants, such as:
Anticonvulsants (seizure medicine)
Antihistamines or medicine for hay fever, other allergies, or colds
Barbiturates
Other narcotics
Prescription pain medicine
Sedatives, tranquilizers, or sleeping medicine

—if you are now taking tricyclic antidepressants, such as:
Amitriptyline
Amoxapine
Clomipramine

Desipramine
Doxepin
Imipramine
Nortriptyline
Protriptyline
Trimipramine

—if you are now taking or have taken within the past 2 weeks monoamine oxidase (MAO) inhibitors, such as:
Furazolidone
Isocarboxazid
Pargyline
Phenelzine
Procarbazine
Tranylcypromine

Proper Use of This Medicine

If this medicine upsets your stomach, your doctor may want you to take it with food.

Take this medicine only as directed by your doctor. Do not take more of it, do not take it more often, and do not take it for a longer period of time than your doctor ordered. If too much is taken, it may become habit-forming, or may cause overdose in a child.

For patients taking the liquid form of this medicine:

• This medicine is to be taken by mouth even though it may come in a dropper bottle. The amount to be taken is to be measured with the specially marked dropper.

If you are taking this medicine on a regular schedule and you miss a dose, take it as soon as possible. However, if it is almost time for your next dose, skip the missed dose and go back to your regular dosing schedule. Do not double doses.

How to store this medicine:

• Store away from heat and direct light.

• **Keep out of the reach of children** since overdose is especially dangerous in children.

• Do not store in the bathroom medicine cabinet because the heat or moisture may cause the medicine to break down.

• Keep the liquid dosage form of this medicine from freezing.

• Do not keep outdated medicine or medicine no longer needed. Flush the contents of the container down the toilet, unless otherwise directed.

Precautions While Using This Medicine

Your doctor should check your progress at regular visits if you will be taking this medicine regularly for a long period of time.

Check with your doctor if your diarrhea does not stop after a few days or if you develop a fever.

This medicine will add to the effects of alcohol and other CNS depressants (medicines that slow down the nervous system, possibly causing drowsiness). Some examples of CNS depressants are antihistamines or medicine for hay fever, other allergies, or colds; sedatives, tranquilizers, or sleeping medicine; prescription pain medicine or narcotics; barbiturates; medicine for seizures; muscle relaxants; or anesthetics, including some dental anesthetics. **Check with your doctor before taking any of the above while you are taking this medicine.**

If you think you may have taken an overdose, get emergency help at once. Taking an overdose of this medicine may lead to unconsciousness and possibly death. Signs of overdose include severe drowsiness; shortness of breath or troubled breathing; unusually fast heartbeat; and unusual warmth, dryness, and flushing of skin.

Before having any kind of surgery (including dental surgery) or emergency treatment, tell the physician or dentist in charge that you are taking this medicine.

This medicine may cause some people to become dizzy, drowsy, or less alert than they are normally. Even if taken at bedtime, it may cause some people to feel drowsy or less alert on arising. **Make sure you know how you react to this medicine before you drive, use machines, or do other jobs that require you to be alert.**

Side Effects of This Medicine

Along with its needed effects, a medicine may cause some unwanted effects. Although not all of these side effects appear very often, when they do occur they may require medical attention. **When this medicine is used for short periods of time at low doses, side effects usually are rare. However, check with your doctor immediately** if any of the following side effects are severe and occur suddenly since they may indicate a more severe and dangerous problem with your bowels:

    Bloating
    Constipation
    Loss of appetite
    Nausea or vomiting
    Stomach pain

Check with your doctor immediately also if the following effects occur, since they may indicate an overdose:

    Blurred vision (continuing) or changes in
        near vision
    Drowsiness (severe)
    Dryness of mouth, nose, and throat
        (severe)
    Shortness of breath or troubled breathing
        (severe)
    Unusual excitement, nervousness, restlessness, or irritability (especially in children)
    Unusually fast heartbeat
    Unusual warmth, dryness, and flushing of skin

Other side effects may occur which usually do not require medical attention. These side effects may go away during treatment as your body adjusts to the medicine. However, check with your doctor if any of the following side effects continue, worsen, or are bothersome:

Less common or rare
    Blurred vision
    Difficult urination
    Dizziness or lightheadedness
    Drowsiness
    Dryness of skin and mouth
    Fever
    Headache
    Mental depression
    Numbness of hands or feet
    Skin rash or itching
    Swelling of the gums

After you stop using this medicine, your body may need time to adjust. The length of time this takes depends on the amount of medicine you were using and how long you used it. During this period of time check with your doctor if you notice any of the following side effects:

    Muscle cramps
    Nausea or vomiting
    Shivering or trembling
    Stomach cramps
    Unusual increase in sweating

The above side effects may be more likely to occur in infants, young children, and children with Down's syndrome. Shortness of breath or troubled breathing may also be more likely to occur in elderly patients.

Other side effects not listed above may also occur in some patients. If you notice any other effects, check with your doctor.

DIPYRIDAMOLE (Systemic)

Some commonly used brand names are Persantine, Pyridamole, and SK-Dipyridamole.

Generic name product may also be available.

Dipyridamole (dye-peer-ID-a-mole) is used to help prevent or reduce the occurrence of angina attacks. It will not relieve the pain of an attack that has already started.

This medicine works by relaxing blood vessels and increasing the supply of blood and oxygen to the heart.

Dipyridamole may also be used for other conditions as determined by your doctor.

Dipyridamole is available only with your doctor's prescription.

Before Using This Medicine

In order to decide on the best treatment for your medical problem, your doctor should be told:

—if you have ever had any unusual or allergic reaction to dipyridamole.

—if you are on a low-salt, low-sugar, or any other special diet, or if you are allergic to any substance, such as sulfites or other preservatives or dyes. Most medicines contain more than their active ingredient. Your doctor or pharmacist can help you avoid products that may cause a problem.

—if you are pregnant or if you intend to become pregnant while taking this medicine. Although dipyridamole has not been shown to cause problems in humans, the chance always exists.

—if you are breast-feeding an infant. Although dipyridamole has not been shown to cause problems in humans, the chance always exists.

—if you are now taking any of the following medicines or types of medicine:

Anticoagulants, oral (blood thinners you take by mouth)
Inflammation medicines, including ibuprofen and aspirin or other salicylates
Sulfinpyrazone
Valproic acid

Proper Use of This Medicine

This medicine works best when there is a constant amount in the blood. To help keep this amount constant, **dipyridamole must be taken in regularly spaced doses,** as ordered by your doctor.

This medicine works best when taken with a full glass (8 ounces) of water at least 1 hour before meals.

For patients taking this medicine for angina:

• Sometimes dipyridamole must be taken regularly for 2 or 3 months before it reaches its full effect in the treatment of angina. If you feel that the medicine is not working, do not stop taking it on your own. Instead, check with your doctor.

If you miss a dose of this medicine, take it as soon as possible. However, if it is within 4 hours of your next scheduled dose, skip the missed dose and go back to your regular dosing schedule. Do not double doses.

How to store this medicine:

• Store away from heat and direct light.

• **Keep out of the reach of children.**

• Do not store in the bathroom medicine cabinet because the heat or moisture may cause the medicine to break down.

• Do not keep outdated medicine or medicine no longer needed. Flush the contents of the container down the toilet, unless otherwise directed.

Precautions While Using This Medicine

For patients taking this medicine for angina:

• Dipyridamole is used to prevent angina attacks. **Do not take this medicine to relieve the pain of an attack** that has already started, because it works too slowly. Check with your doctor if you need a fast-acting medicine such as nitroglycerin to relieve the pain of an angina attack.

Dizziness, lightheadedness, or fainting may occur, especially when you get up from a lying or sitting position. Getting up slowly may help. If this problem continues or gets worse, check with your doctor.

Side Effects of This Medicine

Along with its needed effects, a medicine may cause some unwanted effects. Although not all of these side effects appear very often, when they do occur they may require medical attention. Check with your doctor as soon as possible if the following side effect occurs or gets worse shortly after you start taking this medicine:

Rare

   Chest pain or tightness in chest

Other side effects may occur which usually do not require medical attention. These side effects may go away during treatment as your body adjusts to the medicine. However, check with your doctor if they continue or are bothersome:

Less common

   Dizziness, lightheadedness, or fainting
   Flushing
   Headache
   Nausea or vomiting
   Skin rash
   Stomach cramping
   Weakness

Other side effects not listed above may also occur in some patients. If you notice any other effects, check with your doctor.

DISOPYRAMIDE (Systemic)

Some commonly used brand names are Norpace, Norpace CR, and Rythmodan*.

---

*Not available in the United States.

Disopyramide (dye-soe-PEER-a-mide) is used to correct irregular heartbeats to a normal rhythm and to slow an overactive heart. This allows the heart to work more efficiently.

Disopyramide is available only with your doctor's prescription.

Before Using This Medicine

In order to decide on the best treatment for your medical problem, your doctor should be told:

—if you have ever had any unusual or allergic reaction to disopyramide.

—if you are on a low-salt, low-sugar, or any other special diet, or if you are allergic to any substance, such as sulfites or other preservatives or dyes. Most medicines contain more than their active ingredient and many liquid medicines contain alcohol. Your doctor or pharmacist can help you avoid products that may cause a problem.

—if you are pregnant or if you intend to become pregnant while taking this medicine. Although studies in animals have not shown disopyramide to cause birth defects, studies have not been done in humans. Use in pregnant patients is limited. However, there are some reports that it caused contractions of the uterus when taken during pregnancy.

—if you are breast-feeding an infant. Although this medicine has not been shown to cause problems in humans, the chance always exists because it passes into breast milk.

—if you have any of the following medical problems:

Diabetes mellitus (sugar diabetes)
Difficult urination
Enlarged prostate
Glaucoma (history of)
Kidney disease
Liver disease
Myasthenia gravis

—if you are now taking any of the following medicines or types of medicine:

Anticoagulants, oral (blood thinners)
Antidiabetic agents, oral (diabetes medicine you take by mouth)
Antimuscarinics (medicines for abdominal or stomach spasms or cramps)
Barbiturates
Insulin
Medicine for angina or high blood pressure (such as propranolol or verapamil)
Other heart medicine
Phenytoin
Rifampin

Proper Use of This Medicine

Take disopyramide exactly as directed by your doctor even though you may feel well. Do not take more medicine than ordered and do not miss any doses.

Take disopyramide on an empty stomach, either 1 hour before or 2 hours after meals, unless otherwise directed by your doctor. This will allow it to work better.

If you do miss a dose of this medicine, take it as soon as possible unless the next scheduled dose is in less than 4 hours. If you do not remember until later, skip the missed dose and go back to your regular dosing schedule. Do not double doses.

For patients taking the extended-release capsules:

• Swallow the capsule whole without breaking, crushing, or chewing.

How to store this medicine:

• Store away from heat and direct light.

• **Keep out of the reach of children.**

• Do not store in the bathroom medicine cabinet because the heat or moisture may cause the medicine to break down.

• Do not keep outdated medicine or medicine no longer needed. Flush the contents of the container down the toilet, unless otherwise directed.

Precautions While Using This Medicine

Your doctor should check your progress at regular visits to make sure the medicine is working properly.

Do not stop taking this medicine without first checking with your doctor. Stopping suddenly may cause a serious change in heart function.

Disopyramide may cause hypoglycemia (low blood sugar) in some people. Patients with congestive heart disease or diabetes especially should be aware of the signs of hypoglycemia. (See *Side Effects of This Medicine.*) **If these signs appear, eat or drink a food containing sugar and call your doctor right away.**

Dizziness, lightheadedness, or fainting may occur, especially when you get up from a lying or sitting position. This is due to lowered blood pressure. Getting up slowly may help. This effect does not occur often at doses of disopyramide usually used; however, **make sure you know how you react to this medicine before you drive, use machines, or do other jobs that require you to be alert.** If the problem continues or gets worse, check with your doctor.

Avoid alcoholic beverages until you have discussed their use with your doctor. Alcohol may make the low blood sugar effect worse and/or increase the possibility of dizziness or fainting.

Your eyes, mouth, and nose may feel very dry while you are taking this medicine, especially during the first few weeks. To help relieve mouth dryness, chew sugarless gum or dissolve bits of ice in your mouth.

This medicine will often make you sweat less, allowing your body temperature to increase. **Use extra care not to become overheated during exercise or hot weather while you are taking this medicine** since overheating could possibly result in heat stroke.

Side Effects of This Medicine

Along with its needed effects, a medicine may cause some unwanted effects. Although not all of these side effects appear very often, when they do occur they may require medical attention. Check with your doctor as soon as possible if any of the following side effects occur:

More common
  Difficult urination

Less common
  Chest pains
  Confusion
  Dizziness, lightheadedness, or fainting
  Muscle weakness
  Shortness of breath (unexplained)
  Swelling of feet or lower legs
  Unusually fast or slow heartbeat
  Weight gain (rapid)

Rare
  Eye pain
  Mental depression
  Sore throat and fever
  Yellow eyes and skin

Signs of hypoglycemia (low blood sugar)
  Anxious feeling
  Chills
  Cold sweats
  Confusion
  Cool, pale skin
  Drowsiness
  Headache
  Hunger (excessive)
  Nausea

Nervousness
Rapid heartbeat
Shakiness
Unsteady walk
Unusual tiredness or weakness

Other side effects may occur which usually do not require medical attention. These side effects may go away during treatment as your body adjusts to the medicine. However, check with your doctor if any of the following side effects continue or are bothersome:

More common
  Dry mouth and throat

Less common
  Bloating or stomach pain
  Blurred vision
  Constipation
  Decreased sexual ability
  Dry eyes and nose
  Loss of appetite
  Unusually frequent urge to urinate

Some of the above side effects may be more likely to occur in the elderly, who are usually more sensitive to the effects of disopyramide.

Other side effects not listed above may also occur in some patients. If you notice any other effects, check with your doctor.

DIURETICS, LOOP (Systemic)

This information applies to the following medicines:

Bumetanide (byoo-MET-a-nide)
Ethacrynic acid (eth-a-KRIN-ik AS-id)
Furosemide (fur-OH-se-mide)

Some commonly used brand names are:	Generic names:
Bumex	Bumetanide
Edecrin	Ethacrynic acid

Apo-Furosemide*	
Furoside*	
Lasix	
Neo-Renal*	Furosemide†
Novosemide*	
SK-Furosemide	
Uritol*	

*Not available in the United States.
†Generic name product may also be available.

Loop diuretics are given to help reduce the amount of water in the body. They work by acting on the kidneys to increase the flow of urine.

Furosemide is also used to treat high blood pressure in those patients who are not helped by other medicines or in those patients who have kidney problems. High blood pressure adds to the workload of the heart and arteries. If it continues for a long time, they may not function properly. This can damage the blood vessels of the brain, heart, and kidneys, resulting in a stroke, heart attack, or kidney failure. These problems may be avoided if blood pressure is controlled.

Loop diuretics may also be used for other conditions as determined by your doctor.

This medicine is available only with your doctor's prescription.

Before Using This Medicine

In order to decide on the best treatment for your medical problem, your doctor should be told:

—if you have ever had any unusual or allergic reaction to bumetanide, ethacrynic acid, furosemide, sulfonamides (sulfa drugs), or thiazide diuretics.

—if you are on a low-salt, low-sugar, or any other special diet, or if you are allergic to any substance, such as sulfites or other preservatives or dyes. Most medicines contain more than their active ingredient, and many liquid medicines

contain alcohol. Your doctor or pharmacist can help you avoid products that may cause a problem.

—if you are pregnant or if you intend to become pregnant while taking this medicine. Although studies have not been done in humans, studies in animals have shown this medicine to cause harmful effects on the fetus. Also, ethacrynic acid causes birth defects in animals.

—if you are breast-feeding an infant. Although this medicine has not been shown to cause problems in humans, the chance always exists. Furosemide passes into breast milk; it is not known whether bumetanide or ethacrynic acid passes into breast milk.

—if you have any of the following medical problems:

Diabetes mellitus (sugar diabetes)
Diarrhea
Gout
Hearing problems
Kidney disease (severe)
Liver disease
Lupus erythematosus (history of)
Pancreas disease

—if you have recently had a heart attack.

—if you are now taking any of the following medicines or types of medicine:

Acetazolamide
Adrenocorticoids (cortisone-like medicines)
Allopurinol
Anticoagulants, oral (blood thinners you take by mouth)
Antidiabetic agents, oral (diabetes medicine you take by mouth)
Antihistamines
Antihypertensives (high blood pressure medicine)
Aspirin or other salicylates in very large doses (such as for arthritis)
Barbiturates
Buclizine
Chloral hydrate (for furosemide only)
Chlorprothixene
Clofibrate (for furosemide only)
Colchicine

Cyclizine
Cyclosporine
Dichlorphenamide
Digitalis glycosides (heart medicine)
Inflammation medicine, especially
  indomethacin
Insulin
Lithium
Loxapine
Meclizine
Methazolamide
Narcotics or prescription pain medicine
Other diuretics (water pills)
Phenothiazines
Primidone
Probenecid
Quinine
Sodium bicarbonate
Sulfinpyrazone
Tetracyclines
Thiothixene
Trimethobenzamide

Proper Use of This Medicine

This medicine may cause you to have an unusual feeling of tiredness when you begin to take it. You may also notice an increase in the amount of urine or in your frequency of urination. After taking the medicine for a while, these effects should lessen. In order to keep the increase in urine from affecting your nighttime sleep:

• If you are to take a single dose a day, take it in the morning after breakfast.

• If you are to take more than one dose a day, take the last dose no later than 6 p.m., unless otherwise directed by your doctor.

However, it is best to plan your dose or doses according to a schedule that will least affect your personal activities and sleep. Ask your doctor, nurse, or pharmacist to help you plan the best time to take this medicine.

In order to help remember to take your medicine, try to get into the habit of taking it at the same time each day.

If this medicine upsets your stomach, it may be taken with meals or milk. If stomach upset (nausea, vomiting, or stomach pain) continues or gets worse, or if you suddenly get severe diarrhea, check with your doctor.

If you miss a dose of this medicine, take it as soon as possible. However, if it is almost time for your next dose, skip the missed dose and go back to your regular dosing schedule. Do not double doses.

For patients taking this medicine for high blood pressure:

• Importance of diet—When prescribing medicine for your condition, your doctor may prescribe a personal diet for you. Such a diet may be low in sodium (salt). Most people eat much more sodium than they need and too much sodium in the diet may increase blood pressure. Some foods that contain large amounts of sodium include canned soup, pickles, ketchup, green and ripe olives, relish, frankfurters, soy sauce, and carbonated beverages. Your doctor may want you to limit the amounts of these and other high-sodium foods in your diet. Medicine is usually more effective when such a diet is properly followed.

Also, it may be very important for you to go on a reducing diet. However, check with your doctor before going on any diet.

• Many patients who have high blood pressure will not notice any signs of the problem. In fact, many may feel normal. It is very important that you take your medicine exactly as directed and that you keep your doctor's appointments even if you feel well.

• Remember that this medicine will not cure your high blood pressure but it does help control it. Therefore, you must continue to take it as directed if you expect to lower your blood pressure and keep it down. **You may have to take medicine for** the rest of your life. If high blood pressure is not treated, it can cause serious problems such as heart failure, blood vessel disease, stroke, or kidney disease.

For patients taking the oral liquid form of furosemide:

• This medicine is to be taken by mouth even though it may come in a dropper bottle. If this medicine does not come in a dropper bottle, use a specially marked measuring spoon or other device to measure each dose accurately, since the average household teaspoon may not hold the right amount of liquid.

How to store this medicine:

• Store away from heat and direct light.

• **Keep out of the reach of children.**

• Do not store in the bathroom medicine cabinet because the heat or moisture may cause the medicine to break down.

• Keep the oral liquid form of this medicine from freezing.

• Do not keep outdated medicine or medicine no longer needed. Flush the contents of the container down the toilet, unless otherwise directed.

Precautions While Using This Medicine

It is important that your doctor check your progress at regular visits to make sure that this medicine is working properly.

This medicine may cause a loss of potassium from your body.

• To help prevent this, your doctor may want you to:

—eat or drink foods that have a high potassium content (for example, orange or other citrus fruit juices), or

—take a potassium supplement, or

—take another medicine to help prevent the loss of the potassium in the first place.

• It is very important to follow these directions. Also, it is important not to change your diet on your own. This is more important if you are already on a special diet (as for diabetes), or if you are taking a potassium supplement or a medicine to reduce potassium loss. Extra potassium may not be necessary and, in some cases, too much potassium could be harmful.

To prevent the loss of too much water and potassium, tell your doctor if you become sick, especially with severe or continuing nausea and vomiting or diarrhea.

Before having any kind of surgery (including dental surgery) or emergency treatment, make sure the physician or dentist in charge knows that you are taking this medicine.

Dizziness, lightheadedness, or fainting may occur, especially when you get up from a lying or sitting position. This is more likely to occur in the morning. **Getting up slowly may help** but if the problem continues or gets worse, check with your doctor.

The dizziness, lightheadedness, or fainting is also more likely to occur if you drink alcohol, stand for long periods of time, or exercise, or if the weather is hot. **While you are taking this medicine, be careful of the amount of alcohol you drink. Also, use extra care during exercise or hot weather or if you must stand for long periods of time.**

Diabetics—This medicine may affect blood sugar levels. While you are using this medicine, be especially careful in testing for sugar in your urine.

For patients taking this medicine for high blood pressure:

• **Do not take other medicines unless they have been discussed with your doctor.**

This especially includes over-the-counter (nonprescription) medicines for appetite control, asthma, colds, cough, hay fever, or sinus problems, since they may tend to increase your blood pressure.

For patients taking furosemide:
• A few people who take this medicine may become more sensitive to sunlight than they are normally. When you begin to take this medicine, avoid too much sun or use of a sunlamp until you see how you react, especially if you tend to burn easily. If you have a severe reaction, check with your doctor.

Side Effects of This Medicine

Along with its needed effects, a medicine may cause some unwanted effects. Although not all of these side effects appear very often, when they do occur they may require medical attention. Check with your doctor as soon as possible if any of the following side effects occur:
Rare
　Black tarry stools—for ethacrynic acid injection only
　Blood in urine—for ethacrynic acid injection only
　Joint, flank, or stomach pain
　Ringing or buzzing sound in ears or any loss of hearing—more common with ethacrynic acid
　Skin rash or hives
　Sore throat and fever
　Stomach pain (severe) with nausea and vomiting
　Unusual bleeding or bruising
　Yellowing of the eyes or skin
　Yellow vision—for furosemide only
Signs of loss of too much potassium
　Dryness of mouth
　Increased thirst
　Irregular heartbeats
　Mood or mental changes
　Muscle cramps or pain
　Nausea or vomiting
　Unusual tiredness or weakness
　Weak pulse

Other side effects may occur which usually do not require medical attention. These side effects may go away during treatment as your body adjusts to the medicine. However, check with your doctor if any of the following side effects continue or are bothersome:
More common—less common with bumetanide
　Dizziness or lightheadedness when getting up from a lying or sitting position
Less common
　Blurred vision
　Chest pain—with bumetanide only
　Confusion—with ethacrynic acid only
　Diarrhea—more common with ethacrynic acid
　Headache
　Increased sensitivity of skin to sunlight—with furosemide only
　Loss of appetite—more common with ethacrynic acid
　Nervousness—with ethacrynic acid only
　Premature ejaculation or difficulty in keeping an erection—with bumetanide only
　Redness or pain at the place of injection
　Stomach cramps or pain

Dizziness, lightheadedness, or signs of too much potassium loss may be more likely to occur in the elderly, who are more sensitive to the effects of this medicine.

Other side effects not listed above may also occur in some patients. If you notice any other effects, check with your doctor.

DIURETICS, POTASSIUM-SPARING, AND HYDROCHLOROTHIAZIDE (Systemic)

This information applies to the following medicines:

Amiloride (a-MILL-oh-ride) and Hydrochlorothiazide (hye-droe-klor-oh-THYE-a-zide)

Spironolactone (speer-on-oh-LAK-tone) and Hydrochlorothiazide

Triamterene (trye-AM-ter-een) and Hydrochlorothiazide

Some commonly used brand names are:	Generic names:
Moduretic	Amiloride and Hydrochlorothiazide
Aldactazide	Spironolactone and Hydrochlorothiazide†
Dyazide Maxzide	Triamterene and Hydrochlorothiazide

†Generic name product may also be available.

This medicine is a combination of two diuretics (water pills). It is commonly taken by mouth to help reduce the amount of water in the body.

This combination is also used to treat high blood pressure. High blood pressure adds to the workload of the heart and arteries. If it continues for a long time, they may not function properly. This can damage the blood vessels of the brain, heart, and kidneys, resulting in a stroke, heart attack, or kidney failure. These problems may be avoided if blood pressure is controlled.

Diuretics help to reduce the amount of water in the body by acting on the kidneys to increase the flow of urine. This also helps to lower blood pressure.

This medicine is available only with your doctor's prescription.

Before Using This Medicine

In order to decide on the best treatment for your medical problem, your doctor should be told:

—if you have ever had any unusual or allergic reaction to amiloride, spironolactone, triamterene, sulfonamides (sulfa drugs), or to hydrochlorothiazide or any of the other thiazide diuretics.

—if you are on a low-salt, low-sugar, or any other special diet, or if you are allergic to any substance, such as sulfites or other preservatives or dyes. Most medicines contain more than their active ingredient. Your doctor or pharmacist can help you avoid products that may cause a problem.

—if you are pregnant or if you intend to become pregnant while using this medicine. When hydrochlorothiazide is used during pregnancy, it may cause side effects including jaundice, blood problems, and low potassium in the newborn infant. In addition, although this medicine has not been shown to cause birth defects, the chance always exists.

In general, diuretics are not useful for normal swelling of feet and hands that occurs during pregnancy. They should not be taken during pregnancy unless recommended by your doctor.

—if you are breast-feeding an infant. Although this medicine has not been shown to cause problems in humans, the chance always exists since spironolactone, triamterene, and hydrochlorothiazide may pass into breast milk. It is not known whether amiloride passes into breast milk.

—if you have any of the following medical problems:
  Diabetes mellitus (sugar diabetes)
  Gout
  Kidney disease
  Kidney stones (history of—triamterene only)
  Liver disease
  Lupus erythematosus (history of)
  Menstrual problems or breast enlargement (spironolactone only)
  Pancreas disease

—if you are now taking or using any of the following medicines or types of medicine:

Acetazolamide
Adrenocorticoids (cortisone-like medicine)
Allopurinol
Ammonium chloride (spironolactone only)
Amphotericin B
Anthralin
Anticoagulants, oral (blood thinners you take by mouth)
Antidiabetics, oral (diabetes medicine you take by mouth)
Carbenoxolone (spironolactone only)
Cholestyramine
Coal tar
Colchicine
Colestipol
Corticotropin (ACTH)
Dichlorphenamide
Digitalis glycosides (heart medicine)
Fluorouracil skin solution or cream
Inflammation medicines, especially indomethacin
Insulin
Laxatives
Lithium
Methazolamide
Methenamine
Methoxsalen
Nalidixic acid
Other diuretics (water pills) or antihypertensives (high blood pressure medicine)
Phenothiazines
Potassium-containing medicines or supplements
Probenecid
Salt substitutes
Sodium bicarbonate (baking soda)
Sulfinpyrazone
Sulfonamides (sulfa medicine)
Tetracyclines
Trioxsalen

Proper Use of This Medicine

This medicine may cause you to have an unusual feeling of tiredness when you begin to take it. You may also notice an increase in the amount of urine or in your frequency of urination. After you have taken the medicine for a while, these effects should lessen. In general, in order to keep the increase in urine from affecting your nighttime sleep:

• If you are to take a single dose a day, take it in the morning after breakfast.

• If you are to take more than one dose a day, take the last dose no later than 6 p.m., unless otherwise directed by your doctor.

However, it is best to plan your dose or doses according to a schedule that will least affect your personal activities and sleep. Ask your doctor, nurse, or pharmacist to help you plan the best time to take this medicine.

In order to help remember to take your medicine, try to get into the habit of taking it at the same time each day.

If this medicine upsets your stomach, it may be taken with meals or milk. If stomach upset (nausea, vomiting, stomach pain or cramps) continues, check with your doctor.

For patients taking this medicine for high blood pressure:

• Importance of diet—When prescribing medicine for your condition, your doctor may also prescribe a personal diet for you. Such a diet may be low in sodium (salt). Most people eat much more sodium than they need and too much sodium in the diet may increase blood pressure. Some foods that contain large amounts of sodium include canned soup, pickles, ketchup, green and ripe olives, relish, frankfurters, soy sauce, and carbonated beverages. Your doctor may want you to limit the amounts of these and other high-sodium foods in your diet. Medicine is usually more effective when such a diet is properly followed.

Also, it may be very important for you to go on a reducing diet. However, check with your doctor before going on any diet.

• Many patients who have high blood pressure will not notice any signs of the problem. In fact, many may feel normal. It is very important that you take your medicine exactly as directed and that you keep your doctor's appointments even if you feel well.

• Remember that this medicine will not cure your high blood pressure but it does help control it. Therefore, you must continue to take it as directed if you expect to lower your blood pressure and keep it down. **You may have to take medicine for the rest of your life.** If high blood pressure is not treated, it can cause serious problems such as heart failure, blood vessel disease, stroke, or kidney disease.

If you miss a dose of this medicine, take it as soon as possible. However, if it is almost time for your next dose, skip the missed dose and go back to your regular dosing schedule. Do not double doses.

How to store this medicine:
• Store away from heat and direct light.

• **Keep out of the reach of children.**

• Do not store in the bathroom medicine cabinet because the heat or moisture may cause the medicine to break down.

• Keep the oral liquid form of this medicine from freezing.

• Do not keep outdated medicine or medicine no longer needed. Flush the contents of the container down the toilet, unless otherwise directed.

Precautions While Using This Medicine

It is important that your doctor check your progress at regular visits in order to make sure that this medicine is working properly.

This medicine may cause a loss or increase of potassium in your body. Your doctor may have special instructions about eating or drinking foods or beverages that have a high potassium content (for example, orange or other citrus fruit juices), taking a potassium supplement, or using salt substitutes. It is important not to change your diet on your own. Tell your doctor if you are already on a special diet (as for diabetes), or if you are taking a potassium supplement or using salt substitutes. Check with your doctor, nurse, or pharmacist if you need a list of foods which are high in potassium or if you have any questions.

Check with your doctor if you become sick and have severe or continuing vomiting or diarrhea. These problems may cause you to lose additional water and potassium.

Diabetics—Hydrochlorothiazide may raise blood sugar levels. While you are taking this medicine, be especially careful in testing for sugar in your urine.

A few people who take this medicine may become more sensitive to sunlight than they are normally. When you begin to take this medicine, avoid too much sun or use of a sunlamp until you see how you react, especially if you tend to burn easily. If you have a severe reaction, check with your doctor.

Before having any kind of surgery (including dental surgery) or emergency treatment, tell the physician or dentist in charge that you are taking this medicine.

For patients taking this medicine for high blood pressure:

• **Do not take other medicines unless they have been discussed with your doctor.** This especially includes over-the-counter (nonprescription) medicines for appetite control, asthma, colds, cough, hay fever, or sinus problems, since they may tend to increase your blood pressure.

Side Effects of This Medicine

In rats, spironolactone has been found to increase the risk of development of tumors. The doses given were many times the dose of spironolactone given to humans. It is not known whether spironolactone causes tumors in humans.

Along with its needed effects, a medicine may cause some unwanted effects. Although not all of these side effects appear very often, when they do occur they may require medical attention. Check with your doctor as soon as possible if any of the following side effects occur:

Rare
Joint pain
Skin rash or hives
Sore throat and fever
Stomach pain (severe) with nausea and vomiting
Unusual bleeding or bruising
Yellowing of eyes or skin

Signs of changes in potassium
Dryness of mouth
Increased thirst
Irregular heartbeats
Mood or mental changes
Muscle cramps or pain
Numbness or tingling in hands, feet, or lips
Shortness of breath or difficult breathing
Unusual tiredness or weakness
Weak pulse

Reported for triamterene only (rare)
Bright red tongue
Burning, inflamed feeling in tongue
Cracked corners of mouth

Other side effects may occur which usually do not require medical attention. These side effects may go away during treatment as your body adjusts to the medicine. However, check with your doctor if any of the following side effects continue or are bothersome:

More common (less common with triamterene)
Loss of appetite
Nausea and vomiting
Stomach cramps and diarrhea
Upset stomach

Less common
Decreased sexual ability
Dizziness or lightheadedness when getting up from a lying or sitting position
Increased sensitivity of skin to sunlight

Reported for amiloride and triamterene only (less common)
Constipation
Headache (more common with amiloride)

Reported for spironolactone only (less common)
Breast tenderness in females
Clumsiness
Deepening of voice in females
Enlargement of breasts in males
Increased hair growth in females
Irregular menstrual periods
Unusual sweating

Dizziness or lightheadedness and signs of too much potassium loss may be more likely to occur in the elderly, who are more sensitive to the effects of this medicine.

Spironolactone sometimes causes enlarged breasts in males, especially when they take large doses of it for a long time. Breasts usually decrease in size gradually over several months after this medicine is stopped. If you have any questions about this, check with your doctor.

Other side effects not listed above may also occur in some patients. If you notice any other effects, check with your doctor.

DIURETICS, THIAZIDE
(Systemic)

This information applies to the following medicines:

Bendroflumethiazide (ben-droe-floo-meth-EYE-a-zide)
Benzthiazide (benz-THYE-a-zide)
Chlorothiazide (klor-oh-THYE-a-zide)
Chlorthalidone (klor-THAL-i-doan)
Cyclothiazide (sye-kloe-THYE-a-zide)
Hydrochlorothiazide (hye-droe-klor-oh-THYE-a-zide)
Hydroflumethiazide (hye-droe-floo-meth-EYE-a-zide)
Methyclothiazide (meth-ee-kloe-THYE-a-zide)
Metolazone (me-TOLE-a-zone)
Polythiazide (pol-i-THYE-a-zide)
Quinethazone (kwin-ETH-a-zone)
Trichlormethiazide (trye-klor-meth-EYE-a-zide)

Some commonly used brand names are:	Generic names:
Naturetin	Bendroflume-thiazide
Aquatag Exna Hydrex	Benzthiazide†
Diuril SK-Chlorothiazide	Chlorothiazide†
Hygroton Novothalidone* Thalitone Uridon*	Chlorthalidone†
Anhydron Fluidil	Cyclothiazide
Esidrix Hydrochlorothiazide Intensol HydroDIURIL Mictrin Novohydrazide* Oretic SK-Hydrochlorothiazide Thiuretic	Hydrochloro-thiazide†
Diucardin Saluron	Hydroflume-thiazide†
Aquatensen Duretic* Enduron	Methyclothiazide†
Diulo Zaroxolyn	Metolazone
Renese	Polythiazide
Hydromox	Quinethazone
Metahydrin Naqua	Trichlorme-thiazide†

*Not available in the United States.
†Generic name product may also be available.

Thiazide or thiazide-like diuretics are commonly used to treat high blood pressure. High blood pressure adds to the workload of the heart and arteries. If it continues for a long time, they may not function properly. This can damage the blood vessels of the brain, heart, and kidneys, resulting in a stroke, heart attack, or kidney failure. These problems may be avoided if blood pressure is controlled.

Thiazide diuretics are also used to help reduce the amount of water in the body by increasing the flow of urine. They may also be used for other conditions as determined by your doctor.

Thiazide diuretics are available only with your doctor's prescription.

Before Using This Medicine

In order to decide on the best treatment for your medical problem, your doctor should be told:

—if you have ever had any unusual or allergic reaction to sulfonamides (sulfa drugs) or any of the thiazide diuretics.

—if you are on a low-salt, low-sugar, or any other special diet, or if you are allergic to any substance, such as sulfites or other preservatives or dyes. Most medicines contain more than their active ingredient, and many liquid medicines contain alcohol. Your doctor or pharmacist can help you avoid products that may cause a problem.

—if you are pregnant or if you intend to become pregnant while using this medicine. When this medicine is used during pregnancy, it may cause side effects including jaundice, blood problems, and low potassium in the newborn infant. In addition, although this medicine has not been shown to cause birth defects or other problems in animal studies, studies have not been done in humans.

—if you are breast-feeding an infant. Although thiazide diuretics have not been shown to cause problems in humans, the chance always exists since thiazide diuretics pass into breast milk.

—if you have any of the following medical problems:

Diabetes mellitus (sugar diabetes)
Gout (history of)
Kidney disease (severe)
Liver disease
Lupus erythematosus (history of)
Pancreas disease

—if you are now taking or using any of the following medicines or types of medicine:

Acetazolamide
Adrenocorticoids (cortisone-like medicines)
Allopurinol
Anthralin
Anticoagulants, oral (blood thinners you take by mouth)
Antidiabetics, oral (diabetes medicine you take by mouth)
Cholestyramine
Coal tar
Colchicine
Colestipol
Dichlorphenamide
Digitalis glycosides (heart medicine)
Fluorouracil skin solution or cream
Inflammation medicines, especially indomethacin
Insulin
Lithium
Methazolamide
Methenamine

Methoxsalen
Nalidixic acid
Other diuretics (water pills) or antihypertensives (high blood pressure medicine)
Phenothiazines
Probenecid
Sodium bicarbonate (baking soda)
Sulfinpyrazone
Sulfonamides (sulfa medicine)
Tetracyclines
Trioxsalen

Proper Use of This Medicine

This medicine may cause you to have an unusual feeling of tiredness when you begin to take it. You may also notice an increase in the amount of urine or in your frequency of urination. After taking the medicine for a while, these effects should lessen. In order to keep the increase in urine from affecting your nighttime sleep:

• If you are to take a single dose a day, take it in the morning after breakfast.

• If you are to take more than one dose a day, take the last dose no later than 6 p.m., unless otherwise directed by your doctor.

However, it is best to plan your dose or doses according to a schedule that will least affect your personal activities and sleep. Ask your doctor, nurse, or pharmacist to help you plan the best time to take this medicine.

In order to help remember to take your medicine, try to get into the habit of taking it at the same time each day.

For patients taking this medicine for high blood pressure:

• Importance of diet—When prescribing medicine for your condition, your doctor may also prescribe a personal diet for you. Such a diet may be low in sodium (salt). Most people eat much more sodium than they need and too much sodium in the diet may increase blood pressure. Some foods that contain large amounts of sodium include canned soup, pickles, ketchup, green and ripe olives, relish, frankfurters, soy sauce, and carbonated beverages. Your doctor may want you to limit the amounts of these and other high-sodium foods in your diet. Medicine is usually more effective when such a diet is properly followed.

Also, it may be very important for you to go on a reducing diet. However, check with your doctor before going on any diet.

• Many patients who have high blood pressure will not notice any signs of the problem. In fact, many may feel normal. It is very important that you take your medicine exactly as directed and that you keep your doctor's appointments even if you feel well.

• Remember that this medicine will not cure your high blood pressure but it does control it. Therefore, you must continue to take it as directed if you expect to lower your blood pressure and keep it down. **You may have to take medicine for the rest of your life.** If high blood pressure is not treated, it can cause serious problems such as heart failure, blood vessel disease, stroke, or kidney disease.

For patients taking the oral liquid form of hydrochlorothiazide which comes in a dropper bottle:

• This medicine is to be taken by mouth. The amount you should take is to be measured only with the specially marked dropper.

If you miss a dose of this medicine, take it as soon as possible. However, if it is almost time for your next dose, skip the missed dose and go back to your regular dosing schedule. Do not double doses.

How to store this medicine:

• Store away from heat and direct light.

• **Keep out of the reach of children.**

• Do not store in the bathroom medicine cabinet because the heat or moisture may cause the medicine to break down.

• Keep the oral liquid form of this medicine from freezing.

• Do not keep outdated medicine or medicine no longer needed. Flush the contents of the container down the toilet, unless otherwise directed.

Precautions While Using This Medicine

It is important that your doctor check your progress at regular visits in order to make sure that this medicine is working properly.

This medicine may cause a loss of potassium from your body.

• To help prevent this, your doctor may want you to:

—eat or drink foods that have a high potassium content (for example, orange or other citrus fruit juices), or

—take a potassium supplement, or

—take another medicine to help prevent the loss of the potassium in the first place.

• It is very important to follow these directions. Also, it is important not to change your diet on your own. This is more important if you are already on a special diet (as for diabetes), or if you are taking a potassium supplement or a medicine to reduce potassium loss. Extra potassium may not be necessary and, in some cases, too much potassium could be harmful.

Check with your doctor if you become sick and have severe or continuing vomiting or diarrhea. These problems may cause you to lose additional water and potassium.

Diabetics—Thiazide diuretics may raise blood sugar levels. While you are using this medicine, be especially careful in testing for sugar in your urine. If you have any questions about this, check with your doctor.

A few people who take this medicine may become more sensitive to sunlight than they are normally. When you begin to take this medicine, avoid too much sun or use of a sunlamp until you see how you react, especially if you tend to burn easily. If you have a severe reaction, check with your doctor.

For patients taking this medicine for high blood pressure:

• **Do not take other medicines unless they have been discussed with your doctor.** This especially includes over-the-counter (nonprescription) medicines for appetite control, asthma, colds, cough, hay fever, or sinus problems, since they may tend to increase your blood pressure.

Side Effects of This Medicine

Along with its needed effects, a medicine may cause some unwanted effects. Although not all of these side effects appear very often, when they do occur they may require medical attention. Check with your doctor as soon as possible if any of the following side effects occur:

Rare
> Joint, flank, or stomach pain
> Skin rash or hives
> Sore throat and fever
> Stomach pain (severe) with nausea and vomiting
> Unusual bleeding or bruising
> Yellowing of eyes or skin

Signs of too much potassium loss
> Dryness of mouth
> Increased thirst
> Irregular heartbeats
> Mood or mental changes
> Muscle cramps or pain
> Nausea or vomiting
> Unusual tiredness or weakness
> Weak pulse

Other side effects may occur which usually do not require medical attention. These side effects may go away during treatment as your body adjusts to the medicine. However, check with your doctor if any of the following side effects continue or are bothersome:

Less common
> Decreased sexual ability
> Diarrhea
> Dizziness or lightheadedness when getting up from a lying or sitting position
> Increased sensitivity of skin to sunlight
> Loss of appetite
> Upset stomach

Dizziness or lightheadedness and signs of too much potassium loss may be more likely to occur in the elderly, who are more sensitive to the effects of thiazide diuretics.

Other side effects not listed above may also occur in some patients. If you notice any other effects, check with your doctor.

Additional Information

For patients taking this medicine for diabetes insipidus (water diabetes):

• Some thiazide diuretics are used in the treatment of diabetes insipidus (water diabetes). In patients with water diabetes, this medicine causes a decrease in the flow of urine and helps the body hold water. Thus, the information given above about increased urine flow will not apply to you.

ENALAPRIL (Systemic)

A commonly used brand name is Vasotec.

Enalapril (e-NAL-a-pril) belongs to the general class of medicines called antihypertensives. It is used to treat high blood pressure. High blood pressure adds to the workload of the heart and arteries. If it continues for a long time, they may not function properly. This can damage the blood vessels of the brain, heart, and kidneys, resulting in a stroke, heart attack, or kidney failure. These problems may be avoided if blood pressure is controlled.

The exact way that enalapril works is not known. It blocks an enzyme in the blood that causes blood vessels to tighten. As a result, it probably relaxes blood vessels, which lowers blood pressure and increases the supply of blood and oxygen to the heart.

Enalapril may also be used for other conditions as determined by your doctor.

Enalapril is available only with your doctor's prescription.

Before Using This Medicine

In order to decide on the best treatment for your medical problem, your doctor should be told:

—if you have ever had any unusual or allergic reaction to enalapril or captopril.

—if you are on a low-salt, low-sugar, or any other special diet, or if you are allergic to any substance, such as sulfites or other preservatives or dyes. Most medicines contain more than their active ingredient. Your doctor or pharmacist can help you avoid products that may cause a problem.

—if you are pregnant or if you intend to become pregnant while using this medicine. Studies have not been done in humans. Studies in rats at doses many times the recommended human dose have not shown that enalapril causes problems; however, studies in rabbits have shown that enalapril causes an increase in deaths of the fetus. This medicine has not been shown to cause birth defects in rats or rabbits.

—if you are breast-feeding an infant. Although enalapril has not been shown to cause problems in humans, the chance always exists.

—if you have any of the following medical problems:
  Diabetes mellitus (sugar diabetes)
  Heart or blood vessel disease
  Kidney disease
  Systemic lupus erythematosus
  (SLE)

—if you have recently had a heart attack or stroke.

—if you are now taking any of the following medicines or types of medicine:
  Azathioprine
  Cancer medicines
  Chloramphenicol
  Colchicine
  Diuretics (water pills)
  Flucytosine
  Inflammation medicines, especially indomethacin
  Other antihypertensives (high blood pressure medicine)
  Oxyphenbutazone
  Penicillamine
  Phenylbutazone
  Potassium supplements
  Primaquine
  Pyrimethamine
  Salt substitutes
  Trimethoprim

Proper Use of This Medicine

In order to help remember to take your medicine, try to get into the habit of taking it at the same time each day.

For patients taking enalapril for high blood pressure:

• Importance of diet—When prescribing medicine for your condition, your doctor may also prescribe a personal diet for you. Such a diet may be low in sodium (salt). Most people eat much more sodium than they need and too much sodium in the diet may increase blood pressure. Some foods that contain large amounts of sodium include canned soup, pickles, ketchup, green and ripe olives, relish, frankfurters, soy sauce, and carbonated beverages. Your doctor may want you to limit the amounts of these and other high-sodium foods in your diet. Medicine is usually more effective when such a diet is properly followed.

Also, it may be very important for you to go on a reducing diet. However, check with your doctor before going on any diet.

• Many patients who have high blood pressure will not notice any signs of the problem. In fact, many may feel normal. It is very important that you **take your medicine exactly as directed** and that you keep your doctor's appointments even if you feel well.

• Remember that enalapril will not cure your high blood pressure but it does help control it. Therefore, you must continue to take it as directed if you expect to lower your blood pressure and keep it down. **You may have to take medicine for the rest of your life.** If high blood pressure is not treated, it can cause serious problems such as heart failure, blood vessel disease, stroke, or kidney disease.

If you miss a dose of this medicine, take it as soon as possible. However, if it is almost time for your next dose, skip the missed dose and go back to your regular dosing schedule. Do not double doses.

How to store this medicine:

• Store away from heat and direct light.

• **Keep out of the reach of children.**

• Do not store in the bathroom medicine cabinet because the heat or moisture may cause the medicine to break down.

• Do not keep outdated medicine or medicine no longer needed. Flush the contents of the container down the toilet, unless otherwise directed.

Precautions While Using This Medicine

It is important that your doctor check your progress at regular visits in order to make sure that this medicine is working properly and check for unwanted effects.

Dizziness, lightheadedness, or fainting may occur if you exercise or if the weather is hot. Use extra care during exercise or hot weather.

Check with your doctor right away if you become sick while taking enalapril, especially with severe or continuing nausea and vomiting or diarrhea. These conditions may cause you to lose too much water.

Chest pain resulting from exercise or physical exertion is usually reduced or prevented by enalapril. This may tempt a patient to be overly active. **Make sure you discuss with your doctor a safe amount of exercise for your medical problem.**

Since salt substitutes and low-salt milk may contain potassium, do not use them unless told to do so by your doctor.

Before having any kind of surgery (including dental surgery) or emergency treatment, tell the physician or dentist in charge that you are taking enalapril.

For patients taking enalapril for high blood pressure:

• **Do not take other medicines unless they have been discussed with your doctor.** This especially includes over-the-counter (nonprescription) medicines for appetite control, asthma, colds, cough, hay fever, or sinus problems, since they may tend to increase your blood pressure.

Side Effects of This Medicine

Along with its needed effects, a medicine may cause some unwanted effects. Although not all of these side effects appear very often, when they do occur they may require medical attention. **Check with your doctor immediately if the following side effects occur:**

Rare

Difficult breathing
Fever and chills or sore throat
Swelling of face, mouth, hands, or feet

Check with your doctor as soon as possible if the following side effects occur:

Less common

Chest pain
Dizziness, lightheadedness, or
fainting
Skin rash

Other side effects may occur which usually do not require medical attention. These side effects may go away during treatment as your body adjusts to the medicine. However, check with your doctor if the following side effects continue or are bothersome:

Less common

Cough
Diarrhea
Headache
Loss of taste
Nausea
Unusual tiredness

Dizziness and lightheadedness are more likely to occur in the elderly, who are more sensitive to the effects of enalapril.

Other side effects not listed above may also occur in some patients. If you notice any other effects, check with your doctor.

ERYTHROMYCINS (Systemic)

Some commonly used brand names are:	Generic names:
E-Mycin Eryc Ery-Tab Erythromid* Ilotycin Novorythro* Robimycin RP-Mycin	Erythromycin†
Ilosone Novorythro*	Erythromycin Estolate†
E.E.S. E-Mycin E EryPed Pediamycin Wyamycin E	Erythromycin Ethylsuccinate†
Ilotycin	Erythromycin Gluceptate
Erythrocin	Erythromycin Lactobionate†
Erypar Erythrocin Ethril Novorythro* SK-Erythromycin Wyamycin S	Erythromycin Stearate†

*Not available in the United States.
†Generic name product may also be available.

Erythromycins (eh-rith-roe-MYE-sins) belong to the general family of medicines called antibiotics. They are taken by mouth or given by injection to help the body overcome infections. Erythromycins are also used to prevent "strep" infections in patients with a history of rheumatic heart disease who may be allergic to penicillin. They may also be used in Legionnaires' disease and for other problems as determined by your doctor. They will not work for colds, flu, or other virus infections.

Erythromycins are available only with your doctor's prescription.

Before Using This Medicine

In order to decide on the best treatment for your medical problem, your doctor should be told:

—if you have ever had any unusual or allergic reaction to any of the erythromycins.

—if you are on a low-salt, low-sugar, or any other special diet, or if you are allergic to any substance, such as sulfites or other preservatives or dyes. Most medicines contain more than their active ingredient, and many liquid medicines contain alcohol. Your doctor or pharmacist can help you avoid products that may cause a problem.

—if you are pregnant or if you intend to become pregnant while taking this medicine. Although erythromycins have not been shown to cause birth defects or other problems in humans, the chance always exists.

—if you are breast-feeding an infant. Erythromycins pass into the breast milk. Although erythromycins have not been shown to cause problems in humans, the chance always exists.

—if you have liver disease.

—if you are now taking any of the following medicines or types of medicine:

Aminophylline
Carbamazepine
Chloramphenicol
Clindamycin
Lincomycin
Oxtriphylline
Penicillins
Theophylline
Warfarin

—if you have ever had any problems with erythromycin estolate.

Proper Use of This Medicine

To help clear up your infection completely, **keep taking this medicine for the full time of treatment** even if you begin to feel better after a few days. **If you have a** "strep" infection, you should keep taking this medicine for at least 10 days. This is especially important in "strep" infections since serious heart problems could develop later if your infection is not completely cleared up. Also, if you stop taking this medicine too soon, your symptoms may return.

This medicine works best when there is a constant amount in the blood. **To help keep this amount constant, do not miss any doses. Also, it is best to take each dose at evenly spaced times day and night.** For example, if you are to take 4 doses a day, each dose should be spaced about 6 hours apart. If this interferes with your sleep or other daily activities, or if you need help in planning the best times to take your medicine, check with your doctor, nurse, or pharmacist.

If you do miss a dose of this medicine, take it as soon as possible. This will help to keep a constant amount of medicine in the blood. However, if it is almost time for your next dose and your dosing schedule is:

• 2 doses a day—Space the missed dose and the next dose 5 to 6 hours apart.

• 3 or more doses a day—Space the missed dose and the next dose 2 to 4 hours apart or double your next dose.

Then go back to your regular dosing schedule.

Generally, erythromycins are best taken with a full glass (8 ounces) of water on an empty stomach (for example, 1 hour before or 3 to 4 hours after meals), unless otherwise directed by your doctor. However, certain brands of erythromycin enteric-coated tablets, as well as erythromycin estolate and erythromycin ethylsuccinate, may be taken on a full or empty stomach. In addition, certain brands of erythromycin stearate tablets may be taken on an empty stomach or immediately before meals. If you have any questions about this, check with your doctor or pharmacist.

For patients taking the oral liquid form of this medicine:

• This medicine is to be taken by mouth even though it may come in a dropper bottle. If this medicine does not come in a dropper bottle, use a specially marked measuring spoon or other device to measure each dose accurately since the average household teaspoon may not hold the right amount of liquid.

• Do not use after the expiration date on the label since the medicine may not work as well. Check with your pharmacist if you have any questions about this.

For patients taking the chewable tablet form of this medicine:

• Tablets must be chewed or crushed before they are swallowed.

For patients taking the capsule form (with enteric-coated pellets) or enteric-coated tablet form of this medicine:

• Swallow capsules or tablets whole. Do not break or crush. If you are not sure about the capsule or tablet you are taking, check with your pharmacist.

How to store this medicine:

• Store the liquid form of some erythromycins in the refrigerator because heat will cause this medicine to break down. Follow the directions on the label. However, keep the medicine from freezing.

• **Keep out of the reach of children.**

• Do not keep outdated medicine or medicine no longer needed. Flush the contents of the container down the toilet, unless otherwise directed.

Precautions While Using This Medicine

If your symptoms do not improve within a few days or if they become worse, check with your doctor.

Side Effects of This Medicine

Along with its needed effects, a medicine may cause some unwanted effects. Although not all of these side effects appear very often, when they do occur they may require medical attention. **Stop taking this medicine and check with your doctor immediately** if any of the following side effects occur:

Rare (more common with erythromycin estolate)

    Dark or amber urine
    Pale stools
    Stomach pain (severe)
    Unusual tiredness or weakness
    Yellowing of eyes or skin

Rare (with kidney disease and high doses)

    Loss of hearing (temporary)

Other side effects may occur which usually do not require medical attention. These side effects may go away during treatment as your body adjusts to the medicine. However, check with your doctor if any of the following side effects continue or are bothersome:

Less common

    Diarrhea
    Nausea or vomiting
    Sore mouth or tongue
    Stomach cramping and discomfort

Other side effects not listed above may also occur in some patients. If you notice any other effects, check with your doctor.

ERYTHROMYCIN AND SULFISOXAZOLE (Systemic)

A commonly used brand name is Pediazole.

Erythromycin (eh-rith-roe-MYE-sin) and sulfisoxazole (sul-fi-SOX-a-zole) is a combination antibiotic and sulfa medicine.

Antibiotics and sulfas are used in the treatment of infections caused by bacteria. They work by killing bacteria or preventing their growth.

Erythromycin and sulfisoxazole combination is taken by mouth to help the body's natural defenses overcome ear infections. It may also be used for other problems as determined by your doctor. It will not work for colds, flu, or other virus infections.

Erythromycin and sulfisoxazole combination is available only with your doctor's prescription.

For information about the precautions and side effects of the medicines in this combination, see:

Erythromycins (Systemic)
Sulfonamides (Systemic)

Combination products are designed for specific uses. These uses may not be the same as the uses of the individual ingredients. Therefore, some of the information provided in the individual listings may not be relevant to the combination product. If questions arise, check with your doctor, nurse, or pharmacist.

FLECAINIDE (Systemic)

A commonly used brand name is Tambocor.

Flecainide (FLEK-a-nide) belongs to the group of medicines known as antiarrhythmics. It is taken by mouth to correct irregular heartbeats to a normal rhythm.

Flecainide produces its helpful effects by slowing nerve impulses in the heart and making the heart tissue less sensitive.

This medicine is available only with your doctor's prescription.

Before Using This Medicine

In order to decide on the best treatment for your medical problem, your doctor should be told:

—if you have ever had any unusual or allergic reaction to flecainide or anesthetics.

—if you are on a low-salt, low-sugar, or any other special diet, or if you are allergic to any substance, such as sulfites or other preservatives or dye. Most medicines contain more than their active ingredient. Your doctor or pharmacist can help you avoid products that may cause a problem.

—if you are pregnant or if you intend to become pregnant while using this medicine. Studies have not been done in humans. However, studies in one kind of rabbit given about 4 times the usual human dose have shown that flecainide causes birth defects.

—if you are breast-feeding. Although it is not known whether flecainide passes into breast milk and it has not been shown to cause problems in humans, the chance always exists.

—if you have any of the following medical problems:
Kidney disease
Liver disease

—if you have a pacemaker.

—if you have recently had a heart attack.

—if you are now taking any of the following medicines or types of medicine:
Antineoplastics (cancer medicine)
Azathioprine
Beta-adrenergic blocking agents (acebutolol, atenolol, labetalol, metoprolol, nadolol, oxprenolol, pindolol, propranolol, sotalol, or timolol)
Chloramphenicol
Colchicine
Flucytosine
Other heart medicine
Oxyphenbutazone

Penicillamine
Phenylbutazone
Primaquine
Pyrimethamine
Trimethoprim

Proper Use of This Medicine

Take flecainide exactly as directed by your doctor, even though you may feel well. Do not take more medicine than ordered.

This medicine works best when there is a constant amount in the blood. To help keep this amount constant, do not miss any doses. Also, it is best to take the doses 12 hours apart, in the morning and at night, unless otherwise directed by your doctor. If you need help in planning the best times to take your medicine, check with your doctor or pharmacist.

If you do miss a dose of flecainide and remember within 4 hours, take it as soon as possible. However, if you do not remember until later, skip the missed dose and go back to your regular dosing schedule. Do not double doses.

How to store this medicine:

• Store away from heat and direct light.

• **Keep out of the reach of children.**

• Do not store in the bathroom medicine cabinet because the heat or moisture may cause the medicine to break down.

• Do not keep outdated medicine or medicine no longer needed. Flush the contents of the container down the toilet, unless otherwise directed.

Precautions While Using This Medicine

It is important that your doctor check your progress at regular visits to make sure the medicine is working properly. This will allow for changes to be made in the amount of medicine you are taking, if necessary.

Your doctor may want you to carry a medical identification card or bracelet stating that you are using this medicine.

Before having any kind of surgery (including dental surgery) or emergency treatment, tell the physician or dentist in charge that you are taking this medicine.

Flecainide may cause some people to become dizzy, lightheaded, or less alert than they are normally. Make sure you know how you react to this medicine before you drive, use machines, or do other jobs that require you to be alert.

Side Effects of This Medicine

Along with its needed effects, a medicine may cause some unwanted effects. Although not all of these side effects appear very often, when they do occur they may require medical attention. Check with your doctor as soon as possible if any of the following side effects occur:

Less common
  Chest pain
  Irregular heartbeat
  Shortness of breath
  Swelling of feet or lower legs
  Trembling or shaking
Rare
  Fever, chills, or sore throat
  Unusual bleeding or bruising
  Yellowing of eyes and skin

Other side effects may occur which usually do not require medical attention. These side effects may go away during treatment as your body adjusts to the medicine. However, check with your doctor if any of the following side effects continue or are bothersome:

More common
  Blurred vision
  Dizziness or lightheadedness
Less common
  Anxiety or mental depression
  Constipation
  Headache
  Nausea or vomiting

Skin rash
Stomach pain or loss of appetite
Tiredness or weakness

Dizziness or lightheadedness may be more likely to occur in the elderly, who are usually more sensitive to the effects of flecainide.

Other side effects not listed above may also occur in some patients. If you notice any other effects, check with your doctor.

GOLD COMPOUNDS (Systemic)

This information applies to the following medicines:

Auranofin (au-RANE-oh-fin)
Aurothioglucose (aur-oh-thye-oh-GLOO-kose)
Gold Sodium Thiomalate (gold SO-dee-um thye-oh-MAH-late)

Some commonly used brand names or other names are:	Generic names:
Ridaura	Auranofin
Solganal	Aurothioglucose
Myochrysine Sodium Aurothiomalate	Gold Sodium Thiomalate

The gold compounds are used in the treatment of rheumatoid arthritis. They may also be used for other conditions as determined by your doctor.

In addition to the helpful effects of this medicine in treating your medical problem, it has side effects that could be very serious. Before you take this medicine, you should discuss with your doctor the good that this medicine will do as well as the risks of using it.

Auranofin is taken by mouth and is available only with your doctor's prescription. The other gold compounds are given by injection.

Before Using This Medicine

In order to decide on the best treatment for your medical problem, your doctor should be told:

—if you have ever had any unusual or allergic reaction to gold or other metals.

—if you are on a low-salt, low-sugar, or any other special diet, if you are allergic to sesame seeds or sesame oil, or if you are allergic to any other substance, such as sulfites or other preservatives. Most medicines contain more than their active ingredient. Your doctor or pharmacist can help you avoid products that may cause a problem.

—if you have received a gold compound before and developed serious side effects from it.

—if any medicine you have taken has ever caused an allergy or reaction that affected your blood or lungs.

—if you are pregnant or if you intend to become pregnant while using this medicine. Studies on birth defects with gold compounds have not been done in humans. However, studies in animals have shown that gold compounds may cause birth defects.

—if you are breast-feeding an infant. Aurothioglucose and gold sodium thiomalate pass into the breast milk and may cause unwanted effects in infants of mothers taking this medicine. It is not known whether auranofin passes into the breast milk.

—if you have any of the following medical problems:
Blood or blood vessel disease
Kidney disease (or history of)
Lupus erythematosus
Sjögren's syndrome
Skin disease

—if you are now taking any other arthritis medicine, especially penicillamine.

Proper Use of This Medicine

In order for this medicine to work, it must be taken regularly as ordered by your doctor. Continue receiving the injections or taking auranofin even if you think the medicine is not working. You may not notice the effects of this medicine until after three to six months of regular use.

For patients taking auranofin:

• **Do not take more of this medicine than ordered by your doctor.** Taking too much auranofin may increase the chance of serious unwanted effects.

• If you miss a dose of this medicine, and your dosing schedule is one dose to be taken:

Once a day—Take the missed dose as soon as possible. However, if you do not remember until the next day, skip the missed dose and go back to your regular dosing schedule. Do not double doses.

More than once a day—Take the missed dose as soon as possible. However, if it is almost time for your next dose, skip the missed dose and go back to your regular dosing schedule. Do not double doses.

How to store this medicine:

• Store away from heat and direct light.

• **Keep out of the reach of children.**

• Do not store in the bathroom medicine cabinet because the heat or moisture may cause the medicine to break down.

• Do not keep outdated medicine or medicine no longer needed. Flush the contents of the container down the toilet, unless otherwise directed.

Precautions While Using This Medicine

For patients taking auranofin:

• Your doctor should check your progress at regular visits. Blood and urine tests may be needed to make certain that this medicine is not causing unwanted effects.

For patients receiving gold injections:

• Immediately following an injection of this medicine, side effects such as dizziness, feeling faint, flushing or redness of the face, nausea or vomiting, unusual sweating, or unusual weakness may occur. These will usually go away after you lie down for a few minutes. If any of these effects continue or become worse, check with your doctor.

• Joint pain may occur for 1 or 2 days after you receive an injection of this medicine. This effect usually disappears after the first few injections. However, if this continues or is bothersome, check with your doctor.

Side Effects of This Medicine

Gold compounds have been shown to cause tumors and cancer of the kidney when given to animals in large doses for a long period of time. However, these effects have not been reported in humans receiving gold compounds for arthritis. If you have any questions about this, check with your doctor.

Along with its needed effects, a medicine may cause some unwanted effects. Although not all of these side effects appear very often, they may occur at any time during treatment with this medicine **and up to many months after treatment has ended,** and they may require medical attention. Check with your doctor as soon as possible if any of the following side effects occur:

More common

Irritation or soreness of tongue or gums—less common with auranofin
Metallic taste—less common with auranofin
Skin rash or itching
Ulcers, sores, or white spots in mouth or throat

Less common
  Bloody or cloudy urine
  Hives
  Sore throat and fever
  Unusual bleeding or bruising
  Unusual tiredness or weakness

Rare
  Abdominal or stomach pain (severe)
  Bloody or black tarry stools
  Coughing or shortness of breath
  Yellowing of eyes or skin

With long-term use
  Eye problems
  Numbness, tingling, pain, or weakness in
    hands or feet

Other side effects may occur which usually do not require medical attention. These side effects may go away during treatment as your body adjusts to the medicine. However, check with your doctor if the following side effects continue or are bothersome:

More common with auranofin; rare with injections
  Abdominal or stomach cramps or pain
    (mild or moderate)
  Bloated feeling, gas, or indigestion
  Decrease or loss of appetite
  Diarrhea
  Nausea or vomiting

Less common
  Constipation—with auranofin
  Joint pain—with injections

Some patients receiving auranofin have noticed that certain foods taste different than usual. If you notice a metallic taste while receiving any gold compound, check with your doctor as soon as possible. If you notice any other taste changes while you are taking auranofin, it is not necessary to check with your doctor unless you find this effect especially bothersome.

Other side effects not listed above may also occur in some patients. If you notice any other effects, check with your doctor.

GRISEOFULVIN (Systemic)

Some commonly used brand names are:

Fulvicin P/G	Grisactin Ultra
Fulvicin-U/F	Gris-PEG
Grifulvin V	Grisovin-FP*
Grisactin	

Generic name product may also be available.

* Not available in the United States.

Griseofulvin (gri-see-oh-FUL-vin) belongs to the group of medicines called antifungals. It is taken by mouth to treat fungus infections of the skin, hair, fingernails, and toenails.

Griseofulvin is available only with your doctor's prescription.

Before Using This Medicine

In order to decide on the best treatment for your medical problem, your doctor should be told:

—if you have ever had any unusual or allergic reaction to penicillin or penicillamine.

—if you are pregnant or if you intend to become pregnant while taking this medicine. Although griseofulvin has not been shown to cause birth defects or other problems in humans, the chance always exists. Studies in rats have shown that griseofulvin causes birth defects and other problems.

—if you are breast-feeding an infant. Although griseofulvin has not been shown to cause problems in humans, the chance always exists.

—if you have any of the following medical problems:
  Liver disease
  Lupus erythematosus
  Porphyria

—if you are now taking any of the following medicines or types of medicine:
  Anthralin
  Anticoagulants, coumarin- or indandione-
    type (blood thinners)

Barbiturates
Coal tar
Diuretics (water pills or high blood
    pressure medicine)
Methoxsalen
Nalidixic acid
Oral contraceptives (birth control pills)
Phenothiazines
Primidone
Sulfonamides (sulfa medicine)
Tetracyclines
Trioxsalen

Proper Use of This Medicine

To help clear up your infection completely, **keep taking this medicine for the full time of treatment** even if you begin to feel better after a few days; do not miss any doses.

If you do miss a dose of this medicine, take it as soon as possible. But if it is almost time for your next dose, do not take the missed dose at all and do not double the next one. Instead, go back to your regular dosing schedule.

Griseofulvin is best taken with or after meals, especially fatty ones (for example, whole milk or ice cream). This lessens possible stomach upset and helps to clear up the infection by helping your body absorb the medicine better. **However, if you are on a low-fat diet, check with your doctor.**

For patients taking the oral liquid form of griseofulvin:

• Use a specially marked measuring spoon or other device to measure each dose accurately since the average household teaspoon may not hold the right amount of liquid.

How to store this medicine:

• Store away from heat and direct light, out of the reach of children.

• Do not store in the bathroom medicine cabinet because the heat or moisture may cause the medicine to break down.

• Keep the oral liquid from freezing.

• Do not keep outdated medicine or medicine no longer needed. Flush it down the toilet.

Precautions While Using This Medicine

Your doctor should check your progress at regular visits in order to make sure that griseofulvin does not cause unwanted effects.

Griseofulvin may increase the effects of alcohol. It may also cause unusually fast heartbeat or flushing or redness of the face if taken with alcohol. Therefore, **do not drink alcoholic beverages while you are taking this medicine,** unless you have first checked with your doctor.

A few people who take this medicine may become more sensitive to sunlight than they are normally. When you first begin taking this medicine, avoid too much sun or use of a sunlamp until you see how you react, especially if you tend to burn easily. If you have a severe reaction, check with your doctor.

Side Effects of This Medicine

Along with its needed effects, a medicine may cause some unwanted effects. Although not all of these side effects appear very often, when they do occur they may require medical attention. Check with your doctor as soon as possible if any of the following side effects occur:

Less common
   Confusion
   Skin rash, hives, or itching
   Soreness or irritation of mouth or tongue
Rare
   Numbness, tingling, pain, or weakness in
     hands or feet
   Sore throat and fever

Other side effects may occur which usually do not require medical attention. These side effects may go away during treatment as your body adjusts to the medicine. However, check with your doctor if

any of the following side effects contin-ue or are bothersome:

More common
· Headache

Less common
Diarrhea
Dizziness
Nausea or vomiting
Stomach pain
Trouble in sleeping
Unusual tiredness

Other side effects not listed above may also occur in some patients. If you notice any other effects, check with your doctor.

GUAIFENESIN (Systemic)

[Former name—Glyceryl Guaiacolate]

Some commonly used brand names are:

Anti-Tuss	Guiamid
Baytussin	Guiatuss
Breonesin	Halotussin
Colrex Expectorant	Hytuss
Cremacoat 2	Hytuss-2X
2/G	Malotuss
Gee-Gee	Nortussin
GG-CEN	Peedee Dose
Glyate	Expectorant
Glycotuss	Robafen
Glytuss	Robitussin
	S-T Expectorant

Generic name product may also be available.

Guaifenesin (gwye-FEN-e-sin) is taken by mouth to relieve coughs due to colds or influenza. Guaifenesin works by loosening the mucus or phlegm (pronounced flem) in the lungs.

This medicine is not to be used for the chronic cough that occurs with smoking, asthma, or emphysema or when there is an unusually large amount of mucus or phlegm with the cough.

Guaifenesin is available without a pre-scription; however, your doctor may have special instructions on the proper dose of this medicine for your medical condition.

Before Using This Medicine

Before you use this medicine, check with your doctor or pharmacist:

—if you have ever had any unusual or allergic reaction to guaifenesin.

—if you are on a low-salt, low-sugar, or any other special diet, or if you are aller-gic to any substance, such as sulfites or other preservatives or dyes. Most medi-cines contain more than their active in-gredient, and many liquid medicines contain alcohol. Your doctor or pharma-cist can help you avoid products that may cause a problem.

—if you are pregnant, or if you intend to become pregnant while taking this med-icine. Although guaifenesin has not been shown to cause birth defects or oth-er problems in humans, the chance al-ways exists.

—if you are breast-feeding an infant. Although guaifenesin has not been shown to cause problems in humans, the chance always exists.

Proper Use of This Medicine

To help loosen mucus or phlegm in the lungs, **drink a glass of water after each dose of this medicine,** unless otherwise directed by your doctor.

If you must take this medicine regularly and you miss a dose, take it as soon as possible. However, if it is almost time for your next dose, skip the missed dose and go back to your regular dosing schedule. Do not double doses.

How to store this medicine:

• Store away from heat and direct light.

• **Keep out of the reach of children.**

• Do not store in the bathroom medicine cabinet because the heat or moisture may cause the medicine to break down.

• Do not refrigerate the syrup form of this medicine.

• Do not keep outdated medicine or medicine no longer needed. Flush the contents of the container down the toilet, unless otherwise directed.

Precautions While Using This Medicine

If your cough has not improved after 7 days or if you have a high fever, skin rash, continuing headache, or sore throat with the cough, check with your doctor. These signs may mean that you have other medical problems.

Side Effects of This Medicine

Along with its needed effects, a medicine may cause some unwanted effects. Although no serious side effects have been reported for guaifenesin, the following side effects may be noticed by some patients. Check with your doctor as soon as possible if any of these effects continue or are bothersome:

Less common or rare
   Diarrhea
   Drowsiness
   Nausea or vomiting
   Stomach pain

Other side effects not listed above may also occur in some patients. If you notice any other effects, check with your doctor.

HALOPERIDOL (Systemic)

Some commonly used brand names are Apo-Haloperidol* and Haldol.

---

*Not available in the United States.

Haloperidol (ha-loe-PER-i-dole) is used to treat nervous, mental, and emotional conditions. It is also used to control the symptoms of Tourette's disorder. Haloperidol may also be used for other conditions as determined by your doctor.

Haloperidol is available only with your doctor's prescription.

Before Using This Medicine

In order to decide on the best treatment for your medical problem, your doctor should be told:

—if you have ever had any unusual or allergic reaction to haloperidol.

—if you are on a low-salt, low-sugar, or any other special diet, or if you are allergic to any substance, such as sulfites or other preservatives or dyes. Most medicines contain more than their active ingredient. Your doctor or pharmacist can help you avoid products that may cause a problem.

—if you are pregnant or if you intend to become pregnant while receiving this medicine. Adequate studies have not been done in humans. However, studies in animals given 2 to 20 times the usual maximum human dose of haloperidol have shown reduced fertility, delayed delivery, cleft palate, and an increase in the number of stillbirths and newborn deaths.

—if you are breast-feeding an infant. Haloperidol has not been shown to cause problems in humans. However, animal studies have shown that haloperidol in breast milk causes drowsiness and difficulty with body movements in the nursing offspring. Breast-feeding is not recommended during treatment with haloperidol.

—if you have any of the following medical problems:
   Alcoholism
   Difficult urination
   Epilepsy
   Glaucoma
   Heart or blood vessel disease
   Kidney disease
   Liver disease
   Lung disease

Overactive thyroid
Parkinson's disease

—if you are now taking any of the following medicines or types of medicine:

Amphetamines
Anticoagulants, oral (blood thinners you take by mouth)
Anticonvulsants (seizure medicine)
Antimuscarinics (medicine for stomach ulcers, spasms, or cramps)
Beta-adrenergic blocking agents (acebutolol, atenolol, labetalol, metoprolol, nadolol, oxprenolol, pindolol, propranolol, sotalol, timolol)
Epinephrine
Guanadrel
Guanethidine
Levodopa
Lithium
Methyldopa

—if you are now taking central nervous system (CNS) depressants such as:

Antihistamines or medicine for hay fever, other allergies, or colds
Barbiturates
Narcotics
Prescription pain medicine
Sedatives, tranquilizers, or sleeping medicine

Proper Use of This Medicine

If this medicine upsets your stomach, it may be taken with food or milk to lessen stomach irritation.

For patients taking the liquid form of this medicine:

• This medicine is to be taken by mouth even though it may come in a dropper bottle. Each dose is to be measured with the included, specially marked dropper. Do not use other droppers since they may not deliver the correct amount of medicine.

• This medicine is best taken alone. However, if necessary, it may be mixed with water. If this is done, the mixture should be taken immediately after mixing. Haloperidol should not be taken in

tea or coffee, since they cause the medicine to separate out of the solution.

Take this medicine only as directed by your doctor. Do not take more of it, do not take it more often, and do not take it for a longer period of time than your doctor ordered.

Continue taking this medicine for the full time of treatment. **Sometimes haloperidol must be taken for several days to several weeks before its full effect is reached in the treatment of certain mental and emotional conditions.**

If you miss a dose of this medicine, take it as soon as possible. Then take any remaining doses for that day at regularly spaced intervals. Do not double doses.

How to store this medicine:

• Store away from heat and direct light.

• **Keep out of the reach of children.**

• Do not store in the bathroom medicine cabinet because the heat or moisture may cause the medicine to break down.

• Keep the liquid from freezing.

• Do not keep outdated medicine or medicine no longer needed. Flush the contents of the container down the toilet, unless otherwise directed.

Precautions While Using This Medicine

Your doctor should check your progress at regular visits, especially for the first few months you take this medicine. The amount of haloperidol you take may be changed often to meet the needs of your condition. This also helps to avoid side effects.

Do not suddenly stop taking this medicine without first checking with your doctor. Your doctor may want you to reduce gradually the amount you are taking before stopping completely. This will allow your body time to adjust and help to avoid a worsening of your medical condition.

This medicine will add to the effects of alcohol and other CNS depressants (medicines that slow down the nervous system, possibly causing drowsiness). Some examples of CNS depressants are antihistamines or medicine for hay fever, other allergies, or colds; sedatives, tranquilizers, or sleeping medicine; prescription pain medicine or narcotics; barbiturates; medicine for seizures; or anesthetics, including some dental anesthetics. **Check with your doctor before taking any of the above while you are taking this medicine.**

This medicine may cause some people to become drowsy or less alert than they are normally, especially as the amount of medicine is increased. Even if you take this medicine at bedtime, you may feel drowsy or less alert on arising. **Make sure you know how you react to this medicine before you drive, use machines, or do other jobs that require you to be alert.**

Although not a problem for many patients, dizziness, lightheadedness, or fainting may occur, especially when you get up from a lying or sitting position. Getting up slowly may help. However, if the problem continues or gets worse, check with your doctor.

A few people who take this medicine may become more sensitive to sunlight than they are normally. When you first begin taking this medicine, use sunscreen lotions, or avoid too much sun or too much use of a sunlamp until you see how you react. If you have a severe reaction, check with your doctor.

Your mouth may feel very dry while you are taking haloperidol. To help relieve mouth dryness, chew sugarless gum or melt bits of ice in your mouth.

Side Effects of This Medicine

Along with its needed effects, a medicine may cause some unwanted effects. Although not all of these side effects appear very often, when they do occur they may require medical attention. **Stop taking haloperidol and get emergency help immediately** if any of the following side effects occur:

Rare

    Convulsions (seizures)
    Difficult or unusually fast breathing
    Fever (high) with increased sweating
    Loss of bladder control
    Muscle stiffness (severe)
    Unusual feeling of tiredness or weakness
    Unusually fast heartbeat or irregular pulse

Check with your doctor as soon as possible if any of the following side effects occur:

More common

    Difficulty in speaking or swallowing
    Loss of balance control
    Mask-like face
    Muscle spasms, especially of neck and back
    Restlessness or desire to keep moving (severe)
    Shuffling walk
    Stiffness of arms and legs
    Trembling and shaking of fingers and hands
    Unusual fixation of eyes
    Unusual twisting movements of body

Less common

    Chewing movements
    Decreased feeling of thirst
    Difficulty in urination
    Dizziness, lightheadedness, or fainting
    Lip smacking or puckering
    Puffing of cheeks
    Rapid or worm-like movements of tongue
    Skin rash
    Unusual movements of arms and legs

Rare

    Sore throat and fever
    Yellowing of eyes and skin

Signs of overdose

    Difficulty in breathing (severe)
    Dizziness or lightheadedness (severe)
    Drowsiness (severe)

Muscle trembling, jerking, stiffness, or
uncontrolled movements (severe)
Unusual tiredness or weakness

Other side effects may occur which usually
do not require medical attention. These
side effects may go away during treatment as your body adjusts to the medicine. However, check with your doctor if
any of the following side effects continue or are bothersome:

More common
Blurred vision
Constipation
Dry mouth
Weight gain

Less common
Decreased sexual ability
Drowsiness
Increased sensitivity of skin to sun
Nausea or vomiting

Some side effects, such as dizziness, stomach pain, nausea or vomiting, trembling
of fingers and hands, or uncontrolled
movements of the mouth, tongue, and
jaw, may occur after you have stopped
taking this medicine. If you notice any
of these effects, check with your doctor
as soon as possible.

Side effects are more likely to occur in children and the elderly, who usually are
more sensitive to the effects of haloperidol.

Other side effects not listed above may also
occur in some patients. If you notice any
other effects, check with your doctor.

HYDRALAZINE (Systemic)

Some commonly used brand names are Apreso-
line and Dralzine.

Generic name product may also be available.

Hydralazine (hye-DRAL-a-zeen) belongs to the general class of medicines
called antihypertensives. It is used to treat
high blood pressure.

High blood pressure adds to the workload of the heart and arteries. If it continues
for a long time, they may not function properly. This can damage the blood vessels of
the brain, heart, and kidneys, resulting in a
stroke, heart attack, or kidney failure.
These problems may be avoided if blood
pressure is controlled.

Hydralazine works by relaxing blood
vessels and increasing the supply of blood
and oxygen to the heart while reducing its
work load.

Hydralazine may also be used for other
conditions as determined by your doctor.

Hydralazine is available only with your
doctor's prescription.

Before Using This Medicine

In order to decide on the best treatment for
your medical problem, your doctor
should be told:

—if you have ever had any unusual or
allergic reaction to hydralazine.

—if you are on a low-salt, low-sugar, or
any other special diet, or if you are allergic to any substance, such as sulfites or
other preservatives or dyes. Most medicines contain more than their active ingredient, and many liquid medicines
contain alcohol. Your doctor or pharmacist can help you avoid products that
may cause a problem.

—if you are pregnant or if you intend to
become pregnant while using this medicine. Studies have not been done in humans. However, studies in mice have
shown that hydralazine causes birth defects (cleft palate, defects in head and

face bones); these birth defects may also occur in rabbits, but do not occur in rats.

—if you are breast-feeding an infant. Although hydralazine has not been shown to cause problems, the chance always exists.

—if you have either of the following medical problems:

Heart or blood vessel disease
Kidney disease

—if you have recently had a stroke.

—if you are now taking any of the following medicines or types of medicine:

Diuretics (water pills)
Inflammation medicines, especially indomethacin
Other antihypertensives (high blood pressure medicine)

Proper Use of This Medicine

Importance of diet—When prescribing medicine for your condition, your doctor may also prescribe a personal diet for you. Such a diet may be low in sodium (salt). Most people eat much more sodium than they need and too much sodium in the diet may increase blood pressure. Some foods that contain large amounts of sodium include canned soup, pickles, ketchup, green and ripe olives, relish, frankfurters, soy sauce, and carbonated beverages. Your doctor may want you to limit the amounts of these and other high-sodium foods in your diet. Medicine is usually more effective when such a diet is properly followed.

Also, it may be very important for you to go on a reducing diet. However, check with your doctor before going on any diet.

Many people who have high blood pressure will not notice any signs of the problem. In fact, many may feel normal. It is very important that you **take your medicine exactly as directed** and that you keep your doctor's appointments even if you feel well.

Remember that hydralazine will not cure your high blood pressure but it does help control it. Therefore, you must continue to take it as directed if you expect to lower your blood pressure and keep it down. **You may have to take medicine for the rest of your life.** If high blood pressure is not treated, it can cause serious problems such as heart failure, blood vessel disease, stroke, or kidney disease.

In order to help remember to take your medicine, try to get into the habit of taking it at the same time each day.

If you miss a dose of this medicine, take it as soon as possible. However, if it is almost time for your next dose, skip the missed dose and go back to your regular dosing schedule. Do not double doses.

How to store this medicine:

• Store the tablets away from heat and direct light.

• **Keep out of the reach of children.**

• Do not store in the bathroom medicine cabinet because the heat or moisture may cause the medicine to break down.

• Store the oral solution in the refrigerator. Protect it from freezing.

• Do not keep outdated medicine or medicine no longer needed. Flush the contents of the container down the toilet, unless otherwise directed.

Precautions While Using This Medicine

It is important that your doctor check your progress at regular visits in order to make sure that this medicine is working properly.

Do not take other medicines unless they have been discussed with your doctor. This especially includes over-the-counter (nonprescription) medicines for appetite control, asthma, colds, cough, hay fever, or sinus, since they may tend to increase your blood pressure.

Hydralazine may cause some people to have headaches or to feel dizzy. **Make sure you know how you react to this medicine before you drive, use machines, or do other jobs that require you to be alert.**

Side Effects of This Medicine

Along with its needed effects, a medicine may cause some unwanted effects. Although not all of these side effects appear very often, when they do occur they may require medical attention. In general, side effects with hydralazine are rare at lower doses. However, check with your doctor as soon as possible if any of the following occur:

Less common

Blisters on skin
Chest pain
General feeling of body discomfort or weakness
Joint pain
Numbness, tingling, pain, or weakness in hands or feet
Skin rash or itching
Sore throat and fever
Swelling of feet or lower legs
Swelling of the lymph glands

Other side effects may occur which usually do not require medical attention. These side effects may go away during treatment as your body adjusts to the medicine. However, check with your doctor if any of the following side effects continue or are bothersome:

More common

Diarrhea
Headache
Loss of appetite
Nausea or vomiting
Rapid or irregular heartbeat

Less common

Constipation
Dizziness or lightheadedness
Redness or flushing of the face
Shortness of breath with exercise or work
Stuffy nose
Watering or irritated eyes

Dizziness or lightheadedness may be more likely to occur in the elderly, who are more sensitive to the effects of hydralazine.

Other side effects not listed above may also occur in some patients. If you notice any other effects, check with your doctor.

HYDRALAZINE AND HYDROCHLOROTHIAZIDE
(Systemic)

Some commonly used brand names are:

Apresazide	Apresoline-Esidrix
Apresodex	Hydral

Generic name product may also be available.

Hydralazine (hye-DRAL-a-zeen) and hydrochlorothiazide (hye-droe-klor-oh-THYE-a-zide) combination is taken by mouth to treat high blood pressure.

High blood pressure adds to the workload of the heart and arteries. If it continues for a long time, they may not function properly. This can damage the blood vessels of the brain, heart, and kidneys, resulting in a stroke, heart attack, or kidney failure. These problems may be avoided if blood pressure is controlled.

Hydralazine works by relaxing blood vessels and increasing the supply of blood and oxygen to the heart while reducing its work load. The hydrochlorothiazide in this combination helps reduce the amount of water in the body by acting on the kidneys to increase the flow of urine.

This medicine is available only with your doctor's prescription.

For information about the precautions and side effects of the medicines in this combination, see:

Hydralazine (Systemic)
Diuretics, Thiazide (Systemic)

Combination products are designed for specific uses. These uses may not be the same as the uses of the individual ingredients. Therefore, some of the information provided in the individual listings may not be relevant to the combination product. If questions arise, check with your doctor, nurse, or pharmacist.

HYDROXYZINE (Systemic)

Some commonly used brand names are:

Anxanil	Hyzine
Atarax	Orgatrax
Atozine	Quiess
BayRox	Vamate
Durrax	Vistacon
E-Vista	Vistaject
Hydroxacen	Vistaquel
Hy-Pam	Vistaril
	Vistazine

Generic name product may also be available.

Hydroxyzine (hye-DROX-i-zeen) is used in the treatment of nervous and emotional conditions to help control anxiety. It can also be used to help control anxiety and induce sleep before surgery.

Because hydroxyzine has antihistamine action, it is used to relieve the itching caused by allergic conditions. In addition, hydroxyzine when given by injection can be used to prevent nausea and vomiting.

Hydroxyzine is available only with your doctor's prescription.

Before Using This Medicine

In order to decide on the best treatment for your medical problem, your doctor should be told:

—if you have ever had any unusual or allergic reaction to hydroxyzine.

—if you are on a low-salt, low-sugar, or any other special diet, or if you are allergic to any substance, such as sulfites or other preservatives or dyes. Most medicines contain more than their active ingredient, and many liquid medicines contain alcohol. Your doctor or pharmacist can help you avoid products that may cause a problem.

—if you are pregnant or if you intend to become pregnant while using this medicine. Hydroxyzine is not recommended in the first months of pregnancy since it has been shown to cause birth defects in rats when given in doses up to many times the usual human dose. Be sure you have discussed this with your doctor.

—if you are breast-feeding an infant. Although hydroxyzine has not been shown to cause problems in humans, the chance always exists since hydroxyzine may pass into the breast milk.

—if you are now taking any central nervous system (CNS) depressants, such as:

    Anticonvulsants (seizure medicine)
    Barbiturates
    Clonidine
    Guanabenz
    Methyldopa
    Metyrosine
    Muscle relaxants
    Narcotics
    Other antihistamines or medicine for hay fever, other allergies, or colds
    Prescription pain medicine
    Sedatives, tranquilizers, or sleeping medicine

—if you are now taking tricyclic antidepressants, such as:

    Amitriptyline
    Amoxapine
    Clomipramine
    Desipramine
    Doxepin
    Imipramine
    Nortriptyline
    Protriptyline
    Trimipramine

Proper Use of This Medicine

Take hydroxyzine only as directed by your doctor. Do not take more of it and do not take it more often than your doctor ordered. To do so may increase the chance of side effects.

If you miss a dose of this medicine, take it as soon as possible. However, if it is almost time for your next dose, skip the missed dose and go back to your regular dosing schedule. Do not double doses.

How to store this medicine:

• Store away from heat and direct light.

• **Keep out of the reach of children.**

• Do not store in the bathroom medicine cabinet because the heat or moisture may cause the medicine to break down.

• Keep the liquid form of this medicine from freezing.

• Do not keep outdated medicine or medicine no longer needed. Flush the contents of the container down the toilet, unless otherwise directed.

Precautions While Using This Medicine

Tell the doctor in charge that you are taking this medicine before you have any skin tests for allergies. The results of the test may be affected by this medicine.

Hydroxyzine will add to the effects of alcohol and other CNS depressants (medicines that slow down the nervous system, possibly causing drowsiness). Some examples of CNS depressants are antihistamines or medicine for hay fever, other allergies, or colds; sedatives, tranquilizers, or sleeping medicine; prescription pain medicine or narcotics; barbiturates; medicine for seizures; muscle relaxants; or anesthetics, including some dental anesthetics. **Check with your doctor before taking any of the above while you are using this medicine.**

This medicine may cause some people to become drowsy or less alert than they are normally. Even if taken at bedtime, it may cause some people to feel drowsy or less alert on arising. **Make sure you know how you react to this medicine before you drive, use machines, or do other jobs that require you to be alert.**

Your mouth may feel very dry while you are taking hydroxyzine. To help relieve mouth dryness, chew sugarless gum or dissolve bits of ice in your mouth.

Side Effects of This Medicine

Along with its needed effects, a medicine may cause some unwanted effects. Although not all of these side effects appear very often, when they do occur they may require medical attention. Check with your doctor as soon as possible if any of the following side effects occur:

Rare

    Convulsions (seizures)

    Skin rash

    Trembling or shakiness

Signs of overdose

    Drowsiness (severe)

    Feeling faint

Other side effects may occur which usually do not require medical attention. These side effects may go away during treatment as your body adjusts to the medicine. However, check with your doctor if either of the following side effects continues or is bothersome:

More common

    Drowsiness

Less common

    Dryness of the mouth

Other side effects not listed above may also occur in some patients. If you notice any other effects, check with your doctor.

INDOMETHACIN (Systemic)

Some commonly used brand names and other names are:

Indocid*   Indocin-SR
Indocid SR*   Indometacin
Indocin   Novomethacin*

Generic name product may also be available.

*Not available in the United States.

Indomethacin (in-doe-METH-a-sin) is used to treat the symptoms of many painful conditions, including certain types of arthritis and gout. It may be taken by mouth or used rectally as a suppository to help relieve inflammation, swelling, stiffness, joint pain, and fever.

When used to treat arthritis, indomethacin only relieves the symptoms of the disease. It does not cure arthritis and will help you only as long as you continue to take it.

Indomethacin is also used by injection to treat patent ductus arteriosus (PDA) in premature infants. PDA is a condition that causes heart and breathing problems in some premature infants. Indomethacin helps to correct this condition. However, some premature infants with PDA may need heart surgery if indomethacin does not correct the condition completely or permanently. Because this use of indomethacin by injection is so different from its other uses, the information that follows applies only to the oral and rectal uses of this medicine. If you have any questions about the use of indomethacin to treat PDA, check with your doctor, nurse, or pharmacist.

Indomethacin may also be used for other conditions as determined by your doctor.

This medicine is available only with your doctor's prescription.

Before Using This Medicine

In order to decide on the best treatment for your medical problem, your doctor should be told:

—if you have ever had any unusual or allergic reaction, especially asthma or wheezing, runny nose, or hives, to indomethacin or to any of the following medicines:

Aspirin or other salicylates
Diflunisal
Fenoprofen
Ibuprofen
Meclofenamate
Mefenamic acid
Naproxen
Oxyphenbutazone
Phenylbutazone
Piroxicam
Sulindac
Tolmetin
Zomepirac

—if you are on a low-sugar or any other special diet, or if you are allergic to any substance, such as sulfites or other preservatives or dyes. Most medicines contain more than their active ingredient. Your doctor or pharmacist can help you avoid products that may cause a problem.

—if you are pregnant or if you intend to become pregnant while using this medicine. Studies on birth defects with indomethacin have not been done in humans. However, if indomethacin is used late in pregnancy, it may cause unwanted effects on the heart or blood flow in the fetus or in the newborn infant. Studies in animals have shown that indomethacin causes several unwanted effects such as a lowering of the newborn's weight, slower development of bones, and damage to nerves. Also, studies in animals have shown that indomethacin, if taken late in pregnancy, may increase the length of pregnancy and prolong labor.

—if you are breast-feeding an infant. Indomethacin passes into the breast milk and has been reported to cause unwanted effects in the breast-fed infant. It may be necessary for you to take another medicine or to stop breast-feeding during treatment. Be sure you have discussed the risks and benefits of the medicine with your doctor.

—if you have any of the following medical problems:

Bleeding problems
Colitis, stomach ulcer, or other stomach problems
Epilepsy
Heart disease
High blood pressure
Infection
Kidney disease
Liver disease
Mental illness
Parkinson's disease
Rectal irritation or bleeding, recent (for the suppository only)
Systemic lupus erythematosus (SLE)

—if you are now taking any of the following medicines or types of medicine:

Acetaminophen
Adrenocorticoids (cortisone-like medicine)
Anticoagulants (blood thinners)
Antidiabetics, oral (medicine for sugar diabetes you take by mouth)
Antihypertensives (high blood pressure medicine)
APC and codeine
Aspirin or other salicylates
Corticotropin
Diflunisal
Digitalis glycosides (heart medicine)
Dipyridamole
Diuretics (medicine used to increase the amount of urine or to reduce high blood pressure)
Divalproex
Heparin
Inflammation medicine (for example, other arthritis medicine)
Lithium
Probenecid
Sulfinpyrazone
Valproic acid

Proper Use of This Medicine

Use this medicine only as directed by your doctor. Do not use more of it, do not use it more often, and do not use it for a longer period of time than your doctor ordered. To do so may increase the chance of serious side effects.

If you are using this medicine to relieve arthritis, you must use it regularly as ordered by your doctor. In some types of arthritis, up to 2 weeks may pass before you begin to feel better and up to 1 month may pass before you feel the full effects of this medicine.

For patients taking the capsule forms of indomethacin:

• **Take indomethacin capsules immediately after meals or with food or antacids to lessen stomach upset.** If stomach upset (indigestion, heartburn, nausea, vomiting, stomach pain, or diarrhea) continues, check with your doctor.

• **Take indomethacin capsules with a full glass (8 ounces) of water.** Also, do not lie down for about 15 to 30 minutes after taking this medicine. This helps to prevent irritation that may lead to trouble in swallowing.

For patients using the rectal suppository form of indomethacin:

• If the suppository is too soft to insert because of storage in a warm place, before removing the foil wrapper chill the suppository in the refrigerator for 30 minutes or run cold water over it.

• How to insert the suppository: First, remove the foil wrapper and moisten the suppository with water. Lie down on your side and push the suppository well up into the rectum with the finger.

• Keep the suppository inside the rectum for at least one hour so that all of the medicine can be absorbed by your body. This helps the medicine work better.

If you miss a dose of this medicine and remember within an hour or so of the missed dose, take it right away. But if you do not remember until later, skip the missed dose and go back to your regular dosing schedule. Do not double doses.

How to store this medicine:
- Store away from heat and direct light.
- **Keep out of the reach of children.**
- Do not store in the bathroom medicine cabinet because the heat or moisture may cause the medicine to break down.
- Keep the suppository dosage form of this medicine from freezing.
- Do not keep outdated medicine or medicine no longer needed. Flush the contents of the container down the toilet, unless otherwise directed.

Precautions While Using This Medicine

If you will be using this medicine for a long period of time, your doctor should check your progress at regular visits.

Before having any kind of surgery (including dental surgery), tell the physician or dentist in charge that you are using indomethacin.

Stomach problems may be more likely to occur if you take aspirin or other salicylates, ibuprofen, or other anti-inflammatory analgesics (medicines used to relieve pain and/or inflammation) regularly (for example, every day) or drink alcoholic beverages while being treated with indomethacin. Therefore, **do not take aspirin, ibuprofen, or other anti-inflammatory analgesics regularly or drink alcoholic beverages while taking indomethacin,** unless otherwise directed by your doctor.

Too much use of acetaminophen together with indomethacin may increase the chance of kidney problems. Therefore, do not regularly take acetaminophen together with indomethacin, unless your doctor has directed you to do so.

This medicine may cause some people to become dizzy, lightheaded, drowsy, or less alert than they are normally. **Make sure you know how you react to this medicine before you drive, use machines, or do other jobs that require you to be alert.**

Check with your doctor immediately if chills, fever, muscle aches or pains, or other influenza-like symptoms occur shortly before, or together with, a skin rash. Very rarely, these effects may be the first signs of a serious reaction to this medicine.

Side Effects of This Medicine

Along with its needed effects, a medicine may cause some unwanted effects. Although not all of these side effects appear very often, when they do occur they may require medical attention. **Check with your doctor immediately** if any of the following side effects occur:

Rare
  Convulsions (seizures)
  Shortness of breath, troubled breathing, wheezing, or tightness in chest

Also, check with your doctor as soon as possible if any of the following side effects occur:

More common
  Headache, especially in the morning

Less common
  Bloody or black tarry stools
  Confusion or forgetfulness
  Mental depression or other mood or mental changes
  Rectal irritation, pain, or bleeding, especially with the suppository
  Ringing or buzzing in ears
  Swelling of feet or lower legs
  Unusual weight gain

Rare
  Abdominal or stomach pain, cramping, or burning (severe)
  Bleeding sores on lips
  Bloody urine
  Blurred vision, other vision problems, or eye pain (with prolonged use)
  Decreased hearing, loss of hearing, or any other change in hearing
  Diarrhea (severe and/or bloody)

Fainting

Hallucinations (seeing, hearing, or feeling things that are not there)

Muscle weakness or uncontrollable muscle movements

Numbness, tingling, pain, or weakness in hands or feet

Redness, tenderness, itching, burning, or peeling of skin

Red, thickened, or scaly skin

Skin rash, hives, or itching

Sores, ulcers, or white spots in mouth (painful)

Sore throat and fever

Sudden decrease in amount of urine

Unexplained nosebleeds

Unexplained or unusual vaginal bleeding

Unusual bleeding or bruising

Unusually fast, irregular, or pounding heartbeat

Unusually high blood pressure

Unusual tiredness or weakness

Vomiting blood or material that looks like coffee grounds

Yellowing of eyes or skin

Other side effects may occur which usually do not require medical attention. These side effects may go away during treatment as your body adjusts to the medicine. However, check with your doctor if any of the following side effects continue or are bothersome:

More common

Abdominal or stomach pain (mild to moderate)

Dizziness or lightheadedness

Heartburn or indigestion

Nausea or vomiting

Less common

Constipation

Diarrhea

Drowsiness

General feeling of discomfort or illness

Some of the above side effects, especially confusion, may be more likely to occur in elderly patients, who are usually more sensitive to the effects of indomethacin.

Other side effects not listed above may also occur in some patients. If you notice any other effects, check with your doctor.

INSULIN (Systemic)

This information applies to the following medicines:

Insulin (IN-su-lin)

Isophane Insulin Suspension

Isophane Insulin Suspension and Insulin Injection

Insulin Zinc Suspension

Extended Insulin Zinc Suspension

Prompt Insulin Zinc Suspension

Protamine Zinc Insulin Suspension

Some commonly used brand names and other names are:	Generic names:
Humulin R Novolin R Regular (Concentrated) Iletin II, U-500 Regular Iletin I Regular Iletin II Regular Insulin Velosulin	Insulin Injection
Humulin N Insulatard NPH Novolin N NPH Iletin I NPH Iletin II NPH isophane insulin	Isophane Insulin Suspension
Mixtard	Isophane Insulin Suspension and Insulin Injection
Humulin L Lente Iletin I Lente Iletin II Lente Insulin Novolin L	Insulin Zinc Suspension
Ultralente Iletin I Ultralente Insulin	Extended Insulin Zinc Suspension
Semilente Iletin I Semilente insulin	Prompt Insulin Zinc Suspension
Protamine Zinc & Iletin I Protamine Zinc & Iletin II PZI	Protamine Zinc Insulin Suspension

Insulin (IN-su-lin) belongs to the group of medicines called hormones. It is made naturally by the body to help produce energy from the carbohydrates and sugars in food.

If the body does not make enough insulin to meet its needs, a condition known as diabetes mellitus (sugar diabetes) may develop. Proper diet and exercise may control this condition. If not, your doctor may prescribe insulin along with diet and exercise to help keep your health in balance.

Insulin is obtained from beef or pork sources, or from new processes resulting in biosynthetic or semisynthetic human insulin. Insulin must be injected under the skin because when taken by mouth, it is destroyed by stomach acids.

Although a prescription is not necessary to purchase most insulin, your doctor must first determine your personal insulin needs and provide you with special instructions for control of your diabetic condition.

Before Using This Medicine

Importance of diet—If you have insulin-dependent diabetes (IDDM, type I), your doctor will prescribe both insulin and a personal diabetic meal plan for you. If you have non–insulin-dependent diabetes (NIDDM, type II), before prescribing medicine for your diabetes, your doctor will probably try to control your condition by changing your diet. A diabetic diet is low in refined carbohydrates (foods such as sugar and candy used for quick energy). The daily number of calories in this meal plan should be adjusted to help you reach and maintain your ideal body weight. In addition, meals and snacks are arranged to meet the energy needs of your body at different times of the day. **It is very important that the meal plan prescribed for you is carefully followed.**

Many diabetic patients are able to control their condition by carefully following their doctor's orders for proper diet and exercise. **Medicine is prescribed only when additional help is needed.**

In order to decide on the best treatment for your medical problem, your doctor should be told:

—if you are allergic to beef or pork insulins.

—if you are pregnant.

—if you have any of the following medical problems:
  Infection
  Kidney disease
  Liver disease
  Thyroid disease

—if you are now taking any of the following medicines or types of medicine:
  Acetazolamide
  Adrenocorticoids (cortisone-like medicine)
  Amphetamines
  Anabolic steroids
  Aspirin or other salicylates (in large doses)
  Baclofen
  Beta-adrenergic blocking agents (acebutolol, atenolol, labetalol, metoprolol, nadolol, oxprenolol, pindolol, propranolol, sotalol, timolol)
  Danazol
  Diabetes medicine you take by mouth
  Disopyramide
  Epinephrine
  Estrogens
  Guanethidine
  Nicotine chewing gum or other medicine to help you stop smoking
  Oral contraceptives (birth control pills)
  Phenytoin
  Thyroid medicine
  Water pills (such as chlorthalidone, ethacrynic acid, furosemide, thiazides, triamterene)

—if you are now taking or have taken within the past 2 weeks monoamine oxidase (MAO) inhibitors such as:
  Furazolidone
  Isocarboxazid
  Pargyline
  Phenelzine
  Procarbazine
  Tranylcypromine

Proper Use of This Medicine

Make sure you have the correct type and strength of insulin as ordered for you by your doctor. You may find that keeping an insulin label with you is helpful when buying insulin supplies. The strength (concentration) of insulin is measured by Units and is sometimes expressed in terms such as U-100 insulin instead of insulin 100 Units.

It is very important to use insulin only as directed. Do not change the strength or the formulation type unless told to do so by your doctor.

Each package of insulin contains a patient instruction sheet. Read this sheet carefully for information concerning your syringe and needle and steps to follow when injecting a dose of insulin.

Insulin doses are measured and given with specially marked insulin syringes. For patients using only a few units of U-100 insulin per dose, a special low-dose syringe is available to make dose measurement easier and more accurate. The syringes are marked with a scale in Units that match the Unit strength of insulin being used. For example, a U-100 syringe is used to give U-100 insulin.

For patients using disposable syringes:
• Disposable insulin syringes and needles are presterilized and designed to be used one time only, and then discarded. If you have any questions about the use of disposable syringes, check with your doctor, nurse, or pharmacist.

For patients using a glass syringe and metal needle:
• A glass insulin syringe with a metal needle may be used repeatedly if they are sterilized each time. The patient instruction sheet included in each insulin package will explain how to sterilize the syringe and needle. For more information or for explanation of instructions

you do not understand, ask your doctor, nurse, or pharmacist.

A prescription from your doctor may be required to purchase insulin syringes in some states.

Do not shake the insulin bottle hard before using. Frothing or bubbles can cause an incorrect dose. Mix contents well by rolling the bottle slowly between the palms of the hands or by tipping the bottle end-to-end a few times. Do not use if contents look lumpy or grainy, or stick to the bottle. Do not use regular insulin if it becomes discolored or cloudy. Use regular insulin only when it is clear and colorless.

For patients mixing more than one type of insulin in the same syringe:
• Your doctor may want you to mix two types of insulin in the same syringe to match your needs more closely with one injection.
• When mixing regular insulin with another type of insulin, always draw the regular insulin (the clear one) into the syringe first. When mixing other insulins, it is not critical which type is drawn into the syringe first. However, once you have established an order of mixing, always mix them in that same order.
• Some mixtures of insulins have to be injected immediately after they are mixed. Other mixtures may be stable for a longer period of time. If you have any questions about the stability of the mixture you are using, check with your doctor or pharmacist.
• If your mixture of insulins is stable and mixed for you ahead of time, gently turn the filled syringe back-and-forth to remix the insulins before you inject them. Do not shake the syringe hard.

Storage and expiration date:
• When buying insulin always check the package expiration date to make sure

the insulin will be used before it expires. This expiration date applies only when the insulin has been stored under refrigeration.

• Do not use insulin after the expiration date stated on the label even if the bottle has never been opened. Check with your pharmacist about the possibility of exchanging an outdated bottle not yet opened.

• Insulin should be refrigerated until it is to be used. It should never be frozen. Insulin you are now using regularly may be kept out of the refrigerator at room temperature if it will be used up within a month. Insulin opened and stored at room temperature which has not been used for a month or more should be discarded. Insulin which is used only occasionally is best kept refrigerated.

• Do not expose insulin to extremely hot temperatures or sunlight. Do not leave insulin in the hot summer sun or in a hot, closed automobile. Extreme heat will cause it to spoil more quickly.

Precautions While Using This Medicine

It is very important that your doctor check your progress at regular visits, especially during the first few weeks of insulin treatment.

It is very important to follow carefully any instructions from your doctor such as these for:

• Alcohol. Drinking alcohol may cause severe hypoglycemia (low blood sugar). Discuss the use of alcoholic beverages with your doctor.

• Tobacco. If you have been smoking for a long time and suddenly stop, your dosage of insulin may need to be reduced. If you decide to quit smoking, first check with your doctor.

• Diabetic meal plan. The success of your treatment depends on closely following the diet your doctor or dietitian prescribed for you.

• Exercise. Your doctor will tell you what kind of exercise and how much you should do daily.

• Foot care. Special care of your feet may prevent possible future trouble.

• Urine tests. These tests are used to guide you in the control of your condition and must be done properly. Two urine tests for sugar are widely used: the tablet urine test and the paper-strip urine test. In addition, your doctor may instruct you to test your urine for acetone.

• Blood tests. Many patients have learned to measure their own blood sugar levels and make changes in their insulin dosage as needed. If you are taking blood tests, follow directions carefully.

• Injection sites. Careful selection and rotation of the injection areas on your body, following your doctor's recommendations, may prevent skin problems and difficulties in injecting.

Do not take other medicines unless they have been discussed with your doctor. This especially includes over-the-counter (nonprescription) medicines such as aspirin, and those for appetite control, asthma, colds, cough, hay fever, or sinus.

In case of emergency:

• A medical I.D. bracelet or chain should be worn at all times. In addition, carry a diabetic identification card.

• Keep handy an extra supply of insulin and a syringe with needles.

• Keep handy a glucagon kit with syringe and needle and know how it is used; also, members of your household should know how it is used and when to use it.

• Make sure a source of sugar such as orange juice, non-diet cola or soda, honey, table sugar, corn syrup, sugar cubes, or candy is always available to correct an insulin reaction (hypoglycemia).

• Have on hand several phone numbers you can call for help, such as those of your doctor, the emergency room, your pharmacy, friends, and neighbors.

Check with your doctor immediately if these symptoms of low blood sugar (hypoglycemia or insulin reaction) appear:
> Anxious feeling
> Chills
> Cold sweats
> Confusion
> Cool pale skin
> Difficulty in concentration
> Drowsiness
> Excessive hunger
> Headache
> Nausea
> Nervousness
> Rapid pulse
> Shakiness
> Unusual tiredness or weakness

These symptoms of hypoglycemia (low blood sugar) may develop suddenly and may result from:
—using too much insulin ("insulin reaction").

—delaying or missing a scheduled snack or meal.

—sickness (especially with vomiting).

—exercising more than usual.

Eating some form of sugar when symptoms of hypoglycemia first appear will usually prevent them from getting worse. Good sources include orange juice, corn syrup, honey, and sugar cubes or table sugar (dissolved in water). Also, you should eat some crackers or half a sandwich if you will not be having a snack or a meal for an hour or more.

If you become sick, especially with nausea, vomiting, or fever, you still need insulin. Call your doctor for instructions. Continue taking your insulin and try to stay on your regular diet. However, if you have trouble eating, drink fruit juices, soft drinks, or clear soups, or eat small amounts of bland foods. Test your glucose levels regularly and check your urine for acetone. If acetone is present, call your doctor at once. Even if you control the symptoms of low blood sugar and have no continuing problems, you should keep your doctor informed. If you have severe or prolonged vomiting, check with your doctor. In addition, before you become sick, check with your doctor for instructions regarding sick days.

Check with your doctor right away if the symptoms of high blood sugar (hyperglycemia) occur. These symptoms appear more slowly than those of hypoglycemia, and usually include:
> Drowsiness
> Flushed, dry skin
> Fruit-like breath odor
> Increased urination
> Loss of appetite
> Tiredness
> Unusual thirst

These symptoms may occur if you do not take enough insulin, if you skip a dose, if you do not follow a proper diet or if you overeat, or if you have a fever or infection.

Symptoms of both low blood sugar and high blood sugar must be corrected before they progress to a more serious condition. In either situation, you should check with your doctor immediately.

When traveling:
• Carry a recent prescription from your doctor for your diabetes medicine, and also for the correct syringe and needles, since state and city laws and regulations may vary.

• Do not change your diet or medicine schedule. Before you leave, discuss your trip with your doctor.

• Consider the use of disposable syringes since they are presterilized.

• Carry your diabetic supplies on your person or in a purse or briefcase to reduce the possibility of loss.

• Remember time zone changes and changes in meal times. Such changes may affect your diabetic schedule unless you allow for them.

• In hot climates, consider the use of an insulated container to help maintain the temperature of your insulin. These can be obtained at most pharmacies.

• In foreign countries, it is advisable to carry enough diabetic supplies to last until you return home, although most countries have some form of insulin available.

• When carrying a large quantity of diabetic supplies, divide your insulin supplies equally throughout your pieces of luggage. This will reduce the amount of loss if any of your luggage is lost or delayed.

Fergon Ferralet Fertinic* Novoferrogluc* Simron	Ferrous Gluconate†
Feosol Fer-In-Sol Fer-Iron Fero-Grad* Fero-Gradumet Ferralyn Ferospace Fesofor* Hematinic Iromal Mol-Iron Novoferrosulfa* Slow Fe	Ferrous Sulfate†
Hytinic Niferex Niferex-150 Nu-Iron Nu-Iron 150	Iron-Polysac- charide

*Not available in the United States.
†Generic name product may also be available.

IRON SUPPLEMENTS (Systemic)

This information applies to the following medicines:

Ferrous Fumarate (FER-us FOO-ma-rate)
Ferrous Gluconate (FER-us GLOO-koe-nate)
Ferrous Sulfate (FER-us SUL-fate)
Iron-Polysaccharide (pol-i-SAK-a-ride)

Some commonly used brand names are:	Generic names:
Feco-T Femiron Feostat Fersamal* Fumasorb Fumerin Hemocyte Ircon Palafer* Palmiron	Ferrous Fumarate†

Iron is a mineral used to treat or prevent a condition called iron deficiency (iron shortage) or iron-deficiency anemia. In this condition, the body does not have enough iron to produce the amount of normal red blood cells needed to keep you in good health. Although most people get enough iron from their diet, some must take additional amounts to meet their needs. For example, iron is sometimes lost with slow or small amounts of bleeding in the body that you would not be aware of and which can only be detected by your doctor. Your doctor can determine if you have an iron deficiency, what is causing the deficiency, and if an iron supplement is necessary.

After you start using this medicine continue to return to your doctor to determine if you are benefiting from the iron. Some blood tests may be necessary for this.

Some iron preparations are available only with your doctor's prescription. Others are available without a prescription; however, your doctor may have special instructions on the proper use and dose for your condition.

Before Using This Medicine

In order to decide on the best treatment for your medical problem, your doctor should be told:

—if you have ever had any unusual or allergic reaction to iron medicine.

—if you are pregnant or if you intend to become pregnant while using this medicine. During the first 3 months of pregnancy, a proper diet usually provides enough iron; however, during the last 6 months, in order to meet the increased needs of the developing baby, an iron supplement may be recommended by your doctor.

—if you are breast-feeding an infant. Iron normally is present in breast milk in small amounts. When prescribed by a doctor, iron preparations are not known to cause problems during breast-feeding; however, nursing mothers are advised to check with their doctor before taking iron supplements or any other medication.

—if you have any of the following medical problems:

  Alcoholism
  Blood disease (other than iron-deficiency anemia)
  Infection
  Inflammation of pancreas
  Intestinal disorders
  Liver disease
  Stomach ulcers

—if you are now taking any of the following medicines or types of medicine:

  Acetohydroxamic acid
  Antacids
  Iron by injection
  Pancreatin
  Penicillamine
  Tetracyclines
  Vitamin E

Proper Use of This Medicine

Iron is best taken on an empty stomach, with water or fruit juice (adults: full glass or 8 ounces; children: ½ glass or 4 ounces), about 1 hour before or 2 hours after meals. To lessen the possibility of stomach upset, iron may be taken with food or immediately after meals; however, certain foods should not be taken at the same time as iron (see *Precautions While Using This Medicine*).

For safe and effective use of iron supplements:

• Follow your doctor's instructions if this medicine was prescribed.

• Follow the manufacturer's package directions if you are treating yourself. If you think you still need iron after taking it for 1 or 2 months, check with your doctor.

To prevent, reduce, or remove iron staining of the teeth:

• Liquid dosage forms of iron medicine tend to stain the teeth. This effect may be reduced by mixing each dose in water, fruit juice, or tomato juice. You may use a drinking tube or straw to help keep the medicine from getting on the teeth.

• When doses of liquid iron medicine are to be given by dropper, the dose may be placed well back on the tongue and followed with water or juice.

• Iron stains on teeth can usually be removed by brushing with baking soda (sodium bicarbonate) or medicinal peroxide (hydrogen peroxide 3%).

If you miss a dose of this medicine, skip the missed dose and go back to your regular dosing schedule. Do not double doses.

How to store this medicine:

• Store away from heat and direct light.

• **Keep out of the reach of children because overdose is especially dangerous in** children. As few as 3 or 4 adult iron tablets can cause serious poisoning in small children. Flavored products of vitamins with iron and vitamin-iron products taken during pregnancy often cause iron overdose in small children.

• Do not store in the bathroom medicine cabinet because the heat or moisture may cause the medicine to break down.

• Keep the liquid form of this medicine from freezing.

• Do not keep outdated medicine or medicine no longer needed. Flush the contents of the container down the toilet, unless otherwise directed.

Precautions While Using This Medicine

When iron combines with certain foods it loses much of its value. The following foods should be avoided or taken in very small amounts within 1 hour before or 2 hours after iron:

    Cheese and cottage cheese
    Eggs
    Ice cream
    Milk
    Tea or coffee
    Whole-grain breads and cereals

If you are taking iron medicine without a doctor's prescription:

• Do not take iron medicine by mouth if you are receiving iron injections. To do so may result in iron poisoning.

• Do not regularly take large amounts of iron for longer than 6 months without checking with your doctor. People differ in their need for iron and those with certain medical conditions can gradually become poisoned by taking too much iron over a period of time. Also, unabsorbed iron can mask the presence of blood in the stool which may delay discovery of a serious condition.

• Your total daily intake of iron must be considered, not just the amount contained in iron medicine. Iron-fortified

bread, cereals, and other foods must be added for the total.

Keep a 1 ounce bottle of ipecac *syrup* available at home to be used in case of an emergency when its use is ordered by a doctor, poison control center, or emergency room.

Obtain the telephone numbers of your regional poison control center, nearest hospital emergency room and doctor. Keep these numbers readily available.

If you think an overdose of iron medicine has been taken:

• **Immediate medical attention is very important.**

• **Call your doctor, a poison control center, or the nearest hospital emergency room at once.** Always keep these phone numbers handy.

• **Follow any instructions given to you.** If ipecac syrup has been ordered and given, do not delay going to the emergency room while waiting for the ipecac syrup to empty the stomach, since it may require 20 to 30 minutes to show results.

• **Go to the emergency room without delay.**

• **Take the container of iron medicine with you.**

Early signs of iron overdose may not appear for up to 60 minutes or more. By this time emergency room treatment should be obtained. Do not delay going to the emergency room while waiting for signs to appear.

Side Effects of This Medicine

Along with its needed effects, a medicine may cause some unwanted effects. Although not all of these effects appear very often, when they do occur they may require medical attention. Check with your doctor if any of the following side effects occur:

Less common or rare

Abdominal or stomach pain, cramping, or soreness (prolonged)

Chest or throat pain, especially when swallowing

Stools with signs of blood (red or black color)

Early signs of iron poisoning

Diarrhea (may contain blood)

Nausea

Stomach pain or cramping (sharp)

Vomiting (may contain blood)

Note: May not be noticed for up to 60 minutes or more. By this time emergency room treatment should be obtained. Do not delay going to emergency room while waiting for signs to appear.

Late signs of iron poisoning

Bluish-colored lips, fingernails, and palms of hands

Drowsiness

Pale, clammy skin

Unusual tiredness and/or weakness

Weak and unusually fast heartbeat

Other side effects may occur which usually do not require medical attention. These side effects may go away during treatment as your body adjusts to the medicine. However, check with your doctor if any of the following side effects continue or are bothersome:

Less common

Constipation

Darkened urine

Diarrhea

Heartburn

Nausea

Vomiting

Stools commonly become black when iron preparations are taken by mouth. This is caused by unabsorbed iron and is harmless. However, in rare cases, black stools of a sticky consistency may occur along with other symptoms such as red streaks in the stool, cramping, soreness, or sharp pains in the stomach or abdominal area.

Check with your doctor immediately if these signs appear.

Other side effects not listed above may also occur in some patients. If you notice any other effects, check with your doctor.

ISOTRETINOIN (Systemic)

A commonly used brand name is Accutane.

Isotretinoin (eye-soe-TRET-i-noyn) is taken by mouth and is used in the treatment of severe cystic acne. It is usually used only after other acne medicines have been used and have failed to help the acne. It is not used for other types of acne. Isotretinoin may also be used to treat other skin diseases as determined by your doctor.

This medicine is available only with your doctor's prescription.

Before Using This Medicine

In order to decide on the best treatment for your medical problem, your doctor should be told:

—if you have ever had any unusual or allergic reaction to isotretinoin.

—if you are on a low-salt, low-sugar, or any other special diet, or if you are allergic to any substance, such as sulfites or other preservatives or dyes. Most medicines contain more than their active ingredient. Your doctor or pharmacist can help you avoid products that may cause a problem.

—if you are pregnant or if you intend to become pregnant while taking this medicine. Isotretinoin must not be taken during pregnancy because it has been shown to cause birth defects in humans. Women of childbearing potential should have a pregnancy test within 2 weeks before beginning treatment with isotretinoin to make sure they are not pregnant. Also, isotretinoin should not be taken unless an effective form of contraception (birth control) is used for at least 1 month before beginning treatment. Contraception should be continued during the period of treatment and for 1 month after isotretinoin is stopped. Be sure you have discussed this with your doctor.

—if you are breast-feeding an infant. It is not known whether isotretinoin passes into the breast milk. However, isotretinoin is not recommended during breast-feeding because it may cause unwanted effects in infants of mothers taking this medicine.

—if you have either of the following medical problems:

Diabetes mellitus (sugar diabetes)
(or a family history of)
Overweight (severe)

—if any member of your family has a history of high triglyceride (fat-like substance) levels in the blood.

—if you are now taking either of the following medicines or types of medicine:

Tetracyclines
Vitamin A or any preparation containing vitamin A

—if you are now using any other topical acne preparation or preparation containing a peeling agent, such as benzoyl peroxide, resorcinol, salicylic acid, sulfur, or tretinoin (vitamin A acid).

—if you are now using any topical alcohol-containing preparation such as aftershave lotion, astringent, cologne, perfume, or shaving cream or lotion.

—if you are now using any of the following preparations:

Abrasive soaps or cleansers
Cosmetics or soaps that dry the skin
Medicated cosmetics or "cover-ups"
Other topical medicine for the skin

Proper Use of This Medicine

It is very important that you take isotretinoin only as directed. Do not take more of it, do not take it more often, and do not take it for a longer period of time than your doctor ordered. To do so may increase the chance of side effects.

If you miss a dose of this medicine, take it as soon as possible. However, if it is almost time for your next dose, skip the missed dose and go back to your regular dosing schedule. Do not double doses.

How to store this medicine:

• Store away from heat and direct light.

• **Keep out of the reach of children.**

• Do not store in the bathroom medicine cabinet because the heat or moisture may cause the medicine to break down.

• Do not keep outdated medicine or medicine no longer needed. Flush the contents of the container down the toilet, unless otherwise directed.

Precautions While Using This Medicine

Your doctor should check your progress at regular visits in order to make sure that this medicine does not cause unwanted effects.

Isotretinoin has been shown to cause birth defects in humans if taken during pregnancy. Therefore, if you suspect that you may have become pregnant, stop taking this medicine immediately and check with your doctor.

Do not donate blood to a blood bank while you are taking isotretinoin or for 30 days after you stop taking it. This is to prevent the possibility of a pregnant patient receiving the blood.

Do not take vitamin A or any vitamin supplement containing vitamin A while taking this medicine, unless otherwise directed by your doctor. To do so may increase the chance of side effects.

Drinking too much alcohol while taking this medicine may cause high triglyceride (fat-like substance) levels in the blood and possibly increase the chance of unwanted effects on the heart and blood vessels. Therefore, **while taking this medicine, it is best that you do not drink alcoholic beverages or at least reduce the amount you usually drink.** If you have any questions about this, check with your doctor.

Diabetics—Isotretinoin may cause a change in your blood sugar levels. If you notice a change in the results of your urine sugar test or if you have any questions, check with your doctor.

Isotretinoin may cause dryness of the eyes. Therefore, if you wear contact lenses, your eyes may be more sensitive to them during the time you are taking isotretinoin and for up to about 2 weeks after you stop taking it. To help relieve dryness of the eyes, check with your doctor about using an eye lubricating solution, such as artificial tears. If inflammation of the eyes occurs, check with your doctor.

A few people who take this medicine may become more sensitive to sunlight than they are normally. When you begin to take this medicine, avoid too much sun or overuse of a sunlamp until you see how you react, especially if you tend to burn easily. If you have a severe reaction, check with your doctor.

Your mouth and nose may feel very dry while you are taking this medicine. To help relieve mouth dryness, chew sugarless gum or dissolve bits of ice in your mouth.

For patients taking isotretinoin for acne:
 • When you begin taking isotretinoin, your acne may seem to get worse before it gets better. If irritation or other symptoms of condition become severe, check with your doctor.

Side Effects of This Medicine

Along with its needed effects, a medicine may cause some unwanted effects. Although not all of these side effects appear very often, when they do occur they may require medical attention. Check with your doctor as soon as possible if any of the following side effects occur:

More common
> Burning, redness, itching, or other sign of inflammation of eyes
> Scaling, redness, burning, pain, or other sign of inflammation of lips

Less common
> Skin infection or rash

Rare
> Abdominal or stomach pain (severe)
> Bleeding or inflammation of gums
> Blurred vision or other changes in vision
> Diarrhea (severe)
> Headache (severe or continuing)
> Mood changes
> Nausea and vomiting
> Rectal bleeding

Other side effects may occur which usually do not require medical attention. These side effects may go away during treatment as your body adjusts to the medicine. However, check with your doctor if any of the following side effects continue or are bothersome:

More common
> Dryness or itching of skin
> Dryness of mouth or nose
> Nosebleeds

Less common
> Dryness of eyes
> Headache
> Increased sensitivity of skin to sunlight
> Pain, tenderness, or stiffness in muscles, bones, or joints

Peeling of skin on palms of hands or soles
    of feet
Stomach upset
Thinning of hair
Unusual tiredness

Other side effects not listed above may also
occur in some patients. If you notice any
other effects, check with your doctor.

LAXATIVES, BULK-FORMING
(Oral)

This information applies to the following medicines:

Malt Soup Extract
Methylcellulose (meth-ill-SELL-yoo-lose)
Polycarbophil (pol-i-KAR-boe-fil)
Psyllium (SILL-i-yum)

Some commonly used brand names are:	Generic names:
Maltsupex	Malt Soup Extract
Cologel	Methylcellulose†
Mitrolan	Calcium Polycarbophil
Cillium Effersyllium Fiberall Konsyl Konsyl-D Metamucil Modane Bulk Mucilose Naturacil Perdiem Pro-Lax Regacilium Reguloid Siblin Syllact V-Lax	Psyllium Psyllium Mucilloid

†Generic name product may also be available.

Note: Many laxative formulas include two or
more laxative substances. Only those formulas containing one primary laxative
are listed.

This information does not apply to psyllium or
polycarbophil when prescribed for other than
a laxative use.

Bulk-forming laxatives are medicines
taken by mouth to encourage bowel movements to relieve constipation and to prevent
straining. This type of laxative is not digested but absorbs liquid in the intestines and
swells to form a soft, bulky stool. The bowel
is then stimulated normally by the presence
of the bulky mass.

Some bulk-forming laxatives, like psyllium and polycarbophil, may be prescribed
by your doctor to treat diarrhea.

Laxatives should not be given to young
children (up to 6 years of age) unless prescribed by their doctor. Since children cannot usually describe their symptoms very
well, a doctor should check the child before
giving this medicine. This is to prevent an
unknown condition from getting worse and
to avoid causing unwanted effects in the
child.

Most bulk-forming laxatives are available without a prescription; however, your
doctor may have special instructions for the
proper use and dose for your medical condition.

When indicated, bulk-forming laxatives
may provide relief in a number of situations
such as:

—during pregnancy.

—for a few days after giving birth.

—constipation caused by other medicines.

—to aid in developing normal bowel
function following a period of poor eating habits or a lack of physical exercise.

—following surgery when straining
should be avoided.

—with some medical conditions that may be made worse by straining, for example:

Heart disease
Hemorrhoids
Hernia (rupture)
High blood pressure
History of stroke

Before Using This Medicine

Importance of diet, fluids, and exercise to prevent constipation—Laxatives are to be used to provide short-term relief only, unless otherwise directed by a doctor. A proper diet containing roughage (whole grain breads and cereals, bran, fruit, and green, leafy vegetables), with 6 to 8 full glasses (8 ounces each) of liquids each day, and daily exercise are most important in maintaining a healthy bowel function. Also, for individuals who have problems with constipation, foods such as pastries, puddings, sugar, candy, cake, and cheese may make the constipation worse.

Before you use this medicine, check with your doctor or pharmacist:

—if you have ever had any unusual or allergic reaction to laxatives.

—if you are on a low-salt, low-sugar, or any other special diet, or if you are allergic to any substance, such as sulfites or other preservatives or dyes. Most medicines contain more than their active ingredient. Your doctor or pharmacist can help you avoid products that may cause a problem.

—if you are pregnant. Some bulk-forming laxatives contain a large amount of sodium or sugars, which may have possible unwanted effects such as increasing blood pressure or causing water to be held in the tissues.

—if you have any of the following medical problems:

Appendicitis (or signs of)
Diabetes mellitus (sugar diabetes)
Heart disease

High blood pressure
Intestinal blockage
Laxative habit
Rectal bleeding of unknown cause
Swallowing difficulty

—if you are now taking any of the following medicines or types of medicine:

Amiloride
Anticoagulants, oral (blood thinners you take by mouth)
Aspirin or other salicylates
Digitalis preparations (heart medicine)
Laxatives (other)
Potassium supplements
Spironolactone
Sodium salicylate
Tetracycline antibiotics
Triamterene

Proper Use of This Medicine

For safe and effective use of bulk-forming laxatives:

• Follow your doctor's orders if this laxative was prescribed.

• Follow the manufacturer's package directions if you are treating yourself.

• Do not try to swallow in the dry form. Take with liquid.

To allow bulk-forming laxatives to work properly and to prevent intestinal blockage, it is necessary to drink plenty of fluids during their use. At least six to eight 8-ounce glasses of liquids should be taken each day. Each dose should be taken in or with a full glass (8 ounces) or more of cold water or fruit juice. This will provide enough liquid for the laxative to work properly. A second glass of water or juice by itself is often recommended with each dose for best effect and to avoid side effects.

Results often may be obtained in 12 hours but may not occur for some individuals until after 2 or 3 days.

How to store this medicine:

• Store away from heat and direct light.

• **Keep out of the reach of children.**

• Do not store in the bathroom medicine cabinet because the heat or moisture may cause the medicine to break down.

• Keep the liquid form of this medicine from freezing.

• Do not keep outdated medicine or medicine no longer needed. Flush the contents of the container down the toilet, unless otherwise directed.

Precautions While Using This Medicine

Do not take any type of laxative:

—**if you have signs of appendicitis or inflamed bowel** (such as stomach or lower abdominal pain, cramping, bloating, soreness, nausea, or vomiting). Instead, check with your doctor as soon as possible.

—**for more than 1 week** unless your doctor has prescribed or ordered a special schedule for you. This is true even when you have had no results from the laxative.

—**within 2 hours of taking other medicine** because the desired effect of the other medicine may be reduced.

—**if you do not need it,** as for the common cold, "to clean out your system," or as a "tonic to make you feel better."

—**if you miss a bowel movement for a day or two.**

—**if you develop a skin rash** while taking a laxative or if you had a rash the last time you took it.

If you notice a sudden change in bowel habits or function that lasts longer than 2 weeks, or that keeps returning off and on, check with your doctor before using a laxative. This will allow the cause of your problem to be determined before it becomes more serious.

The "laxative habit"—Laxative products are overused by many people. Such a practice often leads to dependence on the laxative action to produce a bowel movement. In severe cases, overuse of some laxatives has caused damage to the nerves, muscles, and tissues of the intestines and bowel. If you have any questions about the use of laxatives, check with your doctor, nurse, or pharmacist.

Bulk-forming laxatives often contain large amounts of sugars, carbohydrates, and sodium. If you are on a low-sugar, low-caloric, or low-salt diet, check with your doctor, nurse, or pharmacist before using this type of laxative.

Side Effects of This Medicine

Along with its needed effects, a medicine may cause some unwanted effects. Although not all of these side effects appear very often, when they do occur they may require medical attention. Check with your doctor as soon as possible if any of the following side effects occur:

Rare
> Asthma
> Intestinal blockage
> Skin rash or itching
> Swallowing difficulty (feeling of lump in throat)

Other side effects not listed above may also occur in some patients. If you notice any other effects, check with your doctor.

LAXATIVES, EMOLLIENT (Oral)

This information applies to the following medicines:

Docusate (DOK-yoo-sate)
Poloxamer 188 (pol-OX-a-mer)

Some commonly used brand names or other names are:	Generic names:
D-C-S	
Pro-Cal-Sof	Docusate
Surfak	Calcium†
Dialose	
Diocto-K	Docusate
Kasof	Potassium
Afko-Lube	
Bu-Lax	
Colace	
Dilax	
Dioctyl Sodium Sulfosuccinate	
Diocto	
Dioeze	
Diosuccin	
Dio-Sul	
Disonate	
Di-Sosul	Docusate Sodium†
Doss	
Doxinate	
D-S-S	
Duosol	
Laxinate	
Modane Soft	
Molatoc	
Pro-Sof	
Pro-Sof-100	
Regulax SS	
Regutol	
Stulex	
Alaxin	Poloxamer 188

†Generic name product may also be available.

Note: Many laxative formulas include two or more laxative substances. Only those formulas containing one primary laxative are listed.

Emollient laxatives (stool softeners) are medicines taken by mouth to encourage bowel movements by helping liquids mix into the stool and prevent dry, hard stool masses. This type of laxative has been said not to *cause* a bowel movement but instead *allows* the patient to have a bowel movement without straining.

Laxatives should not be given to young children (up to 6 years of age) unless prescribed by their doctor. Since children cannot usually describe their symptoms very well, a doctor should check the child before giving this medicine. This is to prevent an unknown condition from getting worse and to avoid causing unwanted effects in the child.

Emollient laxatives are available without a prescription; however, your doctor may have special instructions for the proper use and dose for your medical condition.

When indicated, emollient laxatives may provide relief when constipation is associated with hard, dry stools such as:

—during pregnancy.

—a few days after giving birth.

—constipation caused by other medicines.

—following surgery when straining should be avoided.

—with some medical conditions that may be made worse by straining, for example:

Heart disease
Hemorrhoids
Hernia (rupture)
High blood pressure
History of stroke

Before Using This Medicine

Importance of diet, fluids, and exercise to prevent constipation—Laxatives are to be used to provide short-term relief only, unless otherwise directed by a doctor. A proper diet containing roughage (whole grain breads and cereals, bran, fruit, and green, leafy vegetables), with 6 to 8 full glasses (8 ounces each) of liquids each day, and daily exercise are most important in maintaining a healthy bowel function. Also, for individuals who have problems with constipation, foods such as pastries, puddings, sugar, candy, cake, and cheese may make the constipation worse.

Before you use this medicine, check with your doctor or pharmacist:

—if you have ever had any unusual or allergic reaction to laxatives.

—if you are on a low-salt, low-sugar, or any other special diet, or if you are allergic to any substance, such as sulfites or other preservatives or dyes. Most medicines contain more than their active ingredient, and many liquid medicines contain alcohol. Your doctor or pharmacist can help you avoid products that may cause a problem.

—if you have any of the following medical problems:
Appendicitis (or signs of)
Diabetes mellitus (sugar diabetes)
Heart disease
High blood pressure
Intestinal blockage
Laxative habit
Rectal bleeding of unknown cause

—if you are now taking any of the following medicines or types of medicine:
Amiloride
Laxatives (other)
Potassium supplements
Spironolactone
Triamterene

Proper Use of This Medicine

For safe and effective use of your laxative, carefully follow:

—your doctor's instructions if this laxative was prescribed.

—the manufacturer's package directions if you are treating yourself.

As with all laxatives, at least 6 to 8 glasses (8 ounces each) of liquids should be taken each day. This will help make the stool softer.

Results may not occur until 1 to 2 days after the first dose but may not occur for some individuals until after 3 to 5 days.

Liquid forms may be taken in milk or fruit juice to improve flavor.

How to store this medicine:

• Store away from heat and direct light.

• **Keep out of the reach of children.**

• Do not store in the bathroom medicine cabinet because the heat or moisture may cause the medicine to break down.

• Keep the liquid form of this medicine from freezing.

• Do not keep outdated medicine or medicine no longer needed. Flush the contents of the container down the toilet, unless otherwise directed.

Precautions While Using This Medicine

Do not take any type of laxative:

—**if you have signs of appendicitis or inflamed bowel** (such as stomach or lower abdominal pain, cramping, bloating, soreness, nausea, or vomiting). Instead, check with your doctor as soon as possible.

—**for more than 1 week** unless your doctor has prescribed or ordered a special schedule for you. This is true even when you have had no results from the laxative.

—**within 2 hours of taking other medicine** because the desired effect of the other medicine may be reduced.

—**if you do not need it,** as for the common cold, "to clean out your system," or as a "tonic to make you feel better."

—**if you miss a bowel movement for a day or two.**

—**if you develop a skin rash** while taking a laxative or if you had a rash the last time you took it.

If you notice a sudden change in bowel habits or function that lasts longer than 2 weeks, or that keeps returning off and on, check with your doctor before using a laxative. This will allow the cause of your problem to be determined before it may become more serious.

The "laxative habit"—Laxative products are overused by many people. Such a practice often leads to dependence on the laxative action to produce a bowel movement. In severe cases, overuse of some laxatives has caused damage to the nerves, muscles, and tissues of the intestines and bowel. If you have any questions about the use of laxatives, check with your doctor, nurse, or pharmacist.

Side Effects of This Medicine

Along with its needed effects, a medicine may cause some unwanted effects. Although not all of these side effects appear very often, when they do occur they may require medical attention. Check with your doctor as soon as possible if the following side effect occurs:

Rare

Skin rash

Other side effects may occur which usually do not require medical attention. These side effects may go away during treatment as your body adjusts to the medicine. However, check with your doctor if any of the following side effects continue or are bothersome:

Less common

Stomach and/or intestinal cramping
Throat irritation (liquid forms only)

Other side effects not listed above may also occur in some patients. If you notice any other effects, check with your doctor.

LAXATIVES, STIMULANT (Oral)

This information applies to the following medicines:

Bisacodyl (bis-a-KOE-dill)
Cascara (kas-KAR-a) Sagrada
Castor (KAS-tor) Oil
Danthron (DAN-thron)
Dehydrocholic (dee-hye-droe-KOE-lik) Acid
Phenolphthalein (fee-nole-THAY-leen)
Senna
Sennosides

Some commonly used brand names or other names are:	Generic names:
Dacodyl Dulcolax Fleet Bisacodyl	Bisacodyl†
Cascara	Cascara Sagrada†
Alphamul Emulsoil Fleet Castor Oil Kellogg's Castor Oil Neoloid Purge	Castor Oil†
Akshun Dorbane Modane Modane Mild	Danthron†
Cholan-DH Decholin Hepahydrin	Dehydrocholic Acid†
Alophen Correctol Espotabs Evac-U-Gen Evac-U-Lax Ex-Lax Feen-A-Mint Feen-A-Mint Gum Phenolax Prulet	Phenolphthalein

Black-Draught	
Senexon	
Senokot	Senna†
Senolax	

Nytilax	Sennosides

†Generic name product may also be available.

Note: Many laxative formulas include two or more laxative substances. Only those formulas containing one primary laxative are listed.

This information does not apply to dehydrocholic acid when prescribed for other than a laxative use.

Stimulant laxatives, also known as contact laxatives, encourage bowel movements by acting on the intestinal wall. They increase the muscle contractions that move along the stool mass. Stimulant laxatives are available in many brand names, package designs, and dosage forms. They are a popular type of laxative for self-treatment. However, they also are more likely to cause side effects.

One of the stimulant laxatives, dehydrocholic acid, may also be used for certain conditions of the biliary tract and is available only with your doctor's prescription.

Laxatives should not be given to young children (up to 6 years of age) unless prescribed by their doctor. Since children cannot usually describe their symptoms very well, a doctor should check the child before giving this medicine. This is to prevent an unknown condition from getting worse and to avoid causing unwanted effects in the child.

Most stimulant laxatives are available without a prescription; however, your doctor may have special instructions for the proper use and dose for your medical condition.

When indicated, stimulant laxatives may provide relief in situations such as:

—constipation caused by other medicines.

—preparation for examination or surgery (castor oil and bisacodyl).

—constipation of bedfast patients.

Before Using This Medicine

Importance of diet, fluids, and exercise to prevent constipation—Laxatives are to be used to provide short-term relief only, unless otherwise directed by your doctor. A proper diet containing roughage (whole grain breads and cereals, bran, fruit, and green, leafy vegetables), with 6 to 8 full glasses (8 ounces each) of liquids each day, and daily exercise are most important in maintaining a healthy bowel function. Also, for individuals who have problems with constipation, foods such as pastries, puddings, sugar, candy, cake, and cheese may make the constipation worse.

Before you use this medicine, check with your doctor or pharmacist:

—if you have ever had any unusual or allergic reaction to laxatives.

—if you are on a low-salt, low-sugar, or any other special diet, or if you are allergic to any substance, such as sulfites or other preservatives or dyes. Most medicines contain more than their active ingredient, and many liquid medicines contain alcohol. Your doctor or pharmacist can help you avoid products that may cause a problem.

—if you are pregnant. Stimulant laxatives may cause unwanted effects in the expectant mother if improperly used. Castor oil in particular should not be used as it may cause contractions of the womb.

—if you are breast-feeding an infant. Laxatives containing cascara, danthron, and phenolphthalein may pass into the breast milk. Although the amount of laxative in the milk is generally thought to be too small to cause problems in the child, your doctor should be told that you plan to use such laxatives. Some reports claim that diarrhea has been caused in the infant.

—if you have any of the following medical problems:

Appendicitis (or signs of)
Colostomy
Diabetes mellitus (sugar diabetes)
Heart disease
High blood pressure
Ileostomy
Intestinal blockage
Laxative habit
Rectal bleeding of unknown cause

—if you are now taking any of the following medicines or types of medicine:

Amiloride
Antacids
Laxatives (other)
Potassium supplements
Spironolactone
Triamterene

Proper Use of This Medicine

For safe and effective use of your laxative, carefully follow:

—your doctor's instructions if this laxative was prescribed.

—the manufacturer's package directions if you are treating yourself.

As with all laxatives, at least 6 to 8 glasses (8 ounces each) of liquids should be taken each day. This will help make the stool softer.

Stimulant laxatives are usually taken on an empty stomach for rapid effect. Results are slowed if taken with food.

Many stimulant laxatives (but not castor oil) are often taken at bedtime to produce results the next morning (although some may require up to 24 hours or more).

For patients taking castor oil:

• Castor oil is not usually taken late in the day because its results occur within 2 to 6 hours.

• The unpleasant taste may be improved by chilling in the refrigerator for at least an hour and then stirring the dose into a full glass of cold orange juice just before it is taken. Also, flavored preparations of castor oil are available.

For patients taking bisacodyl:

• Bisacodyl tablets are specially coated to allow them to work properly without causing irritation and/or nausea. To protect this coating, do not chew, crush, or take the tablets within an hour of milk or antacids.

How to store this medicine:

• Store away from heat and direct light.

• **Keep out of the reach of children.**

• Do not store in the bathroom medicine cabinet because the heat or moisture may cause the medicine to break down.

• Keep the liquid form of this medicine from freezing.

• Do not keep outdated medicine or medicine no longer needed. Flush the contents of the container down the toilet, unless otherwise directed.

Precautions While Using This Medicine

Do not take any type of laxative:

—**if you have signs of appendicitis or inflamed bowel** (such as stomach or lower abdominal pain, cramping, bloating, soreness, nausea, or vomiting). Instead, check with your doctor as soon as possible.

—**for more than 1 week** unless your doctor has prescribed or ordered a special schedule for you. This is true even when you have had no results from the laxative.

—**within 2 hours of taking other medicine** because the desired effect of the other medicine may be reduced.

—**if you do not need it,** as for the common cold, "to clean out your system," or as a "tonic to make you feel better."

—if you miss a bowel movement for a day or two.

—if you develop a skin rash while taking a laxative or if you had a rash the last time you took it.

If you notice a sudden change in bowel habits or function that lasts longer than 2 weeks, or that keeps returning off and on, check with your doctor before using a laxative. This will allow the cause of your problem to be determined before it may become more serious.

The "laxative habit"—Laxative products are overused by many people. Such a practice often leads to dependence on the laxative action to produce a bowel movement. In severe cases, overuse of some laxatives has caused damage to the nerves, muscles, and tissues of the intestines and bowel. If you have any questions about the use of laxatives, check with your doctor, nurse, or pharmacist.

Stimulant laxatives are most often associated with:

—occasional coloration of urine or stool (pink to red is the most common).

—overuse and the laxative habit.

—skin rashes.

—intestinal cramping after dosing (especially if taken on an empty stomach).

—potassium loss.

For patients taking laxative products containing phenolphthalein:

• Because of the way this ingredient works in the body, a single dose may cause a laxative effect in some people for up to 3 days.

Some stimulant laxatives contain large amounts of sugars, carbohydrates, and sodium. If you are on a low-sugar, low-caloric, or low-salt diet, check with your doctor, nurse, or pharmacist before using this type of laxative.

Side Effects of This Medicine

Along with its needed effects, a medicine may cause some unwanted effects. Although not all of these side effects appear very often, when they do occur they may require medical attention. Check with your doctor as soon as possible if any of the following side effects occur:

Rare

Breathing difficulty
Burning on urination
Confusion
Headache
Irregular heartbeat
Irritability
Mood or mental changes
Muscle cramps
Skin rash
Unusual tiredness or weakness

Other side effects may occur which usually do not require medical attention. These side effects may go away during treatment as your body adjusts to the medicine. However, check with your doctor if any of the following side effects continue or are bothersome:

Less common

Belching
Cramping
Diarrhea
Irritation of tissues around the rectal area
Nausea

Other side effects not listed above may also occur in some patients. If you notice any other effects, check with your doctor.

LEVODOPA (Systemic)

This information applies to the following medicines:

Carbidopa and Levodopa (KAR-bi-doe-pa and LEE-voe-doe-pa)
Levodopa

Some commonly used brand names are:	Generic names:
Sinemet	Carbidopa and Levodopa
Dopar Larodopa	Levodopa†

† Generic name product may also be available.

Levodopa used alone or in combination with carbidopa is used to treat Parkinson's disease, sometimes referred to as shaking palsy or paralysis agitans. Some patients require the combination of medicine, while others benefit from levodopa alone. By improving muscle control, this medicine allows more normal movements of the body.

Levodopa alone or in combination is available only with your doctor's prescription.

Before Using This Medicine

In order to decide on the best treatment for your medical problem, your doctor should be told:

—if you have ever had any unusual or allergic reaction to levodopa alone or in combination with carbidopa.

—if you are on a low-salt, low-sugar, or any other special diet, or if you are allergic to any substance, such as sulfites or other preservatives or dyes. Most medicines contain more than their active ingredient. Your doctor or pharmacist can help you avoid products that may cause a problem.

—if you are pregnant or if you intend to become pregnant while taking this medicine. Studies have not been done in humans. However, studies in animals have shown that levodopa affects the baby's growth both before and after birth if given during pregnancy in doses many times the human dose. Also, studies in rabbits have shown that levodopa alone or in combination with carbidopa causes birth defects.

—if you are breast-feeding an infant. Levodopa and carbidopa pass into the breast milk and may cause unwanted side effects in the breast-fed infant. Also, levodopa may reduce the flow of breast milk.

—if you have any of the following medical problems:
Convulsive disorders, such as epilepsy (history of)
Diabetes mellitus (sugar diabetes)
Emphysema, asthma, bronchitis, or other chronic lung disease
Glaucoma
Heart or blood vessel disease
Hormone problems
Kidney disease
Liver disease
Mental illness
Skin cancer (or history of)
Stomach ulcer (history of)

—if you are now taking any of the following medicines or types of medicine:
Amantadine
Amphetamines (for levodopa used alone)
Antacids
Anticonvulsants (for example, ethotoin, mephenytoin, or phenytoin)
Antihypertensives (high blood pressure medicine)
Antimuscarinics (medicine for abdominal or stomach spasms of cramps)
Appetite suppressants (medicine for appetite control) such as phenylpropanolamine-containing diet aids (for levodopa used alone)
Asthma or bronchitis medicine, such as epinephrine, ephedrine, or isoproterenol (for levodopa used alone)
Benztropine
Bromocriptine
Chlorprothixene
Droperidol
Haloperidol
Loxapine
Methyldopa
Metoclopramide
Metyrosine
Papaverine
Procyclidine
Pyridoxine (vitamin B$_6$), present in some foods and vitamin formulas (for levodopa used alone)

Thiothixene
Trihexyphenidyl

—if you are now taking phenothiazine medicines such as:

Acetophenazine
Carphenazine
Chlorpromazine
Fluphenazine
Mesoridazine
Perphenazine
Piperacetazine
Prochlorperazine
Promazine
Promethazine
Thioridazine
Trifluoperazine
Triflupromazine
Trimeprazine

—if you are now taking or have taken within the past 2 weeks monoamine oxidase (MAO) inhibitors such as:

Furazolidone
Isocarboxazid
Pargyline
Phenelzine
Procarbazine
Tranylcypromine

Proper Use of This Medicine

It is best not to take this medicine with or after food, especially high-protein food, since food may decrease levodopa's effect. However, **to lessen possible stomach upset, take food shortly after taking this medicine (about 15 minutes after).** If stomach upset is severe or continues, check with your doctor.

Take this medicine only as directed. Do not take more or less of it, and do not take it more often than ordered.

Some people must take this medicine for several weeks or months before full benefit is received. Do not stop taking it even if you do not think it is working. Instead, check with your doctor.

If you miss a dose of this medicine, take it as soon as possible. However, if your next scheduled dose is within 2 hours, skip the missed dose and go back to your regular dosing schedule. Do not double doses.

How to store this medicine:

• Store away from heat and direct light.

• **Keep out of the reach of children.**

• Do not store in the bathroom medicine cabinet because the heat or moisture may cause the medicine to break down.

• Do not keep outdated medicine or medicine no longer needed. Flush the contents of the container down the toilet, unless otherwise directed.

Precautions While Using This Medicine

Before having any kind of surgery (including dental surgery) or emergency treatment, tell the physician or dentist in charge that you are taking this medicine.

Diabetics—This medicine may cause test results for urine sugar or ketones to be wrong. Check with your doctor before depending on home tests using the paper-strip or tablet method.

This medicine may cause some people to become drowsy or less alert than they are normally. **Make sure you know how you react to this medicine before you drive, use machines, or do other jobs that require you to be alert.**

Dizziness, lightheadedness, or fainting may occur, especially when you get up from a lying or sitting position. Getting up slowly may help. If the problem continues or gets worse, check with your doctor.

For patients taking levodopa by itself:

• Pyridoxine (vitamin B_6) has been found to reduce the effects of levodopa when taken by itself. This does not happen with the combination of carbidopa and levodopa. **If you are taking levodopa by itself, do not take vitamin products containing vitamin B_6 during treatment, unless prescribed by your doctor.**

• Large amounts of pyridoxine are also contained in some foods such as avocado, bacon, beans, beef liver, dry skim milk, oatmeal, peas, pork, sweet potato, tuna, and certain health foods. Check with your doctor about how much of these foods you may have in your diet while you are taking levodopa. Also, ask your doctor or pharmacist for help when selecting vitamin products.

As your condition improves and your body movements become easier, **be careful not to overdo physical activities. Injuries resulting from falls may occur.** Physical activities must be gradually increased to allow your body to adjust to changing balance, circulation, and coordination. **This is especially important in the elderly.**

After taking this medicine for long periods of time, such as a year or more, some patients suddenly lose the ability to move. Their muscles do not seem to work. This loss of movement may last from a few minutes to several hours. The patient then is able to move as before. This condition may unexpectedly occur again and again. If you should have this problem, sometimes called the "on-off" effect, check with your doctor.

Side Effects of This Medicine

Along with its needed effects, a medicine may cause some unwanted effects. Although not all of these side effects appear very often, when they do occur they may require medical attention. Check with your doctor as soon as possible if any of the following side effects occur:

More common

Mental depression

Mood or mental changes (such as aggressive behavior)

Unusual and uncontrolled movements of the body

Less common—more common when levodopa is used alone

Difficult urination

Dizziness or lightheadedness when getting up from a lying or sitting position

Irregular heartbeat

Nausea or vomiting (severe or continuing)

Spasm or closing of eyelid (not more common when levodopa is used alone)

Rare

High blood pressure

Stomach pain

Unusual tiredness or weakness

Other side effects may occur which usually do not require medical attention. These side effects may go away during treatment as your body adjusts to the medicine. However, check with your doctor if any of the following side effects continue or are bothersome:

More common

Anxiety, confusion, or nervousness (especially in elderly patients receiving other medicine for Parkinson's disease)

Less common

Constipation (more common when levodopa is used alone)

Diarrhea

Dry mouth

Flushing of skin

Headache

Loss of appetite

Muscle twitching

Nightmares (more common when levodopa is used alone)

Tiredness

Trouble in sleeping

This medicine may sometimes cause the urine and sweat to be darker in color than usual. The urine may at first be reddish, then turn to nearly black after being exposed to air. Some bathroom cleaning products will produce a similar effect when in contact with urine containing this medicine. This is to be expected during treatment with this medicine.

The above side effects are more likely to occur in elderly patients who are usually more sensitive to the effects of levodopa alone or in combination with carbidopa.

Other side effects not listed above may also occur in some patients. If you notice any other effects, check with your doctor.

LINCOMYCINS (Systemic)

This information applies to the following medicines:

Clindamycin (klin-da-MYE-sin)
Lincomycin (lin-koe-MYE-sin)

Some commonly used brand names are:	Generic names:
Cleocin Dalacin C*	Clindamycin
Lincocin	Lincomycin

*Not available in the United States.

Lincomycins belong to the general family of medicines called antibiotics. They are taken by mouth or given by injection to help the body overcome infections. They will not work for colds, flu, or other virus infections.

Lincomycins are available only with your doctor's prescription.

Before Using This Medicine

In order to decide on the best treatment for your medical problem, your doctor should be told:

—if you have ever had any unusual or allergic reaction to any of the lincomycins.

—if you are pregnant or if you intend to become pregnant while taking this medicine. Although lincomycins have not been shown to cause birth defects or other problems in humans, the chance always exists.

—if you are breast-feeding an infant. Lincomycins pass into the breast milk. Although lincomycins have not been shown to cause problems in humans, the chance always exists.

—if you have any of the following medical problems:

Kidney disease
Liver disease
Stomach or intestinal disease, history of (especially colitis, including colitis caused by antibiotics, or enteritis)

—if you are now taking any of the following medicines or types of medicine:

Ambenonium
Chloramphenicol
Diarrhea medicine
Erythromycins
Narcotics
Neostigmine
Pyridostigmine

—if you have ever had any problems with this medicine.

Proper Use of This Medicine

To help clear up your infection completely, **keep taking this medicine for the full time of treatment** even if you begin to feel better after a few days. **If you have a "strep" infection, you should keep taking this medicine for at least 10 days. This is especially important in "strep" infections since serious heart problems could develop later** if your infection is not completely cleared up. Also, if you stop taking this medicine too soon, your symptoms may return.

This medicine works best when there is a constant amount in the blood. **To help keep this amount constant, do not miss any doses. Also, it is best to take each dose at evenly spaced times day and night.** For example, if you are to take 4 doses a day, each dose should be spaced about 6 hours apart. If this interferes with your sleep or other daily activities, or if you need help in planning the best times to take your medicine, check with your doctor, nurse, or pharmacist.

If you do miss a dose of this medicine, take it as soon as possible. This will help to keep a constant amount of medicine in the blood. However, if it is almost time for your next dose and your dosing schedule is:

• 3 or more doses a day—Space the missed dose and the next dose 2 to 4 hours apart or double your next dose.

Then go back to your regular dosing schedule.

For patients taking the capsule form of clindamycin:
• **The capsule form of clindamycin should be taken with a full glass (8 ounces) of water or with meals** to prevent irritation of the esophagus (tube between the throat and stomach).

Lincomycin is best taken with a full glass (8 ounces) of water on an empty stomach (either 1 hour before or 2 hours after meals), unless otherwise directed by your doctor.

For patients taking the oral liquid form of clindamycin:
• Use a specially marked measuring spoon or other device to measure each dose accurately since the average household teaspoon may not hold the right amount of liquid.

• Do not use after the expiration date on the label since the medicine may not work as well. Check with your pharmacist if you have any questions about this.

How to store this medicine:

• Store away from heat and direct light, out of the reach of children.

• Do not store in the bathroom medicine cabinet because the heat or moisture may cause the medicine to break down.

• Do not refrigerate the oral liquid form of clindamycin. If chilled, the liquid may thicken and be difficult to pour. Follow the directions on the label.

• Do not keep outdated medicine or medicine no longer needed. Flush it down the toilet.

Precautions While Using This Medicine

It is important that your doctor check your progress at regular visits.

If your symptoms do not improve within a few days or if they become worse, check with your doctor.

If diarrhea occurs, do not take any diarrhea medicine without first checking with your doctor or pharmacist. These medicines may make your diarrhea worse or make it last longer.

Before having surgery (including dental surgery) with a general anesthetic, tell the physician or dentist in charge that you are taking a lincomycin.

Side Effects of This Medicine

Along with its needed effects, a medicine may cause some unwanted effects. Although not all of these side effects appear very often, when they do occur they may require medical attention. **Stop taking this medicine and check with your**

doctor immediately if any of the following side effects occur:

More common

Abdominal or stomach cramps, pain, and bloating (severe)

Diarrhea (watery and severe) which may also be bloody

Fever

Nausea or vomiting

Unusual thirst

Unusual tiredness or weakness

Unusual weight loss

(the above side effects may also occur up to several weeks after you stop taking this medicine)

Other side effects may occur which usually do not require medical attention. These side effects may go away during treatment as your body adjusts to the medicine. However, check with your doctor if any of the following side effects continue or are bothersome:

More common

Diarrhea (mild)

Skin rash

Less common

Itching of skin, rectal, or genital areas

Other side effects not listed above may also occur in some patients. If you notice any other effects, check with your doctor.

LITHIUM (Systemic)

Some commonly used brand names are:

Carbolith*	Lithizine*
Cibalith-S	Lithobid
Eskalith	Lithonate
Eskalith CR	Lithotabs
Lithane	

Generic name product may also be available.

---

*Not available in the United States.

Lithium (LITH-ee-um) is taken by mouth to treat the manic stage of manic-depressive illness. Manic-depressive patients experience severe mood changes, ranging from an excitement, or manic state (for example, unusual anger or a false sense of well-being) to depression or sadness. It is also used to reduce the frequency and severity of manic states.

The way lithium works to affect a person's mood is not known. However, it does act on the central nervous system. It helps you to have more stable emotions and be better able to cope with the problems of living.

It is important that you and your family understand all the effects of lithium. These effects depend on your individual condition and response, and the amount of lithium being used. You also must know when to contact your doctor if there are problems with its use. Lithium may also be used for other conditions as determined by your doctor.

This medicine is available only with your doctor's prescription.

Before Using This Medicine

In order to decide on the best treatment for your medical problem, your doctor should be told:

—if you have ever had any unusual or allergic reaction to lithium.

—if you are on a low-salt, low-sugar, or any other special diet, or if you are allergic to any substance, such as sulfites or other preservatives or dyes. Most medicines contain more than their active ingredient. Your doctor or pharmacist can help you avoid products that may cause a problem.

—if you are pregnant or if you intend to become pregnant while using this medicine. Lithium is not recommended for use during pregnancy, especially during the first three months. Studies have shown that lithium may cause thyroid problems and heart or blood vessel defects in the baby. It has also been shown to cause muscle weakness and severe drowsiness in newborns of mothers taking lithium near time of delivery.

—if you are breast-feeding an infant. Lithium passes into the breast milk. It has been reported to cause unwanted effects such as muscle weakness, lowered body temperature, and heart problems in infants of nursing mothers. Before taking this medicine, be sure you have discussed with your doctor the risks and benefits of breast-feeding.

—if you have any of the following medical problems:
  Diabetes mellitus (sugar diabetes)
  Difficult urination
  Epilepsy
  Heart disease
  Infection (severe)
  Kidney disease
  Parkinson's disease
  Thyroid disease

—if you are now taking any of the following medicines or types of medicine:
  Aminophylline
  Amphetamines
  Anti-inflammatory analgesics, such as diflunisal, fenoprofen, ibuprofen, indomethacin, meclofenamate, mefenamic acid, naproxen, oxyphenbutazone, phenylbutazone, piroxicam, sulindac, or tolmetin
  Caffeine
  Carbamazepine
  Chlorpromazine or other phenothiazines (tranquilizers)
  Diuretics (water pills)
  Dyphylline
  Haloperidol
  Medicine for diabetes insipidus (water diabetes)
  Medicine for thyroid disease
  Oxtriphylline
  Sodium bicarbonate (baking soda)
  Sodium chloride (salt)
  Theophylline

—if you drink large amounts of caffeine-containing beverages, such as coffee, tea, or some colas.

—if you are on a low-salt diet.

Proper Use of This Medicine

Take this medicine exactly as directed. Do not take more of it, do not take it more often, and do not take it for a longer period of time than your doctor ordered. To do so may increase the chance of unwanted effects.

If you are taking the long-acting form of this medicine, the tablets are to be swallowed whole. Do not break, crush, or chew them before swallowing.

While taking this medicine, drink 2 or 3 quarts of water or other fluids each day, and use a normal amount of salt in your food, unless otherwise directed by your doctor.

Sometimes lithium must be taken for 1 to several weeks before you begin to feel better.

In order for lithium to work properly, it must be taken every day in regularly spaced doses as ordered by your doctor. This is necessary to keep a constant amount of lithium in your blood. To help keep this amount constant, do not miss any doses and do not stop taking it even if you feel better.

If you do miss a dose of this medicine, take it as soon as possible. However, if it is within 2 hours (6 hours for extended-release tablets) of your next dose, skip the missed dose and go back to your regular dosing schedule. Do not double doses.

How to store this medicine:
  • Store away from heat and direct light.
  • **Keep out of the reach of children.**
  • Do not store in the bathroom medicine cabinet because the heat or moisture may cause the medicine to break down.

• Keep the syrup form of this medicine from freezing.

• Do not keep outdated medicine or medicine no longer needed. Flush the contents of the container down the toilet, unless otherwise directed.

Precautions While Using This Medicine

Your doctor should check your progress at regular visits to make sure that the medicine is working properly and that possible side effects are avoided. Laboratory tests may be necessary.

Lithium may not work as well as it should if you drink large amounts of caffeine-containing coffee, tea, or colas. Check with your doctor before using large amounts of these beverages.

This medicine may cause some people to become dizzy, drowsy, or less alert than they are normally. Make sure you know how you react to this medicine before you drive, use machines, or do other jobs that require you to be alert.

Use extra care in hot weather and during activities that cause you to sweat heavily, such as hot baths, saunas, or exercising. The loss of too much water and salt from your body may lead to serious side effects from this medicine.

If you have an infection or illness that causes heavy sweating, vomiting, or diarrhea, check with your doctor. The loss of too much water and salt from your body may lead to serious side effects from lithium.

Do not go on a diet to lose weight without first checking with your doctor. Improper dieting may cause the loss of too much water and salt from your body and may lead to serious side effects from this medicine.

Side Effects of This Medicine

Along with its needed effects, a medicine may cause some unwanted effects. Although not all of these side effects appear very often, when they do occur they may require medical attention. **Check with your doctor immediately if any of the following side effects occur:**

Early signs of overdose

    Diarrhea
    Drowsiness
    Loss of appetite
    Muscle weakness
    Nausea or vomiting
    Slurred speech
    Trembling

Late signs of overdose

    Blurred vision
    Clumsiness or unsteadiness
    Confusion
    Convulsions (seizures)
    Dizziness
    Trembling (severe)
    Unusual increase in amount of urine

Check with your doctor as soon as possible if any of the following side effects occur:

Less common

    Fainting
    Irregular pulse
    Troubled breathing (especially during hard work or exercise)
    Unusually fast heartbeat
    Unusual tiredness or weakness
    Unusual weight gain

Signs of low thyroid function

    Dry, rough skin
    Hair loss
    Hoarseness
    Swelling of feet or lower legs
    Swelling of neck
    Unusual sensitivity to cold

Other side effects may occur which usually do not require medical attention. These side effects may go away during treatment as your body adjusts to the medicine. However, check with your doctor if

any of the following side effects continue or are bothersome:

More common
- Increased frequency of urination
- Increased thirst
- Nausea (mild)
- Trembling of hands (slight)

Less common
- Acne or skin rash
- Feeling of bloating or pressure in the stomach
- Muscle twitching (slight)

The above side effects, especially the signs of overdose and low thyroid function, are more likely to occur in the elderly, who are usually more sensitive to the effects of lithium.

Other side effects not listed above may also occur in some patients. If you notice any other effects, check with your doctor.

LOPERAMIDE (Oral)
A commonly used brand name is Imodium.

Loperamide (loe-PER-a-mide) is a medicine used along with other measures to treat severe diarrhea.

In infants and children and in persons over 60 years of age, the fluid loss caused by diarrhea may result in a severe condition. These persons should not take any antidiarrhea medicine unless prescribed by their doctor.

Loperamide is available only with your doctor's prescription.

Before Using This Medicine
In order to decide on the best treatment for your medical problem, your doctor should be told:

—if you have ever had any unusual or allergic reaction to loperamide.

—if you are on a low-salt, low-sugar, or any other special diet, or if you are allergic to any substance, such as sulfites or other preservatives or dyes. Most medicines contain more than their active ingredient. Your doctor or pharmacist can help you avoid products that may cause a problem.

—if you are pregnant or if you intend to become pregnant while taking this medicine. Studies have not been done in humans. However, studies in animals have not shown that loperamide causes cancer or birth defects or lessens the chances of becoming pregnant when given in doses many times the human dose.

—if you are breast-feeding an infant. Although loperamide has not been shown to cause problems in humans, the chance always exists.

—if you have either of the following medical problems:
- Colitis (severe)
- Liver disease

—if you are now taking any other medicine, especially the following medicines or types of medicine:
- Cephalosporins (a type of antibiotic)
- Clindamycin
- Lincomycin
- Penicillins

Proper Use of This Medicine
Take this medicine only as directed by your doctor. Do not take more of it, do not take it more often, and do not take it for a longer period of time than your doctor ordered. To do so may increase the chance of side effects.

If you must take this medicine regularly and you miss a dose, skip the missed dose and go back to your regular dosing schedule. Do not double doses.

How to store this medicine:
- Store away from heat and direct light.
- **Keep out of the reach of children.**

• Do not store in the bathroom medicine cabinet because the heat or moisture may cause the medicine to break down.

• Keep the liquid form of this medicine from freezing.

• Do not keep outdated medicine or medicine no longer needed. Flush the contents of the container down the toilet, unless otherwise directed.

Precautions While Using This Medicine

If you will be taking this medicine regularly for a long period of time, your doctor should check your progress at regular visits.

Check with your doctor if your diarrhea doesn't stop after a few days or if you develop a fever.

Side Effects of This Medicine

Along with its needed effects, a medicine may cause some unwanted effects. **When this medicine is used for short periods of time at low doses, side effects usually are rare** and they may go away during treatment as your body adjusts to the medicine. However, check with your doctor as soon as possible if any of the following side effects continue, worsen, or are bothersome:

Rare
  Bloating
  Constipation
  Dizziness
  Drowsiness
  Dry mouth
  Fever
  Loss of appetite
  Nausea and vomiting
  Skin rash
  Stomach pain

Other side effects not listed above may also occur in some patients. If you notice any other effects, check with your doctor.

MAPROTILINE (Systemic)
A commonly used brand name is Ludiomil.

Maprotiline (ma-PROE-ti-leen) belongs to the group of medicines known as tetracyclic antidepressants or "mood elevators." It is used to relieve mental depression, including depression that sometimes occurs with anxiety.

Maprotiline is available only with your doctor's prescription.

Before Using This Medicine

In order to decide on the best treatment for your medical problem, your doctor should be told:

—if you have ever had any unusual or allergic reaction to maprotiline or tricyclic antidepressants.

—if you are on a low-salt, low-sugar, or any other special diet, or if you are allergic to any substance, such as sulfites or other preservatives or dyes. Most medicines contain more than their active ingredient. Your doctor or pharmacist can help you avoid products that may cause a problem.

—if you are pregnant or if you intend to become pregnant while taking this medicine. Although maprotiline has not been shown to cause birth defects or other problems, the chance always exists since studies have not been done in humans.

—if you are breast-feeding an infant. Although this medicine has not been shown to cause problems in humans, the chance always exists since maprotiline passes into the breast milk.

—if you have any of the following medical problems:
  Alcoholism
  Asthma
  Difficult urination
  Enlarged prostate
  Epilepsy or other seizure disorders

Glaucoma
Heart or blood vessel disease
High blood pressure
Liver disease
Mental illness (severe)
Overactive thyroid
Stomach or intestinal problems

--if you are now taking any of the following medicines or types of medicine:

Asthma medicine
Estrogens
High blood pressure medicine
Nasal decongestants (including nose drops and sprays)
Oral contraceptives (birth control pills)
Other medicine for depression
Stomach or intestinal medicine
Thyroid medicine

—if you are now taking central nervous system (CNS) depressants, such as:

Anticonvulsants (seizure medicine)
Antihistamines or medicine for hay fever, other allergies, or colds
Barbiturates
Narcotics
Prescription pain medicine
Sedatives, tranquilizers, or sleeping medicine

—if you are now taking or have taken within the past 2 weeks monoamine oxidase (MAO) inhibitors, such as:

Furazolidone
Isocarboxazid
Pargyline
Phenelzine
Procarbazine
Tranylcypromine

Proper Use of This Medicine

Take this medicine only as directed by your doctor in order to improve your condition as much as possible.

Sometimes this medicine must be taken up to a week or two before you begin to feel better.

If you miss a dose of this medicine and your dosing schedule is:

More than one dose a day—Take the missed dose as soon as possible. Then go back to your regular dosing schedule. However, if it is almost time for your next dose, skip the missed dose and go back to your regular dosing schedule. Do not double doses.

One dose a day at bedtime—Do not take the missed dose in the morning since it may cause disturbing side effects during waking hours. Instead, check with your doctor.

How to store this medicine:

• Store away from heat and direct light.

• **Keep out of the reach of children, since overdose is especially dangerous in children.**

• Do not store in the bathroom medicine cabinet because the heat or moisture may cause the medicine to break down.

• Do not keep outdated medicine or medicine no longer needed. Flush the contents of the container down the toilet, unless otherwise directed.

Precautions While Using This Medicine

It is very important that your doctor check your progress at regular visits. This will allow your dosage to be changed if necessary.

Do not stop taking this medicine without first checking with your doctor. Your doctor may want you to reduce gradually the amount you are taking before stopping completely. This will allow your body to adjust properly and reduce the possibility of unwanted effects.

Before having any kind of surgery (including dental surgery) or emergency treatment, tell the physician or dentist in charge that you are using this medicine.

This medicine will add to the effects of alcohol and other medicines (CNS depressants) that slow down the nervous system. Some examples of CNS depressants are antihistamines or medicine for hay fever, other allergies, or colds; sedatives, tranquilizers, or sleeping medicine; prescription pain medicine or narcotics; barbiturates; medicine for seizures; tricyclic antidepressants (medicine for depression); or anesthetics, including some dental anesthetics. **Check with your doctor before taking any of the above while you are using this medicine.**

Do not take any other medicine, unless prescribed or approved by your doctor. This especially includes over-the-counter (OTC) or nonprescription medicine such as that for colds, cough, asthma, hay fever, or appetite control.

This medicine may cause some people to become drowsy or less alert than they are normally. **Make sure you know how you react to this medicine before you drive, use machines, or do other jobs that require you to be alert.**

Dizziness, lightheadedness, or fainting may occur, especially when you get up from a lying or sitting position. Getting up slowly may help. If this problem continues or gets worse, check with your doctor.

Your mouth may feel very dry while you are taking maprotiline. To keep your mouth comfortably moist, chew sugarless gum, melt bits of ice in your mouth, or use a saliva substitute as often as necessary.

Side Effects of This Medicine

Along with its needed effects, a medicine may cause some unwanted effects. Although not all of these side effects appear very often, when they do occur they may require medical attention. Check with your doctor as soon as possible if any of the following side effects occur:

Less common
   Constipation (severe)
   Convulsions (seizures)
   Nausea or vomiting
   Shakiness or trembling
   Unusual excitement

Rare
   Confusion (especially in the elderly)
   Difficulty in urinating
   Fainting
   Hallucinations (seeing, hearing, or feeling things that are not there)
   Irregular heartbeat (pounding, racing, skipping)
   Sore throat and fever
   Yellowing of eyes and skin

Signs of overdose
   Convulsions (seizures)
   Dizziness (severe)
   Drowsiness (severe)
   Fever
   Muscle stiffness or weakness (severe)
   Restlessness or agitation
   Unusually fast or irregular heartbeat
   Vomiting

Other side effects may occur which usually do not require medical attention. These side effects may go away during treatment as your body adjusts to the medicine. However, check with your doctor if any of the following side effects continue or are bothersome:

More common
   Blurred vision
   Dizziness
   Drowsiness
   Dry mouth
   Skin rash or itching
   Unusual tiredness or weakness

Less common
   Constipation (mild)
   Diarrhea
   Headache
   Heartburn
   Increased sensitivity of skin to sunlight
   Trouble in sleeping
   Unusual increase in sweating

The above side effects, especially drowsiness, dizziness, confusion, vision problems, dry mouth, constipation, and problems in urinating are more likely to occur in elderly patients, who are usually more sensitive to the effects of maprotiline.

After you stop taking this medicine, your body will need time to adjust. This usually takes about 3 to 7 days. Continue to follow the precautions listed above during this period of time.

Other side effects not listed above may also occur in some patients. If you notice any other effects, check with your doctor.

MECLIZINE (Systemic)

This information applies to the following medicines:

Buclizine (BYOO-kli-zeen)
Cyclizine (SYE-kli-zeen)
Meclizine (MEK-li-zeen)

Some commonly used brand names are:	Generic names:
Bucladin-S	Buclizine
Marezine	Cyclizine
Antivert Bonine	Meclizine†

†Generic name product may also be available.

Buclizine, cyclizine, and meclizine are used to prevent motion sickness, nausea, vomiting, and dizziness.

Some of these preparations are available only with your doctor's prescription. Others are available without a prescription; however, your doctor may have special instructions on the proper dose of the medicine for your medical condition.

Before Using This Medicine

Before you use this medicine, check with your doctor, nurse, or pharmacist:

—if you have ever had any unusual or allergic reaction to buclizine, cyclizine, or meclizine.

—if you are on a low-salt, low-sugar, or any other special diet, or if you are allergic to any substance, such as sulfites or other preservatives or dyes. Most medicines contain more than their active ingredient. Your doctor or pharmacist can help you avoid products that may cause a problem.

—if you are pregnant or if you intend to become pregnant while using this medicine. These medicines have not been shown to cause birth defects or other problems in humans. However, studies in animals have shown that buclizine, cyclizine, and meclizine given in doses many times the usual human dose cause birth defects.

—if you are breast-feeding an infant. Although these medicines have not been shown to cause problems in humans, the chance always exists since they may pass into the breast milk. In addition, since these medicines tend to decrease the secretions of the body, it is possible that the flow of breast milk may be reduced in some patients.

—if you have any of the following medical problems:

Enlarged prostate
Glaucoma
Intestinal blockage
Stomach ulcer
Urinary tract blockage

—if you are taking any of the following medicines or types of medicine:

Antimuscarinics (medicine for abdominal or stomach spasms or cramps)
Aspirin or other salicylates (in large doses)
Cisplatin
Clonidine
Guanabenz
Maprotiline
Methyldopa
Metyrosine
Paromomycin
Trazodone
Vancomycin

—if you are now taking any central nervous system (CNS) depressants, such as:

Anticonvulsants (seizure medicine)
Antihistamines or medicine for hay fever, other allergies, or colds
Barbiturates
Medicine for seizures
Narcotics
Prescription pain medicine
Sedatives, tranquilizers, or sleeping medicine

—if you are now taking tricyclic antidepressants, such as:

Amitriptyline
Amoxapine
Desipramine
Doxepin
Imipramine
Nortriptyline
Protriptyline
Trimipramine

Proper Use of This Medicine

If necessary, take this medicine with food or a glass of water or milk to lessen stomach irritation.

This medicine is used to relieve or prevent the symptoms of your medical problem. Take it only as directed. Do not take more of it or take it more often than stated on the label or ordered by your doctor. To do so may increase the chance of side effects.

For patients taking this medicine for motion sickness:

• Take buclizine or cyclizine at least 30 minutes before you begin to travel.

• Take meclizine at least 1 hour before you begin to travel.

If you must take this medicine regularly and you miss a dose, take the missed dose as soon as possible. However, if it is almost time for your next dose, skip the missed dose and go back to your regular dosing schedule. Do not double doses.

How to store this medicine:

• Store away from heat and direct light.

• **Keep out of the reach of children.**

• Do not store in the bathroom medicine cabinet because the heat or moisture may cause the medicine to break down.

• Do not keep outdated medicine or medicine no longer needed. Flush the contents of the container down the toilet, unless otherwise directed.

Precautions While Using This Medicine

Tell the doctor in charge that you are taking this medicine before you have any skin tests for allergies. The results of the test may be affected by this medicine.

Buclizine, cyclizine, or meclizine will add to the effects of alcohol and other CNS depressants (medicines that slow down the nervous system, possibly causing drowsiness). Some examples of CNS depressants are antihistamines or medicine for hay fever, other allergies, or colds; sedatives, tranquilizers, or sleeping medicine; prescription pain medicine or narcotics; barbiturates; medicine for seizures; muscle relaxants; or anesthetics, including some dental anesthetics. **Check with your doctor before taking any of the above while you are using this medicine.**

This medicine may cause some people to become drowsy or less alert than they are normally. **Make sure you know how you react to this medicine before you drive, use machines, or do other jobs that require you to be alert.**

Your mouth may feel very dry while you are taking buclizine, cyclizine, or meclizine. To help relieve this feeling, chew sugarless gum or dissolve bits of ice in your mouth.

When taking this medicine on a regular basis, make sure your doctor knows if you are taking large amounts of aspirin at the same time (as in arthritis or rheumatism). Effects of too much aspirin, such as ringing in the ears, may be covered up by this medicine.

Side Effects of This Medicine

Along with its needed effects, a medicine may cause some unwanted effects. The following side effects may go away during treatment as your body adjusts to the medicine; however, check with your doctor if they continue or are bothersome:

More common
Drowsiness

Less common or rare
Blurred vision
Difficult or painful urination
Dizziness
Dryness of mouth, nose, and throat
Headache
Loss of appetite
Nervousness, restlessness, or trouble in sleeping
Skin rash
Unusually fast heartbeat
Upset stomach

Although not all of the side effects listed above have been reported for all of these medicines, they have been reported for at least one of them. However, since buclizine, cyclizine, and meclizine are very similar, any of the above side effects may occur with any of these medicines.

Other side effects not listed above may also occur in some patients. If you notice any other effects, check with your doctor.

METHYLDOPA (Systemic)

Some commonly used brand names are:
Aldomet   Medimet-250*
Dopamet*   Novomedopa*

Generic name product may also be available.

---

* Not available in the United States.

Methyldopa (meth-ill-DOE-pa) belongs to the general class of medicines called antihypertensives. It is used to treat high blood pressure.

High blood pressure adds to the workload of the heart and arteries. If it continues for a long time, they may not function properly. This can damage the blood vessels of the brain, heart, and kidneys, resulting in a stroke, heart attack, or kidney failure. These problems may be avoided if blood pressure is controlled.

Methyldopa works by controlling impulses along certain nerve pathways. As a result, it relaxes blood vessels so that blood passes through them more easily. This helps to lower blood pressure.

Methyldopa is available only with your doctor's prescription.

Before Using This Medicine

In order to decide on the best treatment for your medical problem, your doctor should be told:

—if you have ever had any unusual or allergic reaction to methyldopa.

—if you are on a low-salt, low-sugar, or any other special diet, or if you are allergic to any substance, such as sulfites or other preservatives or dyes. Most medicines contain more than their active ingredient. Your doctor or pharmacist can help you avoid products that may cause a problem.

—if you are pregnant or if you intend to become pregnant while taking this medicine. Although studies in humans have not shown that methyldopa causes birth defects or other problems, the chance always exists.

—if you are breast-feeding an infant. Although methyldopa has not been shown to cause problems in humans, the chance always exists. Methyldopa passes into breast milk.

—if you have any of the following medical problems:

Angina (chest pain)
Kidney disease
Liver disease
Mental depression (history of)
Parkinson's disease
Pheochromocytoma (PCC)

—if you have taken methyldopa in the past and developed liver problems.

—if you are now taking any of the following medicines or types of medicine:

Anticoagulants, oral (blood thinners you take by mouth)
Appetite suppressants (medicine to help you lose weight)
Diuretics (water pills)
Inflammation medicine, especially indomethacin
Levodopa
Other antihypertensives (high blood pressure medicine)
Tricyclic antidepressants (medicine for depression)

—if you are now taking central nervous system (CNS) depressants such as:

Anticonvulsants (seizure medicine)
Antihistamines or medicine for hay fever, other allergies, or colds
Barbiturates
Muscle relaxants
Narcotics
Prescription pain medicine
Sedatives, tranquilizers, or sleeping medicine

—if you are now taking or have taken within the past 2 weeks monoamine oxidase (MAO) inhibitors such as:

Furazolidone
Isocarboxazid
Pargyline
Phenelzine
Procarbazine
Tranylcypromine

Proper Use of This Medicine

Importance of diet—When prescribing medicine for your condition, your doctor may also prescribe a personal diet for you. Such a diet may be low in sodium (salt). Most people eat much more sodium than they need and too much sodium in the diet may increase blood pressure. Some foods that contain large amounts of sodium include canned soup, pickles, ketchup, green and ripe olives, relish, frankfurters, soy sauce, and carbonated beverages. Your doctor may want you to limit the amounts of these and other high-sodium foods in your diet. Medicine is usually more effective when such a diet is properly followed.

Also, it may be very important for you to go on a reducing diet. However, check with your doctor before going on any diet.

Many patients who have high blood pressure will not notice any signs of the problem. In fact, many may feel normal. It is very important that you take your medicine exactly as directed and that you keep your doctor's appointments even if you feel well.

Remember that methyldopa will not cure your high blood pressure but it does help control it. Therefore, you must continue to take it as directed if you expect to lower your blood pressure and keep it down. **You may have to take medicine for the rest of your life.** If high blood pressure is not treated, it can cause serious problems such as heart failure, blood vessel disease, stroke, or kidney disease.

In order to help remember to take your medicine, try to get into the habit of taking it at the same time each day.

If you miss a dose of this medicine, take it as soon as possible. However, if it is almost time for your next dose, skip the missed dose and go back to your regular dosing schedule. Do not double doses.

How to store this medicine:

- Store away from heat and direct light.
- **Keep out of the reach of children.**
- Do not store in the bathroom medicine cabinet because the heat or moisture may cause the medicine to break down.
- Keep the liquid form of this medicine from freezing.
- Do not keep outdated medicine or medicine no longer needed. Flush the contents of the container down the toilet, unless otherwise directed.

Precautions While Using This Medicine

It is important that your doctor check your progress at regular visits in order to make sure that this medicine is working properly.

If you have a fever and there seems to be no reason for it, check with your doctor. This is especially important during the first few weeks you take methyldopa, since fever may be a sign of a serious reaction to this medicine.

Before having any kind of surgery (including dental surgery) or emergency treatment, make sure the physician or dentist in charge knows that you are taking this medicine.

Methyldopa may cause some people to become drowsy or less alert than they are normally. This is more likely to happen when you begin to take it or when you increase the amount of medicine you are taking. **Make sure you know how you react to this medicine before you drive, use machines, or do other jobs that require you to be alert.**

Dizziness, lightheadedness, or fainting may occur, especially when you get up from a lying or sitting position. Getting up slowly may help but if the problem continues or gets worse, check with your doctor.

Do not take other medicines unless they have been discussed with your doctor. This especially includes over-the-counter (nonprescription) medicines for appetite control, asthma, colds, cough, hay fever, or sinus problems, since they may tend to increase your blood pressure.

Side Effects of This Medicine

Along with its needed effects, a medicine may cause some unwanted effects. Although not all of these side effects appear very often, when they do occur they may require medical attention. **Check with your doctor immediately** if the following side effect occurs:

Less common
> Fever shortly after starting to take this medicine

Check with your doctor as soon as possible if any of the following side effects occur:

More common
> Swelling of feet or lower legs

Less common
> Inability to sleep
> Mental depression or anxiety
> Nightmares or unusually vivid dreams

Rare
> Dark or amber urine
> Diarrhea or stomach cramps (severe or continuing)
> Fever, chills, troubled breathing, and unusually fast heartbeat
> Pale stools
> Shakiness or unusual body movements
> Sore throat and fever
> Stomach pain with nausea and vomiting (severe)
> Tiredness or weakness after having taken this medicine for several weeks (continuing)
> Unusual bleeding or bruising
> Yellowing of eyes and skin

Other side effects may occur which usually do not require medical attention. These side effects may go away during treatment as your body adjusts to the medicine. However, check with your doctor if

any of the following side effects continue or are bothersome:

More common
  Drowsiness
  Dry mouth
  Headache

Less common
  Decreased sexual ability
  Diarrhea
  Dizziness or lightheadedness when getting up from a lying or sitting position
  Fainting
  Nausea or vomiting
  Numbness, tingling, pain, or weakness in hands or feet
  Skin rash
  Stuffy nose
  Swelling of the breasts or unusual milk production
  Unusually slow heartbeat

Dizziness or lightheadedness and drowsiness may be more likely to occur in the elderly, who are more sensitive to the effects of methyldopa.

Other side effects not listed above may also occur in some patients. If you notice any other effects, check with your doctor.

METHYLDOPA AND THIAZIDE DIURETICS (Systemic)

This information applies to the following medicines:

Methyldopa (meth-ill-DOE-pa) and Chlorothiazide (klor-oh-THYE-a-zide)
Methyldopa and Hydrochlorothiazide (hye-droe-klor-oh-THYE-a-zide)

Some commonly used brand names are:	Generic names:
Aldoclor	Methyldopa and Chlorothiazide
Aldoril	Methyldopa and Hydrochlorothiazide

Combinations of methyldopa and a thiazide diuretic are taken by mouth to treat high blood pressure.

High blood pressure adds to the workload of the heart and arteries. If it continues for a long time, they may not function properly. This can damage the blood vessels of the brain, heart, and kidneys, resulting in a stroke, heart attack, or kidney failure. These problems may be avoided if blood pressure is controlled.

Methyldopa works by controlling nerve impulses along certain nerve pathways. As a result, it relaxes blood vessels so that blood passes through them more easily. Thiazide diuretics help reduce the amount of water in the body by increasing the flow of urine. These actions help to lower blood pressure.

This medicine is available only with your doctor's prescription.

For information about the precautions and side effects of the medicines in this combination, see:

  Methyldopa (Systemic)
  Diuretics, Thiazide (Systemic)

Combination products are designed for specific uses. These uses may not be the same as the uses of the individual ingredients. Therefore, some of the information provided in the individual listings may not be relevant to the combination product. If questions arise, check with your doctor, nurse, or pharmacist.

METOCLOPRAMIDE (Systemic)

Some commonly used brand names are Maxeran* and Reglan.

---

*Not available in the United States.

Metoclopramide (met-oh-KLOE-pra-mide) is a medicine that increases the movements or contractions of the stomach and intestines. When given by injection it is used to help diagnose certain problems of the stomach and/or intestines. It is also used by injection to prevent the nausea and vomiting that may occur after treatment with anticancer medicines.

When taken by mouth metoclopramide is used to treat the symptoms of a certain type of stomach problem called diabetic gastroparesis. It relieves symptoms such as nausea, vomiting, continued feeling of fullness after meals, and loss of appetite. Metoclopramide is also used to treat symptoms such as heartburn in patients who regurgitate food.

Metoclopramide may also be used for other conditions as determined by your doctor.

Metoclopramide is available only with your doctor's prescription.

Before Using This Medicine

In order to decide on the best treatment for your medical problem, your doctor should be told:

—if you have ever had any unusual or allergic reaction to metoclopramide, procaine, or procainamide.

—if you are on a low-salt, low-sugar, or any other special diet, or if you are allergic to any substance, such as sulfites or other preservatives or dyes. Most medicines contain more than their active ingredient. Your doctor or pharmacist can help you avoid products that may cause a problem.

—if you are pregnant or if you intend to become pregnant while using this medicine. Not enough studies have been done in humans to determine its safety during pregnancy. However, metoclopramide

has not been shown to cause birth defects or other problems in animal studies.

—if you are breast-feeding an infant. Although metoclopramide has not been shown to cause problems in humans, the chance always exists since it passes into the breast milk.

—if you have any of the following medical problems:
  Abdominal or stomach bleeding
  Epilepsy
  Intestinal blockage
  Kidney disease
  Liver disease
  Parkinson's disease

—if you are now taking any of the following medicines or types of medicine:
  Antimuscarinics (medicine for abdominal or stomach spasms or cramps)
  Bromocriptine
  Chlorprothixene
  Digoxin
  Haloperidol
  Levodopa
  Loxapine
  Metyrosine
  Phenothiazines
  Thiothixene

—if you are now using central nervous system (CNS) depressants such as:
  Anticonvulsants (seizure medicine)
  Antihistamines or medicine for hay fever, other allergies, or colds
  Barbiturates
  Narcotics
  Prescription pain medicine
  Sedatives, tranquilizers, or sleeping medicine

—if you are now taking tricyclic antidepressants (medicine for depression) such as:
  Amitriptyline
  Amoxapine
  Clomipramine
  Desipramine
  Doxepin
  Imipramine
  Nortriptyline
  Protriptyline
  Trimipramine

Proper Use of This Medicine

Take this medicine 30 minutes before meals and at bedtime, unless otherwise directed by your doctor.

Take metoclopramide only as directed. Do not take more of it, do not take it more often, and do not take it for a longer period of time than your doctor ordered. To do so may increase the chance of side effects.

If you miss a dose of this medicine, take it as soon as possible. However, if it is almost time for your next dose, skip the missed dose and go back to your regular dosing schedule. Do not double doses.

How to store this medicine:

• Store away from heat and direct light.

• **Keep out of the reach of children.**

• Do not store in the bathroom medicine cabinet because the heat or moisture may cause the medicine to break down.

• Keep the syrup from freezing.

• Do not keep outdated medicine or medicine no longer needed. Flush the contents of the container down the toilet, unless otherwise directed.

Precautions While Using This Medicine

This medicine will add to the effects of alcohol and other CNS depressants (medicines that slow down the nervous system, possibly causing drowsiness). Some examples of CNS depressants are antihistamines or medicine for hay fever, other allergies, or colds; sedatives, tranquilizers, or sleeping medicine; prescription pain medicine or narcotics; barbiturates; medicine for seizures; muscle relaxants; or anesthetics, including some dental anesthetics. **Check with your doctor before taking any of the above while you are using this medicine.**

This medicine may cause some people to become dizzy, lightheaded, drowsy, or less alert than they are normally. **Make sure you know how you react to this medicine before you drive, use machines, or do other jobs that require you to be alert.**

Side Effects of This Medicine

Along with its needed effects, a medicine may cause some unwanted effects. Although not all of these side effects appear very often, when they do occur they may require medical attention. Check with your doctor as soon as possible if any of the following side effects occur:

Possible signs of overdose—may also occur rarely with usual doses, especially in children and young adults, and with high doses used to treat the nausea and vomiting caused by anticancer medicines
> Confusion
> Drowsiness (severe)
> Muscle spasms (especially of jaw, neck, and back)
> Shuffling walk
> Tic-like (jerky) movements of head and face
> Trembling and shaking of hands

Other side effects may occur which usually do not require medical attention. These side effects may go away during treatment as your body adjusts to the medicine. However, check with your doctor if any of the following side effects continue or are bothersome:

More common
> Drowsiness
> Restlessness
> Unusual tiredness or weakness

Less common or rare
> Breast tenderness and swelling
> Changes in menstruation
> Constipation
> Depression
> Diarrhea
> Dizziness
> Headache
> Increased flow of breast milk

Nausea
Skin rash
Trouble in sleeping
Unusual dryness of mouth
Unusual irritability

Muscle spasms, especially of the jaw, neck, and back, and tic-like (jerky) movements of the head and face are more likely to occur in children. Shuffling walk, trembling, and shaking of hands are more likely to occur in elderly patients, especially after taking metoclopramide over a long period of time.

Other side effects not listed above may also occur in some patients. If you notice any other effects, check with your doctor.

METRONIDAZOLE (Systemic)

Some commonly used brand names are:

Flagyl	Neo-Tric*
Flagyl I.V.	Novonidazol*
Flagyl I.V. RTU	Protostat
Metro I.V.	Satric
Metryl	

Generic name product may also be available.

*Not available in the United States.

Metronidazole (me-troe-NI-da-zole) belongs to the general family of medicines called anti-infectives. It is taken by mouth or given by injection to help the body overcome infections and to help some problems such as dysentery. It may also be used for other problems as determined by your doctor. It will not work for colds, flu, or other virus infections.

Metronidazole is available only with your doctor's prescription.

Before Using This Medicine

Metronidazole has been shown to cause cancer in some animals. Before you take this medicine, be sure that you have discussed this with your doctor.

In order to decide on the best treatment for your medical problem, your doctor should be told:

—if you have ever had any unusual or allergic reaction to metronidazole.

—if you are pregnant or if you intend to become pregnant while taking this medicine. Metronidazole has not been shown to cause birth defects in animal studies. Studies have not been done in humans.

—if you are breast-feeding an infant. Use is not recommended in nursing mothers since metronidazole passes into the breast milk and may cause unwanted effects in the infant. However, in some infections your doctor may want you to stop breast-feeding and take this medicine for a short time. During this time the breast milk should be squeezed out or sucked out with a breast pump and thrown away. One or two days after you finish taking this medicine, you may go back to breast-feeding.

—if you have any of the following medical problems:
Blood disease or a history of blood disease
Central nervous system (CNS) disease, including epilepsy
Heart disease
Liver disease, severe

—if you are now taking any of the following medicines or types of medicine:
Disulfiram
Oral anticoagulants (blood thinners you take by mouth)

Proper Use of This Medicine

To help clear up your infection completely, **keep taking this medicine for the full time of treatment** even if you begin to feel better after a few days. If you stop taking this medicine too soon, your symptoms may return.

In some kinds of infections, this medicine works best when there is a constant amount in the blood. **To help keep this amount constant, do not miss any doses. Also, it is best to take each dose at evenly spaced times day and night.** For example, if you are to take 4 doses a day, each dose should be spaced about 6 hours apart. If this interferes with your sleep or other daily activities, or if you need help in planning the best times to take your medicine, check with your doctor, nurse, or pharmacist.

If you do miss a dose of this medicine, take it as soon as possible. This will help to keep a constant amount of medicine in the blood. However, if it is almost time for your next dose, do not take the missed dose at all and do not double the next one. Instead, go back to your regular dosing schedule.

If this medicine upsets your stomach, it may be taken with meals or a snack. If stomach upset (nausea, vomiting, stomach pain, or diarrhea) continues, check with your doctor.

How to store this medicine:
• Store away from heat and direct light, out of the reach of children.
• Do not store in the bathroom medicine cabinet because the heat or moisture may cause the medicine to break down.
• Do not keep outdated medicine or medicine no longer needed. Flush it down the toilet.

Precautions While Using This Medicine

If your symptoms do not improve within a few days or if they become worse, check with your doctor.

Drinking alcoholic beverages while taking this medicine may cause stomach pain, nausea, vomiting, headache, or flushing or redness of the face. Other alcohol-containing preparations (for example, elixirs, cough syrups, tonics) may also cause problems. Also, this medicine may cause alcoholic beverages to taste different. Therefore, **you should not drink alcoholic beverages or use other alcohol-containing preparations while you are taking this medicine.**

If you are taking this medicine for trichomoniasis (a genital infection in males and females), your doctor may want to treat your sexual partner at the same time you are being treated, even if he has no symptoms. Also, it may be desirable for your partner to wear a condom (prophylactic) during intercourse. These measures will help keep you from getting the infection back again from your partner. If you have any questions about this, check with your doctor.

Side Effects of This Medicine

Along with its needed effects, a medicine may cause some unwanted effects. Although not all of these side effects appear very often, when they do occur they may require medical attention. **Stop taking this medicine and check with your doctor immediately** if any of the following side effects occur:

Less common
Numbness, tingling, pain, or weakness in hands or feet
Seizures

Check with your doctor also if any of the following side effects occur:

Less common
Any irritation, discharge, or dryness of vagina not present before using this medicine
Clumsiness or unsteadiness
Mood or other mental changes
Skin rash, hives, redness, or itching
Sore throat and fever

For injection form
Pain, tenderness, redness, or swelling over vein in which the medicine is given

Other side effects may occur which usually do not require medical attention. These side effects may go away during treatment as your body adjusts to the medicine. However, check with your doctor if

any of the following side effects continue or are bothersome:

More common
Diarrhea
Dizziness or lightheadedness
Headache
Loss of appetite
Nausea or vomiting
Stomach pain or cramps

Less common or rare
Constipation
Dryness of mouth
Unpleasant or sharp metallic taste
Unusual tiredness or weakness

In some patients metronidazole may cause dark urine. This is only temporary and will go away when you stop taking this medicine.

Other side effects not listed above may also occur in some patients. If you notice any other effects, check with your doctor.

NARCOTIC ANALGESICS
(Systemic)

This information applies to the following medicines:

Butorphanol (byoo-TOR-fa-nole)
Codeine (KOE-deen)
Hydrocodone (hye-droe-KOE-done)
Hydromorphone (hye-droe-MOR-fone)
Levorphanol (lee-VOR-fa-nole)
Meperidine (me-PER-i-deen)
Methadone (METH-a-done)
Morphine (MOR-feen)
Nalbuphine (NAL-byoo-feen)
Opium Injection (OH-pee-um)
Oxycodone (ox-i-KOE-done)
Oxymorphone (ox-i-MOR-fone)
Pentazocine (pen-TAZ-oh-seen)
Propoxyphene (proe-POX-i-feen)

This information does *not* apply to Opium Tincture or Paregoric.

Some commonly used brand names or other names are: / Generic names:

Stadol	Butorphanol
Paveral*	Codeine†
Dicodid Hycodan‡ Robidone*	Hydrocodone†
Dihydromorphinone Dilaudid	Hydromorphone†
Levo-Dromoran	Levorphanol
Demer-Idine* Demerol Pethadol Pethidine	Meperidine
Dolophine Methadose	Methadone†
Duramorph PF Epimorph* Morphitec* M.O.S.* M S Contin RMS Uniserts Roxanol Roxanol SR Statex*	Morphine†
Nubain	Nalbuphine
Pantopon	Opium
Supeudol*	Oxycodone†
Numorphan	Oxymorphone
Talwin Talwin-Nx	Pentazocine
Darvon Darvon-N Dolene Doxaphene Novopropoxyn* Profene 642* SK-65	Propoxyphene†

*Not available in the United States.
†Generic name product may also be available.
‡For Canadian product only. In the U.S., *Hycodan* also contains homatropine; in Canada, *Hycodan* contains only hydrocodone.

Narcotic (nar-KOT-ik) analgesics (an-al-JEE-zicks) are medicines used to relieve pain. Some of them are also used just before or during an operation to help the anesthetic work better. Codeine and hydrocodone are also used to relieve coughing. Methadone is also used to help some people control their dependence on heroin or other narcotics. Narcotic analgesics may also be used for other purposes as determined by your doctor.

Narcotic analgesics act in the central nervous system (CNS) to relieve pain. Some of their side effects are also caused by actions in the CNS.

If a narcotic is used for a long time, it may become habit-forming (causing mental or physical dependence). Physical dependence may lead to withdrawal side effects when you stop taking the medicine.

These medicines are available only with your physician's or dentist's prescription. For some of them, prescriptions cannot be refilled and you must obtain a new prescription from your physician or dentist each time you need the medicine. In addition, other rules and regulations may apply when methadone is used to treat narcotic dependence.

Before Using This Medicine

In order to decide on the best treatment for your medical problem, your physician or dentist should be told:

—if you have ever had any unusual or allergic reaction to this medicine.

—if you are on a low-salt, low-sugar, or any other special diet, or if you are allergic to any substance, such as sulfites or other preservatives or dyes. Most medicines contain more than their active ingredient, and many liquid medicines contain alcohol. Your doctor or pharmacist can help you avoid products that may cause a problem.

—if you are pregnant or if you intend to become pregnant while using this medicine. Although studies on birth defects with narcotic analgesics have not been done in humans, these medicines have not been reported to cause birth defects in humans. However, hydrocodone, hydromorphone, and morphine have been shown to cause birth defects in animals when given in very large doses. Codeine has not been shown to cause birth defects in animal studies, but it caused other unwanted effects. Butorphanol, nalbuphine, pentazocine, and propoxyphene have been shown not to cause birth defects in animals. There is no information about whether other narcotic analgesics may cause birth defects, but the chance always exists.

Too much use of narcotics during pregnancy may cause the baby to become dependent on the medicine. This may lead to withdrawal side effects after birth. Also, some of these medicines may cause breathing problems in the newborn infant if taken just before delivery.

—if you are breast-feeding an infant. Although most narcotic analgesics have not been shown to cause problems in humans, the chance always exists, especially if they are taken for a long time or in large amounts. Methadone may cause the baby to become dependent on it. Also, butorphanol, codeine, meperidine, morphine, opium, and propoxyphene have been shown to pass into the breast milk.

—if you have any of the following medical problems:

Brain disease or head injury
Colitis
Convulsions (seizures), history of
Emphysema, asthma, or chronic lung disease
Enlarged prostate or problems with urination
Gallbladder disease or gallstones

Heart disease
Kidney disease
Liver disease
Underactive thyroid

—if you are now taking any of the following medicines or types of medicine:
Amantadine
Anticoagulants (blood thinners)
Antihypertensives (medicine for high
    blood pressure)
Antimuscarinics (medicine for stomach
    spasms or cramps)
Bromocriptine
Carbamazepine
Cephalosporin antibiotics
Clindamycin
Difenoxin and atropine
Diphenoxylate and atropine
Diuretics (water pills or high blood
    pressure medicine)
Levodopa
Lincomycin
Metoclopramide
Naltrexone
Nitrates
Opium tincture
Paregoric
Penicillin antibiotics
Procainamide
Quinidine
Tocainide
Trazodone

—if you are taking methadone and are also taking any of the following medicines or types of medicine:
Phenytoin
Rifampin
Urine acidifiers (medicine to make your
    urine more acid)

—if you are taking propoxyphene and you smoke tobacco, or if you are using nicotine chewing gum or other tobacco substitutes to help you stop smoking.

—if you are now taking central nervous system (CNS) depressants such as:
Anticonvulsants (medicine for seizures)
Antihistamines or medicine for hay fever,
    other allergies, or colds
Barbiturates
Muscle relaxants
Other narcotics, including methadone

Other prescription pain medicine
Sedatives, tranquilizers, or sleeping
    medicine
Tricyclic antidepressants (medicine for
    depression)

—if you are now taking or have taken with the past 2 weeks monoamine oxidase (MAO) inhibitors such as:
Furazolidone
Isocarboxazid
Pargyline
Phenelzine
Procarbazine
Tranylcypromine

Proper Use of This Medicine

Take this medicine only as directed by your physician or dentist. Do not take more of it, do not take it more often, and do not take it for a longer period of time than your physician or dentist ordered. If too much is taken, it may become habit-forming (causing mental or physical dependence) or lead to medical problems because of an overdose.

If you think this medicine is not working as well after you have been taking it for a few weeks, **do not increase the dose.** Instead, check with your doctor.

For patients taking the oral liquid form of meperidine:
• Unless otherwise directed by your physician or dentist, **take this medicine mixed with a half glass (4 ounces) of water** to lessen the numbing effect of the medicine on your mouth and throat.

For patients taking the oral liquid form of methadone available only through a methadone treatment center:
• **This medicine may have to be mixed with water before you take it.** Read the label carefully for directions. If you have any questions about this, check with your doctor, nurse, or pharmacist.

For patients taking the tablets for oral solution form of methadone:
• **These tablets must be dissolved in water or fruit juice before taking. Read the label carefully for directions.** If you have any questions about this, check with your doctor, nurse, or pharmacist.

For patients taking the oral liquid form of morphine:
• This medicine may be mixed with a glass of fruit juice just before you take it, if desired, to improve the taste.

For patients taking the long-acting morphine tablets:
• These tablets must be swallowed whole. Do not break, crush, or chew the tablets.

For patients using a suppository form of a narcotic analgesic:
• How to insert suppository: First remove the foil wrapper and moisten the suppository with water. Lie down on your side and push the suppository well up into rectum with your finger.

If your physician or dentist has ordered you to take this medicine according to a regular schedule and you miss a dose, take it as soon as you remember. However, if it is almost time for your next dose, skip the missed dose and go back to your regular dosing schedule. **Do not double doses.**

How to store this medicine:
• Store away from heat and direct light.

• **Keep out of the reach of children** because overdose is very dangerous in young children.

• Do not store in the bathroom medicine cabinet because the heat or moisture may cause the medicine to break down. Store hydromorphone, oxycodone, or oxymorphone suppositories in the refrigerator.

• Keep the liquid (including injections) and suppository forms of the medicine from freezing.

• Do not keep outdated medicine or medicine no longer needed. Flush the contents of the container down the toilet, unless otherwise directed.

Precautions While Using This Medicine

If you will be taking this medicine for a long period of time (for example, for several months at a time), your doctor should check your progress at regular visits.

Narcotic analgesics will add to the effects of alcohol and other CNS depressants (medicines that slow down the nervous system, possibly causing drowsiness). Some examples of CNS depressants are antihistamines or medicine for hay fever, other allergies, or colds; sedatives, tranquilizers, or sleeping medicine; other prescription pain medicines including other narcotics; barbiturates; medicine for seizures; tricyclic antidepressants (medicine for depression); muscle relaxants; or anesthetics, including some dental anesthetics. **Check with your physician or dentist before taking any of the above while you are using this medicine.**

This medicine may cause some people to become drowsy, dizzy, or lightheaded, or to feel a false sense of well-being. **Make sure you know how you react to this medicine before you drive, use machines, or do other jobs that require you to be alert and clearheaded.**

Dizziness, lightheadedness, or fainting may occur, especially when you get up suddenly from a lying or sitting position. Getting up slowly may help lessen this problem.

Nausea or vomiting may occur, especially after the first couple of doses. This effect may go away if you lie down for a while. However, if nausea or vomiting continues, check with your physician or dentist. Lying down for a while may also help relieve some other side effects, such as dizziness or lightheadedness, that may occur.

Before having any kind of surgery (including dental surgery) or emergency treatment, tell the physician or dentist in charge that you are taking this medicine.

If you have been taking this medicine regularly for several weeks or more, **do not suddenly stop using it without first checking with your doctor.** Your doctor may want you to reduce gradually the amount you are taking before stopping completely, in order to lessen the chance of withdrawal side effects.

If you think you or someone else in your home may have taken an overdose, get emergency help at once. Taking an overdose of this medicine or taking alcohol or CNS depressants with this medicine may lead to unconsciousness or death. Signs of overdose include convulsions, mental confusion, severe nervousness or restlessness, seizures, severe dizziness, severe drowsiness, unusually slow or troubled breathing, and severe weakness.

Side Effects of This Medicine

Along with its needed effects, a medicine may cause some unwanted effects. Although not all of these side effects appear very often, when they do occur they may require medical attention. **Get emergency help immediately if any of the following signs of overdose occur:**

Cold, clammy skin
Confusion
Convulsions (seizures)
Dizziness (severe)
Drowsiness (severe)
Nervousness or restlessness (severe)
Pinpoint pupils of eyes
Unconsciousness

Unusually low blood pressure
Unusually slow heartbeat
Unusually slow or troubled breathing
Weakness (severe)

Also, check with your doctor as soon as possible if any of the following side effects occur:

Less common or rare

Darkening of urine (for propoxyphene only)
Feelings of unreality
Hallucinations (seeing, hearing, or feeling things that are not there)
Hives, itching, or skin rash
Mental depression
Pale stools (for propoxyphene only)
Ringing or buzzing sound in the ears
Shortness of breath or troubled breathing
Swelling of face
Trembling or uncontrolled muscle movements
Unusual excitement, especially in children
Unusually fast, slow, or pounding heartbeat
Unusually slow or irregular breathing
Yellowing of eyes of skin (for propoxyphene only)

Other side effects may occur which usually do not require medical attention. These side effects may go away during treatment as your body adjusts to the medicine. However, check with your doctor if any of the following side effects continue or are bothersome:

More common

Dizziness
Drowsiness
Feeling faint
Lightheadedness
Nausea or vomiting

Less common or rare

Blurred or double vision or other changes in vision
Constipation (more common with long-term use and with codeine)
Difficult or painful urination
Dry mouth
False sense of well-being
Frequent urge to urinate

General feeling of discomfort or illness
Headache
Loss of appetite
Nightmares or unusual dreams
Redness or flushing of face (more common with hydrocodone, meperidine, and methadone)
Redness, swelling, pain, or burning at place of injection
Stomach cramps or pain
Trouble in sleeping
Unusual decrease in amount of urine
Unusual increase in sweating (more common with hydrocodone, meperidine, and methadone)
Unusual nervousness or restlessness
Unusual tiredness or weakness

The above side effects, especially breathing problems, are more likely to occur in very young patients or in elderly patients, who are usually more sensitive to the effects of these medicines.

After you stop using this medicine, your body may need time to adjust. The length of time this takes depends on the amount of medicine you were using and how long you used it. During this period of time check with your doctor if you notice any of the following side effects:

Body aches
Diarrhea
Fever
Gooseflesh
Loss of appetite
Nausea or vomiting
Nervousness or restlessness
Runny nose
Shivering or trembling
Sneezing
Stomach cramps
Trouble in sleeping
Unusual increase in sweating
Unusual increase in yawning
Unusual irritability
Unusually fast heartbeat
Weakness

Other side effects not listed above may also occur in some patients. If you notice any other effects, check with your doctor.

NARCOTIC ANALGESICS AND ACETAMINOPHEN (Systemic)

This information applies to the following medicines:

Acetaminophen (a-seat-a-MEE-noe-fen) and Codeine (KOE-deen)
Hydrocodone (hye-droe-KOE-done) and Acetaminophen
Meperidine (me-PER-i-deen) and Acetaminophen
Oxycodone (ox-i-KOE-done) and Acetaminophen
Pentazocine (pen-TAZ-oh-seen) and Acetaminophen
Propoxyphene (proe-POX-i-feen) and Acetaminophen

Some commonly used brand names are: Generic names:

Aceta with Codeine	
Atasol with Codeine*‡	
Bayapap with Codeine	
Capital with Codeine	
Codap	
Cotabs*	
Empracet with Codeine	Acetaminophen
Exdol with Codeine*‡	and Codeine†
Phenaphen with Codeine‡	
Proval	
SK-APAP with Codeine	
Tylenol with Codeine	
Ty-Tab with Codeine	

Amacodone	
Bancap-HC	
Co-gesic	
Dolo-Pap	
Duradyne DHC	
Hycodaphen	Hydrocodone and
Hydrogesic	Acetaminophen
Lortab 5	
Lortab 7	
Norcet	
T-Gesic Forte	
Vicodin	

Demerol-APAP	Meperidine and Acetaminophen

Oxycocet* Percocet Percocet-Demi* SK-Oxycodone and Acetaminophen Tylox	Oxycodone and Acetamino- phen†
Talacen	Pentazocine and Acetaminophen
Darvocet-N Dolacet Dolene-AP SK-65 APAP Wygesic	Propoxyphene and Acetaminophen†

*Not available in the United States.
†Generic name product may also be available.
‡In Canada, these products also contain other ingredients. Check with your pharmacist for information about these other ingredients.

Combination medicines containing narcotic (nar-KOT-ik) analgesics (an-al-JEE zicks) and acetaminophen are used to relieve pain. A narcotic analgesic and acetaminophen used together may provide better pain relief than either medicine used alone. In some cases, relief of pain may come at lower doses of each medicine.

Narcotic analgesics act in the central nervous system (CNS) to relieve pain. Many of their side effects are also caused by actions in the CNS. When narcotics are used for a long time, your body may get used to them so that larger amounts are needed to relieve pain. This is called tolerance to the medicine. Also, when narcotics are used for a long time or in large doses, they may become habit-forming (causing mental or physical dependence). Physical dependence may lead to withdrawal symptoms when you stop taking the medicine.

Acetaminophen does not become habit-forming when taken for a long time or in large doses, but it may cause other unwanted effects, including liver damage, if too much is taken.

In the United States, these medicines are available only with your physician's or dentist's prescription. In Canada, some of these medicines may be available without a prescription.

For information about the precautions and side effects of the medicines in this combination, see:

Narcotic Analgesics (Systemic)
Acetaminophen (Systemic)

Combination products are designed for specific uses. These uses may not be the same as the uses of the individual ingredients. Therefore, some of the information provided in the individual listings may not be relevant to the combination product. If questions arise, check with your doctor, nurse, or pharmacist.

NARCOTIC ANALGESICS AND ASPIRIN (Systemic)

This information applies to the following medicines:

Aspirin (AS-pir-in) and Codeine (KOE-deen)
Drocode (DROE-kode) and Aspirin
Hydrocodone (hye-droe-KOE-done), Aspirin, and Caffeine (KAF-een)
Oxycodone (ox-i-KOE-done) and Aspirin
Pentazocine (pen-TAZ-oh-seen) and Aspirin
Propoxyphene (proe-POX-i-feen) and Aspirin

Some commonly used brand names are:	Generic names:
Coryphen with Codeine* Emcodeine Empirin with Codeine	Aspirin and Codeine†

A.C.&C.* A&C with Codeine* Ancasal* Anexsia with Codeine A.S.A. and Codeine Compound C2 with Codeine* Instantine Plus* Novo AC&C* 222* 282* 292*	Aspirin, Codeine, and Caffeine
Ascriptin with Codeine	Buffered Aspirin and Codeine
Synalgos-DC	Drocode, Aspirin, and Caffeine
Anexsia-D Damason-P	Hydrocodone, Aspirin, and Caffeine
Codoxy Oxycodan* Percodan Percodan-Demi SK-Oxycodone with Aspirin	Oxycodone and Aspirin†
Talwin Compound	Pentazocine and Aspirin
Darvon with A.S.A. Darvon-N with A.S.A.	Propoxyphene and Aspirin
Bexophene Darvon Compound Dolene Compound Doxaphene Compound SK-65 Compound	Propoxyphene, Aspirin, and Caffeine†

*Not available in the United States.
†Generic name product may also be available.

Combination medicines containing narcotic (nar-KOT-ik) analgesics (an-al-JEE-zicks) and aspirin are used to relieve pain. A narcotic analgesic and aspirin used together may provide better pain relief than either medicine used alone. In some cases, relief of pain may come at lower doses of each medicine.

Narcotic analgesics act in the central nervous system (CNS) to relieve pain. Many of their side effects are also caused by actions in the CNS. When narcotics are used for a long time, your body may get used to them so that larger amounts are needed to relieve pain. This is called tolerance to the medicine. Also, when narcotics are used for a long time or in large doses, they may become habit-forming (causing mental or physical dependence). Physical dependence may lead to withdrawal symptoms when you stop taking the medicine.

Aspirin does not become habit-forming when taken for a long time or in large doses, but it may cause other unwanted effects if too much is taken.

There have been reports suggesting that use of aspirin (contained in this combination medicine) in children with fever due to a viral infection (especially flu or chicken pox) may cause a serious illness called Reye's syndrome. Do not give this medicine to a child or a teenager with symptoms of flu or chicken pox unless you have first discussed this with your child's doctor.

In the United States, these medicines are available only with your physician's or dentist's prescription. In Canada, some of these medicines may be available without a prescription.

For information about the precautions and side effects of the medicines in this combination, see:

Narcotic Analgesics (Systemic)
Salicylates (Systemic)

Combination products are designed for specific uses. These uses may not be the same as the uses of the individual ingredients. Therefore, some of the information provided in the individual listings may not be relevant to the combination product. If questions arise, check with your doctor, nurse, or pharmacist.

NICOTINE (Systemic)

A commonly used brand name is Nicorette.

Nicotine (NIK-o-teen) in a flavored chewing gum is used to help you stop smoking. It is used for up to 3 months as part of a supervised stop-smoking program.

As you chew nicotine gum, nicotine passes through the lining of your mouth and into your body. This nicotine takes the place of nicotine that you would otherwise get from smoking. In this way, the withdrawal effects of not smoking are less severe. Then, as your body adjusts to not smoking, the use of the nicotine gum is decreased gradually. Finally, its use is stopped altogether.

Children and nonsmokers should not use nicotine gum because of unwanted side effects.

Nicotine gum is available only with your doctor's prescription.

Before Using This Medicine

In order to decide on the best treatment for your medical problem, your doctor should be told:

—if you have ever had any unusual or allergic reaction to nicotine.

—if you are pregnant or if you intend to become pregnant while using this medicine. Nicotine, whether from smoking or the gum, is not recommended during pregnancy. Studies in humans show that nicotine when used during the last 3 months of pregnancy causes breathing problems in the fetus.

—if you are breast-feeding an infant. Nicotine passes into breast milk and may cause unwanted effects in the breast-fed infant. It may be necessary for you to stop breast-feeding during treatment.

—if you have any of the following medical problems:

    Dental problems
    Diabetes mellitus (sugar diabetes)
    Heart or blood vessel disease
    High blood pressure

    Inflammation of mouth or throat
    Temperomandibular (jaw muscle) joint
      disease (TMJ)
    Overactive thyroid
    Stomach ulcer

—if you are now taking any of the following medicines or types of medicine:

    Asthma medicines (such as aminophylline, oxtriphylline, and theophylline)
    Insulin
    Propoxyphene
    Propranolol

Proper Use of This Medicine

Nicotine gum usually comes with patient directions. **Read the directions carefully before using this medicine.**

When you feel the urge to smoke, chew one piece of gum very slowly until you taste it or feel a slight tingling in your mouth. Stop chewing until the taste or tingling is almost gone. Then chew slowly until you taste it again. Continue chewing and stopping in this way for about 30 minutes in order to get the full dose of nicotine.

Do not chew too fast, do not chew more than one piece at a time, and do not chew a piece of gum too soon after another. To do so may cause unwanted side effects or an overdose. Also, slower chewing will reduce the possibility of belching.

Use nicotine gum exactly as directed by your doctor. Remember that it is also important to participate in a stop-smoking program during treatment. This may make it easier for you to stop smoking.

As your urge to smoke becomes less frequent **gradually reduce the number of pieces of gum you chew each day** until you are chewing one or two pieces a day. This may be possible within 2 to 3 months.

Remember to carry nicotine gum with you at all times in case you feel the sudden urge to smoke. One cigarette may be enough to start you on the smoking habit again.

Using hard sugarless candy between doses of gum may help to relieve the discomfort in your mouth.

How to store this medicine:
• Store away from heat and direct light.

• **Keep out of the reach of children** because children are more sensitive to the unwanted effects of even small doses of nicotine.

• Do not store in the bathroom medicine cabinet because the heat or moisture may cause the medicine to break down.

• Do not keep outdated medicine or medicine no longer needed. Flush the contents of the container down the toilet, unless otherwise directed.

Precautions While Using This Medicine

Your doctor should check your progress at regular visits to make sure that nicotine gum is working properly and that possible side effects are avoided.

Do not chew more than 30 pieces of gum a day. Chewing too many pieces may be harmful because of the risk of overdose or toxicity.

Do not smoke during treatment with nicotine gum because of the risk of nicotine overdose or toxicity.

If the gum sticks to your dental work, stop using it and check with your physician or dentist. Dentures or other dental work may be damaged because nicotine gum is stickier and harder to chew than ordinary gum.

Nicotine should not be used in pregnancy. If there is a possibility you might become pregnant, you may want to use some type of birth control. If you think you may have become pregnant, stop taking

this medicine immediately and check with your doctor.

Side Effects of This Medicine

Along with its needed effects, a medicine may cause some unwanted effects. Although not all of these side effects appear very often, when they do occur they may require medical attention. Check with your doctor as soon as possible if any of the following side effects occur:
More common
   Injury to mouth, teeth, or dental work
Rare
   Irregular heartbeat
Signs of overdose (may occur in the following order)
   Nausea or vomiting
   Increased watering of mouth (severe)
   Abdominal or stomach pain (severe)
   Diarrhea
   Cold sweat
   Headache (severe)
   Dizziness (severe)
   Disturbed hearing and vision
   Confusion
   Weakness (severe)
   Fainting
   Difficulty in breathing (severe)
   Rapid, weak, or irregular pulse
   Convulsions (seizures)

Other side effects may occur which usually do not require medical attention. These side effects may go away during treatment as your body adjusts to the medicine. However, check with your doctor if any of the following side effects continue or are bothersome:
More common
   Belching
   Headache (mild)
   Hiccups
   Increased appetite
   Increased watering of mouth (mild)
   Jaw muscle ache
   Rapid heartbeat
   Sore mouth or throat
Less common or rare
   Constipation
   Coughing

Dizziness or lightheadedness (mild)
Dry mouth
Hoarseness
Laxative effect
Loss of appetite
Stomach upset or indigestion (mild)
Trouble in sleeping
Unusual irritability

Other side effects not listed above may also occur in some patients. If you notice any other effects, check with your doctor.

NITRATES (Systemic—Oral)

This information applies to the following medicines:

Erythrityl Tetranitrate (e-RI-thri-till tet-ra-NYE-trate)

Isosorbide Dinitrate (eye-soe-SOR-bide dye-NYE-trate)

Nitroglycerin (nye-troe-GLI-ser-in)

Pentaerythritol Tetranitrate (pen-ta-er-ITH-ri-tole tet-ra-NYE-trate)

This information does *not* apply to amyl nitrite or mannitol hexanitrate.

Some commonly used brand names or other names are:	Generic names:
Cardilate Erythritol Tetranitrate	Erythrityl Tetranitrate

Coronex* Dilatrate SR Iso-Bid Isochron Isonate Isonate TR Isordil Isotrate Sorate Sorbide T.D. Sorbitrate Sorbitrate SA	Isosorbide Dinitrate†

Ang-O-Span Glyceryl Trinitrate Klavikordal N-G-C Niong Nitro-Bid Nitrobon Nitrocap Nitrocap T.D. Nitroglyn Nitrolin Nitro-Long Nitronet Nitrong Nitrospan Nitrostat SR Nitro-Time Trates Sustachron	Nitroglycerin†

Duotrate Naptrate Pentol Pentol S.A. Pentraspan SR Pentritol Pentylan Peritrate Peritrate SA P.E.T.N. Vaso-80	Pentaerythritol Tetranitrate†

*Not available in the United States.
†Generic name product may also be available.

Nitrates are used for angina. Depending on the dosage form, they are used either to relieve the pain of angina attacks (fast-acting dosage forms) or to prevent angina attacks from occurring (slower-acting dosage forms).

Oral nitrates come in the form of regular tablets, chewable tablets, or extended-release capsules or tablets. When taken orally and swallowed, nitrates are used to prevent angina attacks. They do not act fast enough to relieve the pain of an angina attack.

Nitrates relax blood vessels and increase the supply of blood and oxygen to the heart while reducing its work load.

Nitrates may also be used for other conditions as determined by your doctor.

Nitrates are available only with your doctor's prescription.

Before Using This Medicine

In order to decide on the best treatment for your medical problem, your doctor should be told:

—if you have ever had any unusual or allergic reaction to nitrates or nitrites.

—if you are on a low-salt, low-sugar, or any other special diet, or if you are allergic to any substance, such as sulfites or other preservatives or dyes. Most medicines contain more than their active ingredient. Your doctor or pharmacist can help you avoid products that may cause a problem.

—if you are pregnant or if you intend to become pregnant while using this medicine. Although nitrates have not been shown to cause problems in humans, studies in rabbits given large doses of isosorbide dinitrate have shown adverse effects on the fetus. Studies have not been done with erythrityl tetranitrate, nitroglycerin, or pentaerythrityl tetranitrate.

—if you are breast-feeding an infant. Although this medicine has not been shown to cause problems in humans, the chance always exists.

—if you have any of the following medical problems:
Anemia (severe)
Glaucoma
Intestinal problems
Overactive thyroid

—if you have recently had a heart attack, stroke, or head injury.

—if you are now taking any of the following medicines or types of medicine:
Antihypertensives (high blood pressure medicine)
Asthma or hay fever medicine
Cold medicine

Decongestants
Medicine for appetite or diet control
Narcotics or prescription pain medicine
Sinus congestion medicine

Proper Use of This Medicine

Take this medicine exactly as directed by your doctor. It will work only if taken correctly.

This form of nitrate is used to prevent angina attacks. In most cases, it will not relieve an attack that has already started, because it works too slowly (the extended-release form releases medicine gradually over a 6-hour period to provide its effect for 8 to 10 hours). Check with your doctor if you need a fast-acting medicine to relieve the pain of an angina attack.

Take this medicine with a full glass (8 ounces) of water on an empty stomach. If taken either 1 hour before or 2 hours after meals, it will start working sooner.

Extended-release capsules and tablets are not to be broken, crushed, or chewed before they are swallowed. If broken up, they will not release the medicine properly.

If you are taking this medicine regularly and you miss a dose, take it as soon as possible. However, if the next scheduled dose is within 2 hours (or within 6 hours for extended-release capsules or tablets), skip the missed dose and go back to your regular dosing schedule. Do not double doses.

How to store this medicine:
• Store away from heat and direct light.
• **Keep out of the reach of children.**
• Do not store in the bathroom medicine cabinet because the heat or moisture may cause the medicine to break down.

• Do not keep outdated medicine or medicine no longer needed. Flush the contents of the container down the toilet, unless otherwise directed.

Precautions While Using This Medicine

If you have been taking this medicine regularly for several weeks or more, do not suddenly stop using it. Stopping suddenly may bring on attacks of angina. Check with your doctor for the best way to reduce gradually the amount you are taking before stopping completely.

Dizziness, lightheadedness, or a fainting feeling may occur, especially when you get up quickly from a lying or sitting position. Getting up slowly may help. If you feel dizzy, sit or lie down.

The dizziness, lightheadedness, or fainting is also more likely to occur if you drink alcohol, stand for long periods of time, exercise, or if the weather is hot. While you are taking this medicine, be careful in the amount of alcohol you drink. Also, use extra care during exercise or hot weather or if you must stand for long periods of time.

After taking a dose of this medicine you may get a headache that lasts for a short time. This is a common side effect which should become less noticeable after you have taken the medicine for a while. If this effect continues, or if the headaches are severe, check with your doctor.

For patients taking the extended-release dosage forms of isosorbide dinitrate or pentaerythritol tetranitrate:

• Partially dissolved tablets have been found in the stools of a few patients taking the extended-release tablets of this medicine. Be alert to this possibility especially if you have frequent bowel movements, diarrhea, or digestive problems. Notify your doctor if any such tablets are discovered. The tablets must be properly digested in order to provide the correct dose of medicine.

Side Effects of This Medicine

Along with its needed effects, a medicine may cause some unwanted effects. Although not all of these side effects appear very often, when they do occur they may require medical attention. Check with your doctor as soon as possible if any of the following side effects occur:

Rare

> Blurred vision
> Dry mouth
> Skin rash

Possible signs of overdose (in the order in which they may occur)

> Bluish-colored lips, fingernails, or palms of hands
> Dizziness (extreme) or fainting
> Feeling of extreme pressure in head
> Shortness of breath
> Unusual tiredness or weakness
> Weak and unusually fast heartbeat
> Fever
> Convulsions (seizures)

Other side effects may occur which usually do not require medical attention. These side effects may go away during treatment as your body adjusts to the medicine. However, check with your doctor if any of the following side effects continue or are bothersome:

More common

> Dizziness, lightheadedness, or fainting
> Flushing of face and neck
> Headache (severe or prolonged)
> Nausea or vomiting
> Rapid pulse
> Restlessness

Other side effects not listed above may also occur in some patients. If you notice any other effects, check with your doctor.

NITRATES (Systemic—Sublingual, Chewable, or Buccal)

This information applies to the following medicines:

Erythrityl Tetranitrate (e-RI-thri-till tet-ra-NYE-trate)

Isosorbide Dinitrate (eye-soe-SOR-bide dye-NYE-trate)

Nitroglycerin (nye-troe-GLI-ser-in)

This information does *not* apply to amyl nitrite, mannitol hexanitrate, or pentaerythritol tetranitrate.

Some commonly used brand names or other names are:	Generic names:
Cardilate Erythritol Tetranitrate	Erythrityl Tetranitrate
Coronex* Iso-Bid Isonate Isordil Onset Sorate Sorbitrate	Isosorbide Dinitrate†
Glyceryl Trinitrate Nitrostat Sustachron	Nitroglycerin†

*Not available in the United States.
†Generic name product may also be available.

Nitrates are used for angina. Depending on the dosage form, they are used either to relieve the pain of angina attacks (fast-acting dosage forms) or to prevent angina from occurring (slower-acting dosage forms).

Sublingual or chewable isosorbide dinitrate and sublingual or buccal nitroglycerin are used either to relieve the pain of angina attacks or to prevent such attacks from occurring. Sublingual or chewable erythrityl tetranitrate is used only to prevent angina attacks from occurring.

Sublingual nitrates are generally placed under the tongue where they dissolve and are absorbed through the lining of the mouth. However, they can also be used buccally, being placed under the lip or in the cheek. A buccal extended-release nitroglycerin tablet is also available. The chewable dosage forms, after being chewed and held in the mouth before swallowing, are absorbed in the same way.

Nitrates relax blood vessels and increase the supply of blood and oxygen to the heart while reducing its work load.

Nitrates may also be used for other conditions as determined by your doctor.

Nitrates are available only with your doctor's prescription.

Before Using This Medicine

In order to decide on the best treatment for your medical problem, your doctor should be told:

—if you have ever had any unusual or allergic reaction to nitrates or nitrites.

—if you are on a low-salt, low-sugar, or any other special diet, or if you are allergic to any substance, such as sulfites or other preservatives or dyes. Most medicines contain more than their active ingredient. Your doctor or pharmacist can help you avoid products that may cause a problem.

—if you are pregnant or if you intend to become pregnant while using this medicine. Although nitrates have not been shown to cause problems in humans, studies in rabbits given large doses of isosorbide dinitrate have shown adverse effects on the fetus. Studies have not been done with erythrityl tetranitrate or nitroglycerin.

—if you are breast-feeding an infant. Although this medicine has not been shown to cause problems in humans, the chance always exists.

—if you have any of the following medical problems:
Anemia (severe)
Glaucoma
Intestinal problems
Overactive thyroid

—if you have recently had a heart attack, stroke, or head injury.

—if you are now taking any of the following medicines or types of medicine:

Antihypertensives (high blood pressure medicine)
Asthma or hay fever medicine
Cold medicine
Decongestants
Medicine for appetite or diet control
Narcotics or prescription pain medicine
Sinus congestion medicine

Proper Use of This Medicine

Take this medicine exactly as directed by your doctor. It will work only if taken correctly.

Sublingual tablets should not be chewed, crushed, or swallowed. They work much faster when absorbed through the lining of the mouth. Place the tablet under the tongue, between the lip and gum, or between the cheek and gum and let it dissolve there. Do not eat, drink, or smoke while a tablet is dissolving.

Buccal extended-release tablets should not be chewed, crushed, or swallowed. They are designed to release a dose of nitroglycerin over a period of hours, not all at one time. Allow the tablet to dissolve slowly in place between lip and gum, or cheek and gum. If food or drink is to be taken during the 3 to 5 hours the tablet is dissolving, place the tablet between the *upper* lip and gum.

Chewable tablets must be chewed well and held in the mouth for about 2 minutes before swallowing. This will allow the medicine to be absorbed through the lining of the mouth.

For patients using nitroglycerin or isosorbide dinitrate to relieve the pain of an angina attack:

• **When you begin to feel an attack of angina starting (chest pains or a tightness or squeezing in the chest), sit down.**

Then place a tablet in your mouth, either sublingually or buccally, or chew a chewable tablet. This medicine works best when you are standing or sitting. However, since you may become dizzy, lightheaded, or faint soon after using a tablet, it is safer to sit rather than stand while the medicine is working. If you become dizzy or faint while sitting, take several deep breaths and bend forward with your head between your knees.

• Remain calm and you should feel better in a few minutes.

• **This medicine usually gives relief in 1 to 5 minutes.** However, if the pain is not relieved, and you are using:

—Sublingual tablets, either sublingually or buccally: Use a second tablet. If the pain continues for another 5 minutes, a third tablet may be used. **If you still have the chest pains after a total of 3 tablets in a 15-minute period, contact your doctor or go to a hospital emergency room immediately.**

—Buccal extended-release tablets: **Check with your doctor.** Do not use another tablet since the effects of a buccal tablet last for several hours.

For patients using nitroglycerin, erythrityl tetranitrate, or isosorbide dinitrate to prevent an anticipated angina attack:

• You may prevent anginal chest pains for up to 1 hour (6 hours for the extended-release nitroglycerin tablet) by using a buccal or sublingual tablet or chewing a chewable tablet 5 to 10 minutes before expected emotional stress or physical exertion that in the past seemed to bring on an attack.

For patients using erythrityl tetranitrate, isosorbide dinitrate, or extended-release buccal nitroglycerin regularly to prevent angina attacks:

• **Erythrityl tetranitrate is used to prevent angina attacks. It will not relieve an attack that has already started,** because it works too slowly. Check with your doctor if you need a fast-acting medicine to relieve the pain of an angina attack.

• Chewable isosorbide dinitrate and buccal extended-release nitroglycerin tablets can be used either to prevent angina attacks or to help relieve an attack that has already started.

• If you miss a dose of this medicine, use it as soon as possible. However, if the next scheduled dose is within 2 hours, skip the missed dose and go back to your regular dosing schedule. Do not double doses.

Stability and storage of sublingual nitroglycerin:

• When properly stored, sublingual nitroglycerin tablets retain their strength until the expiration date printed on the original label. However, because of patient usage, changing temperature and moisture, shaking, and repeated bottle opening, the tablets may be good for only 3 to 6 months. The "stabilized" sublingual tablets may stay good for a longer period of time but require the same care in storage and use.

• Some people think they should test the strength of their sublingual nitroglycerin tablets by looking for a tingling or burning sensation, a feeling of warmth or flushing, or a headache, after a tablet has been dissolved under the tongue. This kind of testing is not completely reliable since some patients may be unable to detect these effects. In addition, newer, stabilized sublingual nitroglycerin tablets are less likely to produce these detectable effects.

• To help keep the nitroglycerin tablets at full strength:

—keep the medicine in the original glass, screw-cap bottle. For patients who may wish to carry a small number of tablets with them for emergency use, a specially designed container

is available. However, only containers specifically labeled as being suitable for use with nitroglycerin sublingual tablets should be used.

—remove the cotton plug that comes in the bottle and *do not* put it back.

—**put the cap on the bottle quickly and tightly after each use.**

—to select a tablet for use, pour several into the bottle cap, take one, and pour the others back into the bottle. Try not to hold them in the palm of your hand because they may pick up moisture and crumble.

—do not keep other medicines in the same bottle with the nitroglycerin since they will weaken the nitroglycerin effect.

—keep the medicine handy at all times but try not to carry the bottle close to the body. Medicine may lose strength because of body warmth. Instead, carry the tightly closed bottle in your purse, jacket pocket, or other loose-fitting clothing whenever possible.

—store the bottle of nitroglycerin tablets in a cool, dry place. Average room temperature away from direct heat or direct sunlight is best. Do not store in the refrigerator or in a bathroom medicine cabinet because the moisture usually present in these areas may cause the tablets to crumble if the container is not tightly closed. Do not keep the tablets in your automobile glove compartment.

• **Keep out of the reach of children.**

• Do not keep outdated medicine or medicine no longer needed. Flush the contents of the container down the toilet, unless otherwise directed.

Stability and storage of erythrityl tetranitrate, isosorbide dinitrate, and buccal extended-release nitroglycerin:

• These forms of nitrates are more stable than sublingual nitroglycerin.

• Store away from heat and direct light.

• **Keep out of the reach of children.**

• Do not store in the bathroom medicine cabinet because the heat or moisture may cause the medicine to break down.

• Do not keep outdated medicine or medicine no longer needed. Flush the contents of the container down the toilet, unless otherwise directed.

Precautions While Using This Medicine

If you have been taking this medicine regularly for several weeks, do not suddenly stop using it. Stopping suddenly may bring on attacks of angina. Check with your doctor for the best way to reduce gradually the amount you are taking before stopping completely.

Dizziness, lightheadedness, or a fainting feeling may occur, especially when you get up quickly from a lying or sitting position. Getting up slowly may help. If you feel dizzy, sit or lie down.

The dizziness, lightheadedness, or fainting is also more likely to occur if you drink alcohol, stand for long periods of time, exercise, or if the weather is hot. **While you are taking this medicine, be careful in the amount of alcohol you drink. Also, use extra care during exercise or hot weather or if you must stand for long periods of time.**

After taking a dose of this medicine you may get a headache that lasts for a short time. This is a common side effect which should become less noticeable after you have taken the medicine for a while. If this effect continues or if the headaches are severe, check with your doctor.

Side Effects of This Medicine

Along with its needed effects, a medicine may cause some unwanted effects. Although not all of these side effects appear very often, when they do occur they may require medical attention. Check with your doctor as soon as possible if any of the following side effects occur:

Rare
>   Blurred vision
>   Dry mouth
>   Skin rash

Possible signs of overdose (in the order in which they may occur)
>   Bluish-colored lips, fingernails, or palms of hands
>   Dizziness (extreme) or fainting
>   Feeling of extreme pressure in head
>   Shortness of breath
>   Unusual tiredness or weakness
>   Weak and unusually fast heartbeat
>   Fever
>   Convulsions (seizures)

Other side effects may occur which usually do not require medical attention. These side effects may go away during treatment as your body adjusts to the medicine. However, check with your doctor if any of the following side effects continue or are bothersome:

More common
>   Dizziness or lightheadedness
>   Flushing of face and neck
>   Headache (severe or prolonged)
>   Nausea or vomiting
>   Rapid pulse
>   Restlessness

Other side effects not listed above may also occur in some patients. If you notice any other effects, check with your doctor.

NITRATES (Systemic—Topical)

This information applies to nitroglycerin ointment and transdermal patches.

Some commonly used brand names or other names are:

Glyceryl Trinitrate	Nitrol
Nitro-Bid	Nitrong
Nitrodisc	Nitrostat
Nitro-Dur	Transderm-Nitro

Generic name product may also be available.

Nitrates (NYE-trates) are used for angina. Depending on the dosage form, they are used either to relieve the pain of angina attacks (fast-acting dosage forms) or to prevent angina attacks from occurring (slower-acting dosage forms).

When applied to the skin, nitrates are used to prevent angina attacks. The only nitrate available for this purpose is topical nitroglycerin (nye-troe-GLI-ser-in). It is available either as an ointment or a transdermal (stick-on) patch.

Topical nitroglycerin is absorbed through the skin. It relaxes blood vessels and increases the supply of blood and oxygen to the heart while reducing its work load. This helps prevent future angina attacks from occurring.

Topical nitroglycerin may also be used for other conditions as determined by your doctor.

Nitroglycerin is available only with your doctor's prescription.

Before Using This Medicine

In order to decide on the best treatment for your medical problem, your doctor should be told:

—if you have ever had any unusual or allergic reaction to nitrates or nitrites.

—if you are allergic to any substance, such as certain preservatives or dyes. Most medicines contain more than their active ingredient. Your doctor or pharmacist can help you avoid products that may cause a problem.

—if you are pregnant or if you intend to become pregnant while using this medicine. Although nitroglycerin has not been shown to cause problems, the chance always exists. Studies have not been done in humans.

—if you are breast-feeding an infant. Although this medicine has not been shown to cause problems in humans, the chance always exists.

—if you have any of the following medical problems:
  Anemia (severe)
  Glaucoma
  Intestinal problems
  Overactive thyroid

—if you have recently had a heart attack, stroke, or head injury.

—if you are now taking any of the following medicines or types of medicine:
  Antihypertensives (high blood pressure medicine)
  Asthma or hay fever medicine
  Cold medicine
  Decongestants
  Medicine for appetite or diet control
  Narcotics or prescription pain medicine
  Sinus congestion medicine

Proper Use of This Medicine

Use nitroglycerin exactly as directed by your doctor. It will work only if applied correctly.

The ointment and transdermal forms of nitroglycerin are used to prevent angina attacks. They will not relieve an attack that has already started because they work too slowly. Check with your doctor if you need a fast-acting medicine to relieve the pain of an angina attack.

This medicine usually comes with patient instructions. Read them carefully before using.

For patients using the ointment form of this medicine:

• Before applying a new dose of ointment, remove any ointment remaining on the skin from a previous dose; this will allow the fresh ointment to release the nitroglycerin properly.

• This medicine comes with dose-measuring papers. Use them to measure the length of ointment squeezed from the tube and to apply the ointment to the skin. **Do not rub or massage the ointment on the skin; just spread in a thin, even layer, covering an area of the same size each time it is applied.**

• Apply the ointment to skin that has little or no hair.

• Each dose of ointment is best applied to a different area of skin to prevent irritation or other skin problems.

• If your doctor has ordered an occlusive dressing (for example, kitchen plastic wrap) to be applied over this medicine, make sure you know how to apply it. Since occlusive dressings increase the amount of medicine absorbed through the skin and the possibility of side effects, use them only as directed. If you have any questions about this, check with your doctor, nurse, or pharmacist.

• If you miss a dose of this medicine, apply it as soon as possible unless the next scheduled dose is within 2 hours. Then go back to your regular dosing schedule. Do not increase the amount used.

• How to store this medicine:

—Store the tube of nitroglycerin ointment in a cool place and keep it tightly closed.

—**Keep out of the reach of children.**

For patients using the transdermal (stick-on patch) system:

• Do not try to trim or cut the adhesive patch to adjust the dosage. Check with your doctor if you think the medicine is not working as it should.

• Apply the patch to a clean, dry skin area with little or no hair and free of scars, cuts, or irritation.

• Apply a new patch if the first one becomes loose or falls off.

• Each dose is best applied to a different area of skin to prevent skin problems or other irritation.

• If you miss a dose of this medicine, apply it as soon as possible. Then go back to your regular dosing schedule.

• How to store this medicine:

—Store away from heat and direct light.

—**Keep out of the reach of children.**

—Do not store in the bathroom medicine cabinet because the heat or moisture may cause the medicine to break down.

Precautions While Using This Medicine

If you have been using nitroglycerin regularly for several weeks or more, do not suddenly stop using it. Stopping suddenly may bring on attacks of angina. Check with your doctor for the best way to reduce gradually the amount you are using before stopping completely.

Dizziness, lightheadedness, or a fainting feeling may occur, especially when you get up quickly from a lying or sitting position. Getting up slowly may help. If you feel dizzy, sit or lie down.

The dizziness, lightheadedness, or fainting is also more likely to occur if you drink alcohol, stand for long periods of time, exercise, or if the weather is hot. **While you are taking this medicine, be careful in the amount of alcohol you drink. Also, use extra care during exercise or hot weather or if you must stand for long periods of time.**

After using a dose of this medicine you may get a headache that lasts for a short time. This is a common side effect, which should become less noticeable after you have used the medicine for a while. If this effect continues, or if the headaches are severe, check with your doctor.

Side Effects of This Medicine

Along with its needed effects, a medicine may cause some unwanted effects. Although not all of these side effects appear very often, when they do occur they may require medical attention. Check with your doctor as soon as possible if any of the following side effects occur:

Rare

  Blurred vision
  Dry mouth

Possible signs of overdose (in the order in which they may occur)

  Bluish-colored lips, fingernails, or palms of hands
  Dizziness (extreme) or fainting
  Feeling of extreme pressure in head
  Shortness of breath
  Unusual tiredness or weakness
  Weak and unusually fast heartbeat
  Fever
  Convulsions (seizures)

Other side effects may occur which usually do not require medical attention. These side effects may go away during treatment as your body adjusts to the medicine. However, check with your doctor if any of the following side effects continue or are bothersome:

More common

  Dizziness or lightheadedness
  Flushing of face and neck
  Headache (severe or prolonged)
  Nausea or vomiting
  Rapid heartbeat
  Restlessness

Less common

  Sore, reddened skin

Other side effects not listed above may also occur in some patients. If you notice any other effects, check with your doctor.

NITROFURANTOIN (Systemic)

Some commonly used brand names are:

Furadantin	Nephronex*
Furalan	Nifuran*
Macrodantin	Novofuran*

Generic name product may also be available.

---

*Not available in the United States.

Nitrofurantoin (nye-troe-fyoor-AN-toyn) belongs to the general family of medicines called anti-infectives. It is taken by mouth to treat infections of the urinary tract. It may also be used for other problems as determined by your doctor.

Nitrofurantoin is available only with your doctor's prescription.

Before Using This Medicine

In order to decide on the best treatment for your medical problem, your doctor should be told:

—if you have ever had any unusual or allergic reaction to any related medicines such as furazolidone or nitrofurazone.

—if you are pregnant and within a week or two of your delivery date. Nitrofurantoin should not be used during the last part of pregnancy since it may cause problems in the infant.

—if you are breast-feeding an infant. Nitrofurantoin passes into the breast milk in small amounts and may cause problems in an infant with glucose-6-phosphate dehydrogenase (G6PD) deficiency.

—if you have any of the following medical problems:

  Glucose-6-phosphate dehydrogenase (G6PD) deficiency
  Kidney disease (other than infection)
  Lung disease
  Nerve damage

—if you are now taking any of the following medicines or types of medicine:

Dapsone
Dipyrone
Furazolidone
Primaquine
Probenecid
Sulfinpyrazone
Sulfonamides (sulfa medicine)
Sulfoxone
Vitamin K

Proper Use of This Medicine

Nitrofurantoin is best taken with food or milk. This may lessen stomach upset and help your body absorb the medicine better.

For patients taking the oral liquid form of this medicine:

• Shake the oral liquid sharply (forcefully) before each dose to help make it pour more smoothly and to be sure the medicine is evenly mixed.

• Use a specially marked measuring spoon or other device to measure each dose accurately since the average household teaspoon may not hold the right amount of liquid.

• May be mixed with water, milk, fruit juices, or infants' formulas. If mixed with other liquids, take immediately after mixing. Be sure to drink all the liquid in order to get the full dose of medicine.

• To help keep this medicine from staining the teeth, rinse the mouth with water after swallowing the oral liquid form. The stain is not permanent, however.

To help clear up your infection completely, **keep taking this medicine for the full time of treatment** even if you begin to feel better after a few days; **do not miss any doses.**

If you do miss a dose of this medicine, take it as soon as possible. However, if it is almost time for your next dose and your dosing schedule is:

• 3 or more doses a day—Space the missed dose and the next dose 2 to 4 hours apart or double your next dose.

Then go back to your regular dosing schedule.

Do not give this medicine to infants under 1 month of age.

How to store this medicine:

• Store away from heat and direct light, out of the reach of children.

• Do not store in the bathroom medicine cabinet because the heat or moisture may cause the medicine to break down.

• Keep the oral liquid form of this medicine from freezing.

• Do not keep outdated medicine or medicine no longer needed. Flush it down the toilet.

Precautions While Using This Medicine

If your symptoms do not improve within a few days or if they become worse, check with your doctor.

Diabetics—This medicine may cause false test results with some urine sugar tests. Check with your doctor before changing your diet or the dosage of your diabetes medicine.

Side Effects of This Medicine

Along with its needed effects, a medicine may cause some unwanted effects. Although not all of these side effects appear very often, when they do occur they may require medical attention. **Stop taking this medicine and check with your doctor immediately** if any of the following side effects occur:

More common
Chest pain
Chills
Cough

Fever
Troubled breathing
Less common
Dizziness
Drowsiness
Headache
Numbness, tingling, or burning of face
or mouth
Pale skin
Unusual tiredness or weakness
Rare
Yellowing of eyes or skin

Other side effects may occur which usually
do not require medical attention. These
side effects may go away during treatment as your body adjusts to the medicine. However, check with your doctor if
any of the following side effects continue or are bothersome:

More common
Diarrhea
Loss of appetite
Nausea or vomiting
Less common
Discoloration of infants' or children's
teeth (oral liquid only)
Itching
Skin rash

This medicine may cause the urine to become rust-yellow to brown. This side effect does not require medical attention.

Other side effects not listed above may also
occur in some patients. If you notice any
other effects, check with your doctor.

ORPHENADRINE (Systemic)
Some commonly used brand names are:

Banflex	Neocyten
Disipal	Norflex
Flexoject	O-Flex
Flexon	Orflagen
K-Flex	Orphenate
Myolin	X-Otag
	X-Otag S.R.

Generic name product may also be available.

Orphenadrine (or-FEN-a-dreen) is a
medicine that is used to help relax certain
muscles in your body and relieve the pain
and discomfort caused by strains, sprains,
or other injury to your muscles. Orphenadrine is also used to relieve trembling
caused by Parkinson's disease. However,
this medicine does not take the place of
rest, exercise or physical therapy, or other
treatment that your doctor may recommend for your medical problem.

Orphenadrine acts in the central nervous system (CNS) to produce its muscle
relaxant effects. Orphenadrine also has other actions (antimuscarinic) which produce
its helpful effects in Parkinson's disease. Orphenadrine's CNS and antimuscarinic actions may also be responsible for some of its
side effects.

This medicine is available only with
your doctor's prescription.

Before Using This Medicine
In order to decide on the best treatment for
your medical problem, your doctor
should be told:

—if you have ever had any unusual or
allergic reaction to orphenadrine.

—if you are on a low-salt, low-sugar, or
any other special diet, or if you are allergic to any substance, such as sulfites or
other preservatives or dyes. Most medicines contain more than their active ingredient. Your doctor or pharmacist can
help you avoid products that may cause
a problem.

—if you are pregnant or if you intend to
become pregnant while using this medicine. Although orphenadrine has not
been shown to cause birth defects or other problems in humans, the chance always exists.

—if you are breast-feeding an infant.
Although orphenadrine has not been
shown to cause problems in humans, the
chance always exists. It is not known
whether orphenadrine passes into the
breast milk.

—if you have any of the following medical problems:

Disease of the digestive tract, especially esophagus disease, stomach ulcer, or intestinal blockage
Enlarged prostate
Glaucoma
Heart disease
Kidney disease
Liver disease
Myasthenia gravis
Unusually fast or irregular heartbeat
Urinary tract blockage

—if you are now taking antimuscarinics (medicine for abdominal or stomach cramps or spasms).

—if you are now taking other central nervous system (CNS) depressants, such as:

Anticonvulsants (seizure medicine)
Antihistamines or medicine for hay fever, other allergies, or colds
Barbiturates
Narcotics
Other muscle relaxants
Prescription pain medicine
Sedatives, tranquilizers, or sleeping medicine
Tricyclic antidepressants (medicine for depression)

—if you are now taking or have taken within the past 2 weeks monoamine oxidase (MAO) inhibitors, such as:

Furazolidone
Isocarboxazid
Pargyline
Phenelzine
Procarbazine
Tranylcypromine

Proper Use of This Medicine

If you miss a dose of this medicine and remember within an hour or so of the missed dose, take it right away. But if you do not remember until later, skip the missed dose and go back to your regular dosing schedule. Do not double doses.

How to store this medicine:

• Store away from heat and direct light.

• **Keep out of the reach of children.**

• Do not store in the bathroom medicine cabinet because the heat or moisture may cause the medicine to break down.

• Do not keep outdated medicine or medicine no longer needed. Flush the contents of the container down the toilet, unless otherwise directed.

Precautions While Using This Medicine

If you will be taking this medicine for a long period of time (for example, more than a few weeks), your doctor should check your progress at regular visits.

This medicine may add to the effects of alcohol and other CNS depressants (medicines that slow down the nervous system, possibly causing drowsiness). Some examples of CNS depressants are antihistamines or medicine for hay fever, other allergies, or colds; sedatives, tranquilizers, or sleeping medicine; prescription pain medicine or narcotics; barbiturates; medicine for seizures; tricyclic antidepressants (medicine for depression); other muscle relaxants; or anesthetics, including some dental anesthetics. **Check with your doctor before taking any of the above while you are using this medicine.**

This medicine may cause some people to have blurred vision or to become drowsy, dizzy, lightheaded, faint, or less alert than they are normally. It may also cause muscle weakness in some people. **Make sure you know how you react to this medicine before you drive, use machines, or do other jobs that require you to be alert.**

Dryness of the mouth may occur while you are taking this medicine. Sucking on sugarless hard candy or ice chips or chewing sugarless gum may help relieve the dry mouth.

Side Effects of This Medicine

Along with its needed effects, a medicine may cause some unwanted effects. Although not all of these side effects appear very often, when they do occur they may require medical attention. Check with your doctor as soon as possible if any of the following side effects occur:

Less common
  Fainting
  Unusually fast or pounding heartbeat

Rare
  Hallucinations (seeing, hearing, or feeling things that are not there)
  Skin rash, hives, itching, or redness
  Unusual tiredness or weakness

Other side effects may occur which usually do not require medical attention. These side effects may go away during treatment as your body adjusts to the medicine. However, check with your doctor if any of the following side effects continue or are bothersome:

More common
  Dryness of mouth

Less common
  Abdominal or stomach cramps or discomfort
  Blurred or double vision or other vision problems
  Confusion
  Constipation
  Difficult urination
  Dizziness or lightheadedness
  Drowsiness
  Headache
  Nausea or vomiting
  Trembling
  Unusual excitement, irritability, nervousness or restlessness
  Unusual muscle weakness

Other side effects not listed above may also occur in some patients. If you notice any other effects, check with your doctor.

ORPHENADRINE, ASPIRIN, AND CAFFEINE (Systemic)

Some commonly used brand names are Back-Ese*, Norgesic, and Norgesic Forte.

---

*Not available in the United States.

Orphenadrine (or-FEN-a-dreen), aspirin (AS-pir-in), and caffeine (KAF-een) is a combination medicine used to help relax certain muscles in your body and relieve the pain and discomfort caused by strains, sprains, or other injury to your muscles. However, this medicine does not take the place of rest, exercise, or other treatment that your doctor may recommend for your medical problem.

In the United States, this combination medicine is available only with your doctor's prescription. In Canada, it is available without a prescription.

For information about the precautions and side effects of the medicines in this combination, see:

  Orphenadrine (Systemic)
  Salicylates (Systemic)

Combination products are designed for specific uses. These uses may not be the same as the uses of the individual ingredients. Therefore, some of the information provided in the individual listings may not be relevant to the combination product. If questions arise, check with your doctor, nurse, or pharmacist.

OXTRIPHYLLINE AND GUAIFENESIN (Systemic)

Some commonly used brand names are Brondecon and Brondelate.

Oxtriphylline (ox-TRYE-fi-lin) and guaifenesin (gwye-FEN-e-sin) combination is used to treat the symptoms of bronchial asthma, chronic bronchitis, emphysema, and other lung diseases. This medicine relieves cough, wheezing, shortness of breath, and troubled breathing. It works by opening up the bronchial tubes or air passages of the lungs and increasing the flow of air through them.

This medicine is available only with your doctor's prescription.

For information about the precautions and side effects of the medicines in this combination, see:

Xanthine-derivative Bronchodilators (Systemic)

Guaifenesin (Systemic)

Combination products are designed for specific uses. These uses may not be the same as the uses of the individual ingredients. Therefore, some of the information provided in the individual listings may not be relevant to the combination product. If questions arise, check with your doctor, nurse, or pharmacist.

PENICILLINS (Systemic)

This information applies to the following medicines:

Amdinocillin (am-DEE-noe-sill-in)
Amoxicillin (a-mox-i-SILL-in)
Amoxicillin and Clavulanate (klav-yoo-LAN-ate)
Ampicillin (am-pi-SILL-in)
Azlocillin (az-loe-SILL-in)
Bacampicillin (ba-kam-pi-SILL-in)
Carbenicillin (kar-ben-i-SILL-in)
Cloxacillin (klox-a-SILL-in)
Cyclacillin (sye-kla-SILL-in)
Dicloxacillin (dye-klox-a-SILL-in)
Methicillin (meth-i-SILL-in)
Mezlocillin (mez-loe-SILL-in)
Nafcillin (naf-SILL-in)
Oxacillin (ox-a-SILL-in)
Penicillin G (pen-i-SILL-in)
Penicillin V
Piperacillin (pi-PER-a-sill-in)
Ticarcillin (tye-kar-SILL-in)
Ticarcillin and Clavulanate

Some commonly used brand names and other names are:	Generic names:
Coactin Mecillinam	Amdinocillin
Amoxil Moxilean* Novamoxin* Polymox Sumox Trimox Utimox Wymox	Amoxicillin†
Augmentin	Amoxicillin and Clavulanate
Amcill Ampicin* Ampilean* NaMPICIL Omnipen Omnipen-N Penbritin* Polycillin Polycillin-N Principen SK-Ampicillin SK-Ampicillin-N Supen Totacillin Totacillin-N	Ampicillin†
Azlin	Azlocillin
Spectrobid	Bacampicillin
Geocillin Geopen Pyopen	Carbenicillin
Cloxapen Cloxilean* Novocloxin* Orbenin* Tegopen	Cloxacillin†
Cyclapen-W	Cyclacillin
Dycill Dynapen Pathocil	Dicloxacillin†
Staphcillin	Methicillin
Baypen* Mezlin	Mezlocillin

Nafcil Nallpen Unipen	Nafcillin
Bactocill Prostaphlin	Oxacillin†
Ayercillin* Bicillin Bicillin L-A Crystapen* Crysticillin Duracillin A.S. Megacillin* Novopen-G* Pentids Permapen Pfizerpen Pfizerpen-AS Pfizerpen G SK-Penicillin G Wycillin	Penicillin G†
Beepen-VK Betapen-VK Ledercillin VK Nadopen-V* Novopen-VK* Penapar VK Pen Vee K Robicillin VK SK-Penicillin VK Uticillin VK V-Cillin K Veetids	Penicillin V†
Pipracil	Piperacillin
Ticar	Ticarcillin
Timentin	Ticarcillin and Clavulanate

*Not available in the United States.
†Generic name product may also be available.

Penicillins belong to the general family of medicines called antibiotics. Antibiotics are medicines used in the treatment of infections caused by bacteria. They work by killing bacteria or preventing their growth.

There are several different kinds of penicillins. Each is used to treat different kinds of infections. One kind of penicillin usually may not be used in place of another. None of the penicillins will work for colds, flu, or other virus infections.

Penicillins are taken by mouth or given by injection to treat infections in many different parts of the body. They are sometimes given with other antibiotics. Carbenicillin taken by mouth is used only to treat infections of the urinary tract and prostate gland. Penicillin G and penicillin V are also used to prevent "strep" infections in patients with a history of rheumatic heart disease. Piperacillin is also given by injection to prevent infections before, during, and after surgery. Some of the penicillins may also be used for other problems as determined by your doctor.

Penicillins are available only with your doctor's prescription.

Before Using This Medicine

In order to decide on the best treatment for your medical problem, your doctor should be told:

—if you have ever had any unusual or allergic reaction to any of the penicillins, cephalosporins, griseofulvin, or penicillamine. Serious reactions may occur in patients who are allergic to penicillins.

—if you are on a low-salt, low-sugar, or any other special diet, or if you are allergic to any substance, such as sulfites or other preservatives or dyes. Most medicines contain more than their active ingredient, and many liquid medicines contain alcohol. Your doctor or pharmacist can help you avoid products that may cause a problem.

—if you are receiving penicillin G procaine and have ever had any unusual or allergic reaction to procaine or other "caine-type" anesthetics (medicines which cause numbing).

—if you are pregnant or if you intend to become pregnant while taking this medicine. Studies have not been done in humans. However, penicillins have not been shown to cause birth defects or other problems in animals given more than 25 times the usual human dose.

—if you are breast-feeding an infant. Most penicillins (except amdinocillin) pass into the breast milk. Even though only small amounts may pass, allergic reaction, diarrhea, fungal infection, and skin rash may occur in the infant.

—if you have any of the following medical problems (may not apply to all penicillins):

Allergy (general), history of (such as asthma, eczema, hay fever, hives)
Bleeding problems, history of
Kidney disease
Liver disease
Mononucleosis ("mono")
Stomach or intestinal disease, history of (especially colitis, including colitis caused by antibiotics, or enteritis)

—if you are now taking any of the following medicines or types of medicine (may not apply to all penicillins):

Allopurinol
Amiloride
Anticoagulants (blood thinners)
Aspirin or other salicylates
Captopril
Chloramphenicol
Cholestyramine
Colestipol
Diarrhea medicine
Diflunisal
Dipyridamole
Disulfiram
Divalproex
Erythromycins
Fenoprofen
Heparin
Ibuprofen
Indomethacin
Meclofenamate
Mefenamic acid
Naproxen
Neomycin (by mouth)
Oral contraceptives (birth control pills)
Oxyphenbutazone

Phenylbutazone
Piroxicam
Plicamycin
Potassium-containing medicines
Potassium supplements
Probenecid
Spironolactone
Streptokinase
Sulfinpyrazone
Sulfonamides (sulfa medicine)
Sulindac
Tetracyclines
Tolmetin
Triamterene
Urokinase
Valproic acid

Proper Use of This Medicine

To help clear up your infection completely, **keep taking this medicine for the full time of treatment** even if you begin to feel better after a few days. **If you have a "strep" infection, you should keep taking this medicine for at least 10 days. This is especially important in "strep" infections since serious heart problems could develop later** if your infection is not cleared up completely. Also, if you stop taking this medicine too soon, your symptoms may return.

This medicine works best when there is a constant amount in the blood or urine. **To help keep this amount constant, do not miss any doses. Also, it is best to take each dose at evenly spaced times day and night.** For example, if you are to take 4 doses a day, each dose should be spaced about 6 hours apart. If this interferes with your sleep or other daily activities, or if you need help in planning the best times to take your medicine, check with your doctor, nurse, or pharmacist.

If you do miss a dose of this medicine, take it as soon as possible. This will help to keep a constant amount of medicine in the blood or urine. However, if it is almost time for your next dose and your dosing schedule is:

• 2 doses a day—Space the missed dose and the next dose 5 to 6 hours apart.

• 3 or more doses a day—Space the missed dose and the next dose 2 to 4 hours apart or double your next dose. Then go back to your regular dosing schedule.

Penicillins (except bacampicillin tablets, amoxicillin, and amoxicillin and clavulanate combination) are best taken with a full glass (8 ounces) of water on an empty stomach (either 1 hour before or 2 hours after meals) unless otherwise directed by your doctor.

For patients taking amoxicillin and amoxicillin and clavulanate combination:

• Amoxicillin and amoxicillin and clavulanate combination may be taken on a full or empty stomach.

• The liquid form of amoxicillin may also be taken straight or mixed with formulas, milk, fruit juice, water, ginger ale, or other cold drinks. If mixed with other liquids, take immediately after mixing. Be sure to drink all the liquid in order to get the full dose of medicine.

For patients taking bacampicillin:

• The liquid form of this medicine is best taken with a full glass (8 ounces) of water on an empty stomach (either 1 hour before or 2 hours after meals) unless otherwise directed by your doctor.

• The tablet form of this medicine may be taken on a full or empty stomach.

For patients taking carbenicillin by mouth:

• This medicine usually comes with a drying agent in a small packet to help keep the tablets from taking on water and breaking down. **Do not swallow the drying agent;** keep it in the bottle with the tablets until they are used up and then throw it away.

For patients taking penicillin G by mouth:

• Do not take acidic fruit juices (for example, orange or grapefruit juice) or other acidic beverages within 1 hour of the time you take penicillin G since this may keep the medicine from working as well.

For patients taking the oral liquid form of this medicine:

• This medicine is to be taken by mouth even though it may come in a dropper bottle. If this medicine does not come in a dropper bottle, use a specially marked measuring spoon or other device to measure each dose accurately since the average household teaspoon may not hold the right amount of liquid.

• Do not use after the expiration date on the label since the medicine may not work as well. Check with your pharmacist if you have any questions about this.

For patients taking the chewable tablet form of this medicine:

• Tablets should be chewed or crushed before they are swallowed.

How to store this medicine:

• Store the liquid form of most penicillins in the refrigerator because heat will cause this medicine to break down. Follow the directions on the label. However, keep the medicine from freezing.

• **Keep out of the reach of children.**

• Do not keep outdated medicine or medicine no longer needed. Flush the contents of the container down the toilet, unless otherwise directed.

Precautions While Using This Medicine

If your symptoms do not improve within a few days or if they become worse, check with your doctor.

If you have ever had an allergic reaction to any of the penicillins, your doctor may want you to carry a medical identification (ID) card or wear a medical ID bracelet stating this.

If diarrhea occurs, do not take any diarrhea medicine without first checking with your doctor or pharmacist. These medicines may make your diarrhea worse or make it last longer.

Oral contraceptives (birth control pills) may not work as well if you take them while you are taking ampicillin, bacampicillin, or penicillin V. Unplanned pregnancies may occur. You should use a different means of birth control while you are taking any of these penicillins. If you have any questions about this, check with your doctor or pharmacist.

Diabetics—Amoxicillin, amoxicillin and clavulanate combination, ampicillin, bacampicillin, and penicillin G may cause false test results with some urine sugar tests. Check with your doctor before changing your diet or the dosage of your diabetes medicine.

Side Effects of This Medicine

Along with its needed effects, a medicine may cause some unwanted effects. Although not all of these side effects appear very often, when they do occur they may require medical attention. **Stop taking this medicine and check with your doctor immediately** if any of the following side effects occur:

More common (may be less common with some penicillins)

Skin rash, hives, itching, or wheezing
    Note: Skin rash may occur much more commonly in patients with mononucleosis ("mono") who are taking amoxicillin, ampicillin, or bacampicillin.

Rare (may be more common with some penicillins)

Abdominal or stomach cramps, pain, and bloating (severe)
Diarrhea (watery and severe) which may also be bloody
Fever
Nausea or vomiting
Unusual thirst

Unusual tiredness or weakness
Unusual weight loss
    (the above side effects may also occur up to several weeks after you stop taking any of these medicines)
Seizures
Unusual bleeding or bruising

In addition to the side effects mentioned above, **check with your doctor immediately** if any of the following side effects also occur:

Less common (may be more common with some penicillins)

Blood in urine
Passage of large amounts of light-colored urine
Swelling of the face and ankles
Troubled breathing
Unusual tiredness or weakness

For patients receiving azlocillin, mezlocillin, or piperacillin:

• In addition to the side effects mentioned above, **check with your doctor immediately** if any of the following side effects also occur:

Less common

Dark or amber urine
Pale stools
Stomach pain
Yellowing of eyes or skin

Other side effects may occur which usually do not require medical attention. These side effects may go away during treatment as your body adjusts to the medicine. However, check with your doctor if any of the following side effects continue or are bothersome:

More common (may be less common with some penicillins)

Bitter, unpleasant, or unusual taste in mouth (for carbenicillin by mouth and mezlocillin only)
Diarrhea (mild)
Nausea, vomiting, or stomach upset
Sore mouth or tongue (for amoxicillin, amoxicillin and clavulanate combination, ampicillin, azlocillin, and bacampicillin only)

Less common or rare

  Changes in sense of taste and smell
    (for azlocillin and ticarcillin and
    clavulanate only)
  Dizziness (for amdinocillin and azlocillin
    only)
  Muscle weakness

In some patients amoxicillin, amoxicillin
and clavulanate combination, ampicillin, bacampicillin, penicillin G, and
penicillin V may cause the tongue to become darkened or discolored. These
changes are only temporary and will go
away when you stop taking these medicines.

Overdose is very unlikely to occur with
penicillins. However, if you think that
you or someone else, especially a child,
has taken too much, check with your
doctor. Severe diarrhea, nausea, or vomiting may need to be treated.

Other side effects not listed above may also
occur in some patients. If you notice any
other effects, check with your doctor.

PENTOXIFYLLINE (Systemic)

A commonly used brand name is Trental.

Pentoxifylline (pen-tox-IF-i-lin) is a
medicine that improves the flow of blood
through blood vessels. It is taken by mouth
to reduce leg pain caused by poor blood
circulation. Pentoxifylline makes it possible
to walk further before having to rest because of leg cramps.
  Pentoxifylline is available only with
your doctor's prescription.

Before Using This Medicine

In order to decide on the best treatment for
your medical problem, your doctor
should be told:

—if you have ever had any unusual or
allergic reaction to pentoxifylline or to
other xanthines such as aminophylline,
caffeine, dyphylline, ethylenediamine
(contained in aminophylline), oxtriphylline, theobromine, or theophylline.

—if you are on a low-salt, low-sugar, or
any other special diet, or if you are allergic to any substance, such as sulfites or
other preservatives or dyes. Most medicines contain more than their active ingredient. Your doctor or pharmacist can
help you avoid products that may cause
a problem.

—if you are pregnant or if you intend to
become pregnant while using this medicine. Studies have not been done in humans. Although pentoxifylline has not
been shown to cause birth defects in animals, it has caused other harmful effects
in rats given doses 25 times the maximum human dose.

—if you are breast-feeding an infant.
Although it is not known whether pentoxifylline passes into the breast milk
and this medicine has not been shown to
cause problems in humans, the chance
always exists.

—if you are now taking antihypertensives (high blood pressure medicine).

—if you smoke tobacco.

—if you have kidney disease.

Proper Use of This Medicine

Swallow the tablet whole. Do not crush,
break, or chew before swallowing.

**Pentoxifylline should be taken with meals so
that it will not upset your stomach.**

If you miss a dose of this medicine, take it
as soon as possible. However, if it is almost time for your next dose, skip the

missed dose and go back to your regular dosing schedule. Do not double doses.

How to store this medicine:
- Store away from heat and direct light.
- **Keep out of the reach of children.**
- Do not store in the bathroom medicine cabinet because the heat or moisture may cause the medicine to break down.
- Do not keep outdated medicine or medicine no longer needed. Flush the contents of the container down the toilet, unless otherwise directed.

Precautions While Using This Medicine

It may take several weeks for this medicine to work. If you feel that pentoxifylline is not working, do not stop taking it on your own. Instead, check with your doctor.

Smoking tobacco may worsen your condition since nicotine may further narrow your blood vessels. Therefore, it is best to avoid smoking.

Side Effects of This Medicine

Along with its needed effects, a medicine may cause some unwanted effects. Although not all of these side effects appear very often, when they do occur they may require medical attention. Check with your doctor as soon as possible if any of the following side effects occur:

Rare
   Chest pain
   Irregular heartbeat
Possible signs of overdose (usually occur in the following order)
   Drowsiness
   Flushing
   Faintness
   Unusual excitement
   Convulsions (seizures)

Other side effects may occur which usually do not require medical attention. These side effects may go away during treatment as your body adjusts to the medicine. However, check with your doctor if any of the following side effects continue or are bothersome:

Less common
   Dizziness
   Headache
   Nausea or vomiting
   Stomach discomfort

The above side effects may be more likely to occur in the elderly, who are usually more sensitive to the effects of pentoxifylline.

Other side effects not listed above may also occur in some patients. If you notice any other effects, check with your doctor.

PERPHENAZINE AND AMITRIPTYLINE (Systemic)

Some commonly used brand names are Etrafon and Triavil.

Perphenazine (per-FEN-a-zeen) and amitriptyline (a-mee-TRIP-ti-leen) combination is taken by mouth to treat certain mental and emotional conditions.

This combination is available only with your doctor's prescription.

For information about the precautions and side effects of the medicines in this combination, see:

Phenothiazines (Systemic)
Antidepressants, Tricyclic (Systemic)

Combination products are designed for specific uses. These uses may not be the same as the uses of the individual ingredients. Therefore, some of the information provided in the individual listings may not be relevant to the combination product. If questions arise, check with your doctor, nurse, or pharmacist.

PHENAZOPYRIDINE
(Systemic)

Some commonly used brand names are:

Azo-Standard	Phenazodine
Baridium	Pyridiate
Di-Azo	Pyridium
Phenazo*	Pyronium*

Generic name product may also be available.

---

*Not available in the United States.

Phenazopyridine (fen-az-oh-PEER-i-deen) is a medicine used to relieve the pain, burning, and discomfort caused by infection or irritation of the urinary tract. It is not an antibiotic and will not cure the infection itself.

Phenazopyridine is available only with your doctor's prescription.

Before Using This Medicine

In order to decide on the best treatment for your medical problem, your doctor should be told:

—if you have ever had any unusual or allergic reaction to phenazopyridine.

—if you are on a low-salt, low-sugar, or any other special diet, or if you are allergic to any substance, such as sulfites or other preservatives or dyes. Most medicines contain more than their active ingredient. Your doctor or pharmacist can help you avoid products that may cause a problem.

—if you are pregnant or if you intend to become pregnant while taking this medicine. Studies on birth defects with phenazopyridine have not been done in humans. However, the medicine has not been shown to cause birth defects in animal studies.

—if you are breast-feeding an infant. Although phenazopyridine has not been shown to cause problems in humans, the chance always exists.

—if you have either of the following medical problems:
Hepatitis
Kidney disease

Proper Use of This Medicine

This medicine is best taken with meals or following meals to lessen stomach upset.

Do not use any leftover medicine for future urinary tract problems without first checking with your doctor. An infection may require additional medicine.

If you miss a dose of this medicine, take it as soon as you remember. However, if it is almost time for your next dose, skip the missed dose and go back to your regular dosing schedule. Do not double doses.

How to store this medicine:

• Store away from heat and direct light.

• **Keep out of the reach of children.**

• Do not store in the bathroom medicine cabinet because the heat or moisture may cause the medicine to break down.

• Do not keep outdated medicine or medicine no longer needed. Flush the contents of the container down the toilet, unless otherwise directed.

Precautions While Using This Medicine

Check with your doctor if symptoms such as bloody urine, difficult or painful urination, frequent urge to urinate, or sudden decrease in the amount of urine appear or become worse while you are taking this medicine.

This medicine causes the urine to turn reddish orange. This is to be expected while you are using this medicine. Also, the medicine may stain clothing.

For diabetics—This medicine may cause false test results with urine sugar tests and urine ketone tests. If you have any questions about this, check with your doctor, nurse, or pharmacist, especially if your diabetes is not well controlled.

Side Effects of This Medicine

Along with its needed effects, a medicine may cause some unwanted effects. Although not all of these side effects appear very often, when they do occur they may require medical attention. Check with your doctor as soon as possible if any of the following side effects occur:

> Blue or blue-purple color of skin
> Unusual tiredness or weakness
> Yellowing of eyes or skin

Other side effects may occur which usually do not require medical attention. These side effects may go away during treatment as your body adjusts to the medicine. However, check with your doctor if any of the following side effects continue or are bothersome:

> Dizziness
> Headache
> Indigestion
> Stomach cramps or pain

Other side effects not listed above may also occur in some patients. If you notice any other effects, check with your doctor.

PHENOTHIAZINES (Systemic)

This information applies to the following medicines:

Acetophenazine (a-set-oh-FEN-a-zeen)
Chlorpromazine (klor-PROE-ma-zeen)
Fluphenazine (floo-FEN-a-zeen)
Mesoridazine (mez-oh-RID-a-zeen)
Perphenazine (per-FEN-a-zeen)
Prochlorperazine (proe-klor-PAIR-a-zeen)
Promazine (PROE-ma-zeen)
Thioridazine (thye-oh-RID-a-zeen)
Trifluoperazine (trye-floo-oh-PAIR-a-zeen)
Triflupromazine (trye-floo-PROE-ma-zeen)

This information does *not* apply to the following medicines:

Ethopropazine
Methdilazine
Methotrimeprazine
Promethazine
Propiomazine
Thiethylperazine
Thiopropazate
Trimeprazine

Some commonly used brand names are:	Generic names:
Tindal	Acetophenazine
Clorazine Largactil* Ormazine Promapar Promaz Thorazine Thor-Prom	Chlorpromazine†
Modecate* Moditen* Permitil Prolixin Prolixin Decanoate Prolixin Enanthate	Fluphenazine
Serentil	Mesoridazine
Phenazine* Trilafon	Perphenazine
Chlorazine Compazine Stemetil*	Prochlorperazine†
Prozine Sparine	Promazine†
Mellaril Mellaril-S Millazine Novoridazine*	Thioridazine†
Novoflurazine* Solazine* Stelazine Suprazine Terfluzine*	Trifluoperazine†

Vesprin	Triflupromazine

*Not available in the United States.
†Generic name product may also be available.

Phenothiazines (fee-noe-THYE-a-zeens) are a family of medicines used to treat nervous, mental, and emotional conditions. Some are used also to control anxiety, nausea and vomiting, and severe hiccups.

Phenothiazines are available only with your doctor's prescription.

Before Using This Medicine

In order to decide on the best treatment for your medical problem, your doctor should be told:

—if you have ever had any unusual or allergic reaction to phenothiazine medicines.

—if you are on a low-salt, low-sugar, or any other special diet, or if you are allergic to any substance, such as sulfites or other preservatives or dyes. Most medicines contain more than their active ingredient, and many liquid medicines contain alcohol. Your doctor or pharmacist can help you avoid products that may cause a problem.

—if you are pregnant or if you intend to become pregnant while using this medicine. Although phenothiazines have not been shown to cause birth defects, some side effects such as jaundice and muscle tremors have occurred in a few newborns whose mothers received phenothiazines during pregnancy.

—if you are breast-feeding an infant. Phenothiazines have not been shown to cause problems during breast-feeding but the chance does exist since some phenothiazines are known to pass into the breast milk.

—if you have any of the following medical problems:
    Alcoholism
    Blood disease
    Difficult urination
    Enlarged prostate
    Glaucoma
    Heart or blood vessel disease
    Liver disease
    Lung disease
    Parkinson's disease
    Reye's syndrome
    Stomach ulcers

—if you are now taking any of the following medicines or types of medicine:
    Amantadine
    Amphetamines
    Antacids
    Anthralin
    Antibiotics (by injection)
    Anticoagulants, oral (blood thinners you take by mouth)
    Anticonvulsants (seizure medicine)
    Antidyskinetics (medicine for Parkinson's disease)
    Antihypertensives (high blood pressure medicine)
    Antimuscarinics (medicine for abdominal or stomach spasms or cramps)
    Appetite suppressants
    Asthma medicine
    Beta-adrenergic blocking agents (acebutolol, atenolol, labetalol, metoprolol, nadolol, oxprenolol, pindolol, propranolol, sotalol, timolol)
    Bromocriptine
    Coal tar
    Epinephrine
    Griseofulvin
    Levodopa
    Lithium
    Medicine for diarrhea
    Methoxsalen
    Metoclopramide
    Metyrosine
    Nalidixic acid
    Papaverine
    Quinidine
    Sulfonamides
    Tetracyclines
    Thiazide diuretics
    Trioxsalen

—if you are now taking central nervous system (CNS) depressants, such as:
    Antihistamines or medicine for hay fever, other allergies, or colds

Barbiturates
Narcotics
Prescription pain medicine
Sedatives, tranquilizers, or sleeping
  medicine

—if you are now taking tricyclic antidepressants (medicine for depression),
such as:

Amitriptyline
Amoxapine
Clomipramine
Desipramine
Doxepin
Imipramine
Nortriptyline
Protriptylne
Trimipramine

—if you are now taking or have taken
within the past 2 weeks monoamine oxidase (MAO) inhibitors, such as:

Furazolidone
Isocarboxazid
Pargyline
Phenelzine
Procarbazine
Tranylcypromine

—if you are planning to have a myelo-
gram.

Proper Use of This Medicine

For patients taking this medicine by mouth:
• This medicine may be taken with food
or a full glass (8 ounces) of water or milk
to reduce stomach irritation.

• Do not take this medicine within two
hours of taking antacids or medicine for
diarrhea. Taking them too close together
may make this medicine less effective.

• **If your medicine comes in a dropper
bottle,** it must be diluted before you take
it. Just before taking, measure each dose
with the specially marked dropper and
dilute it in ½ glass (4 ounces) of orange
or grapefruit juice or distilled water.

• If you are taking the extended-release
tablet form of this medicine, each dose
should be swallowed whole. Do not
break, crush, or chew before swallowing.

For patients using the suppository form of
this medicine:
• To insert suppository: First remove the
foil wrapper and moisten the suppository with water. Lie down on left side with
right knee bent, and push the suppository well up into the rectum with finger.

• If the suppository is too soft to insert
because of storage in a warm place, before removing the foil wrapper chill the
suppository in the refrigerator for 30
minutes or run cold water over it.

**Do not take more of this medicine or take it
more often than your doctor ordered.**
This is particularly important when it is
given to children, since they may react
very strongly to the effects of the medicine.

**Sometimes this medicine must be taken for
several weeks before its full effect is
reached in the treatment of certain mental and emotional conditions.**

Do not stop taking this medicine without
first checking with your doctor. Your
doctor may want you to reduce gradually the amount you are taking before
stopping completely. This is to prevent
side effects or to prevent your condition
from becoming worse.

If you miss a dose of this medicine and your
dosing schedule is one dose to be taken:
Once a day—Take the missed dose as
  soon as possible. Then go back to
  your regular dosing schedule. But if
  you do not remember the missed
  dose until the next day, skip it and go
  back to your regular dosing schedule.
  Do not double doses.

Two times a day—Take the missed dose
  as soon as possible. Then go back to
  your regular dosing schedule. However, if it is almost time for your next
  dose, skip the missed dose and go
  back to your regular dosing schedule.
  Do not double ⁴oses.

More than two times a day—If you remember within an hour or so of the missed dose, take it right away. But if you do not remember until later, skip the missed dose and go back to your regular dosing schedule. Do not double doses.

How to store this medicine:

- Store away from heat and direct light.
- **Keep out of the reach of children.**
- Do not store in the bathroom medicine cabinet because the heat or moisture may cause the medicine to break down.
- Keep the liquid medicine from freezing.
- Do not keep outdated medicine or medicine no longer needed. Flush the contents of the container down the toilet, unless otherwise directed.

Precautions While Using This Medicine

Your doctor should check your progress at regular visits, especially for the first few months you take this medicine. This will allow your dosage to be changed if necessary to meet your needs.

This medicine will add to the effects of alcohol and other CNS depressants (medicines that slow down the nervous system, possibly causing drowsiness). Some examples of CNS depressants are antihistamines or medicine for hay fever, other allergies, or colds; sedatives, tranquilizers, or sleeping medicine; prescription pain medicine or narcotics; barbiturates; medicine for seizures; tricyclic antidepressants (medicine for depression); muscle relaxants; or anesthetics, including some dental anesthetics. **Check with your doctor before taking any of the above while you are using this medicine.**

This medicine may cause some people to become drowsy or less alert than they are normally, especially during the first few weeks the medicine is being taken. Even if you take this medicine only at bedtime, you may feel drowsy or less alert on arising. **Make sure you know how you react to this medicine before you drive, use machines, or do other jobs that require you to be alert.**

Dizziness, lightheadedness, or fainting may occur, especially when you get up from a lying or sitting position. Getting up slowly may help. If the problem continues or gets worse, check with your doctor.

Sometimes, patients may show signs of restlessness and excitement after taking this medicine. If this occurs, stop taking the medicine and check with your doctor.

This medicine will often make you sweat less, allowing your body temperature to increase. **Use extra care not to become overheated during exercise or hot weather while you are taking this medicine,** since overheating could possibly result in heat stroke. Also, hot baths or saunas may make you feel dizzy or faint while you are taking this medicine.

A few people who take this medicine may become more sensitive to sunlight than they are normally. When you first begin taking this medicine, use sun screen lotions, or avoid too much sun or too much use of a sunlamp until you see how you react. If you have a severe reaction, check with your doctor.

Your mouth may feel very dry while you are taking phenothiazines. To keep your mouth comfortably moist, chew sugarless gum, melt bits of ice in your mouth, or use a saliva substitute as often as necessary.

If you are taking a liquid form of this medicine, try to avoid getting it on your skin or clothing because it may cause a skin rash or other irritation.

If you are receiving this medicine by injection:

• The effects of the long-acting injection form of this medicine may last for up to 6 weeks. The precautions and side effects information for this medicine applies during this period of time.

Side Effects of This Medicine

Along with its needed effects, a medicine may cause some unwanted effects. Although not all of these side effects appear very often, when they do occur they may require medical attention. **Stop taking this medicine and check with your doctor immediately** if any of the following side effects occur:

Rare

Convulsions (seizures)
Difficulty in breathing
Fever
High or low blood pressure
Increase in sweating
Loss of bladder control
Muscle stiffness (severe)
Unusual feeling of tiredness or weakness
Unusually fast heartbeat or irregular pulse

Also, check with your doctor as soon as possible if any of the following side effects occur:

More common

Blurred vision or any change in vision
Difficulty in speaking or swallowing
Fainting
Loss of balance
Mask-like face
Muscle spasms, especially of face, neck, and back
Restlessness or desire to keep moving
Shuffling walk
Stiffness of arms or legs
Trembling and shaking of fingers and hands
Unusual twisting movements of body

Less common

Chewing movements
Difficult urination
Lip smacking or puckering
Puffing of cheeks
Rapid or fine, worm-like movements of tongue
Skin rash
Uncontrolled movements of arms or legs

Rare

Skin discoloration (after prolonged use)
Sore throat and fever
Yellowing of eyes and skin

Other side effects may occur which usually do not require medical attention. These side effects may go away during treatment as your body adjusts to the medicine. However, check with your doctor if any of the following side effects continue or are bothersome:

More common

Constipation
Decreased sweating
Dizziness
Drowsiness
Dry mouth
Nasal congestion

Less common

Changes in menstrual period
Decreased sexual ability
Increased sensitivity of skin to sun
Swelling of breasts

Although not all of the side effects listed above have been reported for all of these medicines, they have been reported for at least one of the phenothiazines are very similar, any of the above side effects may occur with any of these medicines.

The above side effects, especially constipation, dizziness or fainting, drowsiness, dry mouth, uncontrolled movements of the mouth and tongue, and trembling of fingers and hands are more likely to occur in the elderly, who are usually more sensitive to the effects of phenothiazines.

Other side effects not listed above may also occur in some patients. If you notice any other effects, check with your doctor.

PHENYLBUTAZONE (Systemic)

This information applies to the following medicines:

Oxyphenbutazone (ox-i-fen-BYOO-ta-zone)
Phenylbutazone (fen-ill-BYOO-ta-zone)

Some commonly used brand names are:	Generic names:
Oxalid Oxybutazone* Tandearil*	Oxyphenbutazone

Algoverine* Apo-Phenylbutazone* Azolid Butazolidin Neo-Zoline* Novobutazone*	Phenylbutazone†

*Not available in the United States.
†Generic name product may also be available.

Oxyphenbutazone and phenylbutazone are used to treat the symptoms of certain types of arthritis or rheumatism and to relieve attacks of gout. They help relieve inflammation, swelling, stiffness, joint pain, and fever.

Oxyphenbutazone and phenylbutazone are very strong medicines. In addition to their helpful effects in treating your medical problem, they have side effects that could be very serious. Before you take either one of these medicines, be sure that you have discussed the use of it with your doctor. **Also, do not use either of these medicines to treat any painful condition other than the one for which it was prescribed by your doctor.**

These medicines are available only with your doctor's prescription.

Before Using This Medicine

In order to decide on the best treatment for your medical problem, your doctor should be told:

—if you have ever had any unusual or allergic reaction to oxyphenbutazone or phenylbutazone or to any other medicine, especially aspirin, dipyrone, or sulfinpyrazone.

—if you are on a low-salt, low-sugar, or any other special diet, or if you are allergic to any substance, such as sulfites or other preservatives or dyes. Most medicines contain more than their active ingredient. Your doctor or pharmacist can help you avoid products that may cause a problem.

—if you are pregnant or if you intend to become pregnant while using this medicine. Studies on birth defects have not been done in humans. However, studies in animals have shown that phenylbutazone and oxyphenbutazone may cause unwanted effects in the unborn infant.

—if you are breast-feeding an infant. Phenylbutazone passes into the breast milk and may cause blood problems in infants of mothers taking this medicine. Although oxyphenbutazone has not been shown to cause problems in humans, the chance always exists since it may also pass into the breast milk.

—if you have any of the following medical problems:
Asthma
Blood disease
Edema (swelling of feet or lower legs)
Heart disease
High blood pressure
Kidney disease
Liver disease
Polymyalgia rheumatica or temporal arteritis
Stomach ulcer, other stomach problems, or colitis
Ulcers, sores, or white spots in mouth

—if you regularly take acetaminophen.

—if you regularly take any of the following medicines for pain, inflammation, or gout:
Aspirin or other salicylates
Colchicine

Other anti-inflammatory analgesics, such as diflunisal, fenoprofen, ibuprofen, indomethacin, meclofenamate, mefenamic acid, naproxen, piroxicam, sulindac, or tolmetin
Sulfinpyrazone

—if you are now taking **any** other medicines or types of medicine, especially:

Adrenocorticoids (cortisone-like medicine)
Anticoagulants (blood thinners)
Anticonvulsants, hydantoin (medicine for seizures)
Antidiabetics, oral (medicine for sugar diabetes you take by mouth)
Antineoplastics (medicine for cancer)
Azathioprine
Captopril
Chloramphenicol
Chloroquine
Contraceptives, estrogen-containing (birth control pills)
Corticotropin
Digitalis glycosides (heart medicine)
Flucytosine
Gold compounds
Heparin
Hydroxychloroquine
Lithium
Methimazole
Methylphenidate
Penicillamine
Phenothiazines
Primaquine
Pyrimethamine
Sulfonamides (sulfa medicines)
Trimethoprim

Proper Use of This Medicine

This medicine is intended to treat your current medical problem only. **Do not take it for any other aches or pains.**

Take this medicine only as directed by your doctor. Do not take more of it, do not take it more often, and do not take it for a longer period of time than your doctor ordered. To do so may cause serious side effects.

Take this medicine with meals to lessen stomach upset. If stomach upset (nausea, vomiting, stomach pain, or diarrhea) continues, check with your doctor.

Take this medicine with a full glass (8 ounces) of water. Also, do not lie down for about 15 to 30 minutes after taking this medicine. This helps to prevent irritation that may lead to trouble in swallowing.

If you miss a dose of this medicine and your dosing schedule is one dose to be taken:

Once or twice a day—Take the missed dose as soon as possible. But if you do not remember the missed dose until it is almost time for your next dose or until the next day, skip the missed dose and go back to your regular dosing schedule. Do not double doses.

Three or more times a day—If you remember within an hour or so of the missed dose, take it right away. But if you do not remember until later, skip the missed dose and go back to your regular dosing schedule. Do not double doses.

How to store this medicine:

• Store away from heat and direct light.

• **Keep out of the reach of children.**

• Do not store in the bathroom medicine cabinet because the heat or moisture may cause the medicine to break down.

• Do not keep outdated medicine or medicine no longer needed. Flush the contents of the container down the toilet, unless otherwise directed.

Precautions While Using This Medicine

Your doctor should check your progress at regular visits in order to make sure that this medicine does not cause unwanted effects.

This medicine may cause some people to become confused, drowsy, or less alert than they are normally. **Make sure you know how you react to this medicine before you drive, use machines, or do other jobs that require you to be alert.**

Stomach problems may be more likely to occur if you drink alcoholic beverages while being treated with this medicine. Also, alcohol may add to the depressant side effects of this medicine. Therefore, **do not drink alcoholic beverages while taking this medicine,** unless otherwise directed by your doctor.

Too much use of certain other medicines together with oxyphenbutazone or phenylbutazone may increase the chance of stomach or kidney problems. Therefore, do not regularly take any of the following medicines together with oxyphenbutazone or phenylbutazone, unless your doctor has directed you to do so:

    Acetaminophen
    Aspirin or other salicylates
    Diflunisal
    Fenoprofen
    Ibuprofen
    Indomethacin
    Meclofenamate
    Mefenamic acid
    Naproxen
    Piroxicam
    Sulindac
    Tolmetin

Check with your doctor immediately if chills, fever, muscle aches or pains, or other influenza-like symptoms occur shortly before, or together with, a skin rash. Very rarely, these effects may be the first signs of a serious reaction to this medicine.

Side Effects of This Medicine

Along with its needed effects, a medicine may cause some unwanted effects. Although not all of these side effects appear very often, when they do occur they may require medical attention. **Stop taking this medicine and check with your doctor immediately** if any of the following side effects occur·

More common
    Swelling of feet or lower legs
    Unusual weight gain

Rare
    Abdominal or stomach pain (severe)
    Bloody or black, tarry stools
    Sore throat and fever
    Ulcers, sores, or white spots in mouth
    Unusual bleeding or bruising
    Unusual tiredness or weakness
    Vomiting of blood or material that looks like coffee grounds

Also, check with your doctor as soon as possible if any of the following side effects occur:

Less common
    Skin rash

Rare
    Bleeding sores on lips
    Bloody or cloudy urine
    Burning feeling in throat, chest, or stomach
    Confusion
    Difficult or painful urination
    Eye pain, blurred vision, or any change in vision
    Fever and joint pain
    Hives or itching of skin
    Mental depression, especially in elderly patients
    Red eyes
    Redness, tenderness, burning, or peeling of skin
    Ringing or buzzing in ears or any loss of hearing
    Shortness of breath, troubled breathing, wheezing, or tightness in chest
    Sudden decrease in amount of urine
    Swelling of neck or throat
    Thickened or scaly skin
    Yellowing of eyes or skin

Possible signs of overdose
    Blood in urine or sudden decrease in amount of urine
    Bluish color of fingernails, lips, or skin
    Convulsions (seizures), especially in children
    Difficulty in hearing or ringing or buzzing sound in the ears
    Dizziness or lightheadedness
    Hallucinations (seeing, hearing, or feeling things that are not there)
    Headache (severe and continuing)
    Increase or decrease in blood pressure
    Mood or mental changes

Nausea, vomiting, or stomach pain
(severe)
Shortness of breath, troubled breathing,
or unusually slow, fast, or irregular
breathing
Swelling of feet or lower legs

Other side effects may occur which usually
do not require medical attention. Those
side effects may go away during treatment as your body adjusts to the medicine. However, check with your doctor if
any of the following side effects continue or are bothersome:

More common
Nausea
Less common or rare
Bloated feeling or gas
Constipation
Diarrhea
Drowsiness
Feeling of numbness
Headache
Indigestion
Irritability
Stomach pain (mild)
Swelling of stomach
Trembling
Unusual nervousness or restlessness
Vomiting

The above side effects are more likely to
occur in patients 40 years of age or older.
These patients, especially if they are 60
years of age or older, are usually more
sensitive to the effects of phenylbutazone and oxyphenbutazone.

Some side effects may occur many days or
weeks after you have stopped using this
medicine. During this period of time
check with your doctor immediately if
you notice any of the following side
effects:
Sore throat and fever
Ulcers, sores, or white spots in mouth
Unusual bleeding or bruising
Unusual tiredness or weakness

Other side effects not listed above may also
occur in some patients. If you notice any
other effects, check with your doctor.

PHENYLPROPANOLAMINE
(Systemic)

Some commonly used brand names or other
names are:

Acutrim Maximum	Propagest
Strength	Resolution I
Control	Maximum
Decongestant-P	Strength
Dex-A-Diet	Resolution II Half
Dexatrim Extra	Strength
Strength	Rhindecon
Dexatrim-15	Unitrol
Diadax	Westrim
PPA	Westrim LA 75
Prolamine	

Phenylpropanolamine (fen-ill-proe-pa-
NOLE-a-meen) or PPA is used as a nasal
decongestant and as an appetite suppres-
sant. It acts on many different parts of the
body. PPA's actions produce effects which
may be helpful or harmful. This depends on
a patient's individual condition and response and the amount taken.

PPA is taken by mouth. It produces two
effects which are used in medicine: constriction of blood vessels and decrease in
appetite.

Blood vessel constriction leads to clearing of nasal congestion (stuffy nose). However, the same effect may cause an increase
in blood pressure in patients who have hy-
pertension (high blood pressure).

The way PPA and similar medicines decrease appetite is unclear. Stimulation of
the central nervous system (CNS) may be a
major reason. The decrease in appetite is
temporary—no more than a few weeks—
and requires a change in diet for best effect.
The continuous use of PPA for dieting is not
recommended.

The misuse of PPA has caused serious
side effects (even death) when too much
was taken.

There are a number of products on the
market that contain only phenylpropanolamine. Other products contain PPA along
with added ingredients. The information
that follows is for PPA alone. There may be

additional information for the combination products. Read the label of the product you are using. If you have questions or if you want more information about the other ingredients, check with your doctor or pharmacist.

Some preparations containing PPA are available only with your doctor's prescription. Others are available without a prescription; however, your doctor may have special instructions on the proper use of this medicine.

Before Using This Medicine

Before you use phenylpropanolamine, your doctor should be told:

—if you have ever had any unusual or allergic reaction to phenylpropanolamine or to amphetamine, dextroamphetamine, ephedrine, epinephrine, isoproterenol, metaproterenol, methamphetamine, norepinephrine, phenylephrine, pseudoephedrine, or terbutaline.

—if you are on a low-salt, low-sugar, or any other special diet, or if you are allergic to any substance, such as sulfites or other preservatives or dyes. Most medicines contain more than their active ingredient, and many liquid medicines contain alcohol. Your doctor or pharmacist can help you avoid products that may cause a problem.

—if you are pregnant or if you intend to become pregnant while taking this medicine. Although phenylpropanolamine has not been shown to cause birth defects or other problems in humans, the chance always exists.

—if you are breast-feeding an infant. Although phenylpropanolamine has not been shown to cause problems in humans, the chance always exists.

—if you have any of the following medical problems:
    Diabetes mellitus (sugar diabetes)
    Heart or blood vessel disease
    High blood pressure
    Overactive thyroid

—if you have suffered a heart attack or stroke.

—if you are now taking any of the following medicines or types of medicine:
    Amphetamines
    Antihypertensives (high blood pressure medicine)
    Beta-adrenergic blocking agents (acebutolol, atenolol, labetalol, metoprolol, nadolol, oxprenolol, pindolol, propranolol, sotalol, timolol)
    Caffeine
    Digitalis (heart medicine)
    Levodopa
    Medicine for asthma or breathing problems
    Medicine for hay fever, other allergies, or colds (including nose drops or sprays)
    Methylphenidate
    Pemoline
    Other appetite suppressants

—if you are now taking tricyclic antidepressants (medicine for depression), such as:
    Amitriptyline
    Amoxapine
    Clomipramine
    Desipramine
    Doxepin
    Imipramine
    Nortriptyline
    Protriptyline
    Trimipramine

—if you are now taking or have taken within the past 2 weeks monoamine oxidase (MAO) inhibitors, such as:
    Furazolidone
    Isocarboxazid
    Pargyline
    Phenelzine
    Procarbazine
    Tranylcypromine

Proper Use of This Medicine

If you are taking an extended-release form of this medicine:

• Swallow the capsule or tablet whole.

• Do not break, crush, or chew before swallowing.

• Take only once a day.

Take phenylpropanolamine (PPA) only as directed. Do not take more of it, do not take it more often, and do not take it for a longer period of time than directed. To do so may increase the chance of side effects.

If PPA causes trouble in sleeping, take the last dose for each day a few hours before bedtime. If you are taking an extended-release form of this medicine, take your daily dose at least 12 hours before bedtime.

Phenylpropanolamine should not be used for weight control in children unless directed by their doctor.

For patients taking phenylpropanolamine for nasal congestion:

• If you miss a dose, take it as soon as possible. However, if it is within 2 hours (or 12 hours for extended-release forms) of your next dose, skip the missed dose and go back to your regular dosing schedule. Do not double doses.

How to store this medicine:

• Store away from heat and direct light.

• **Keep out of the reach of children.**

• Do not store in the bathroom medicine cabinet because the heat or moisture may cause the medicine to break down.

• Keep the liquid medicine from freezing.

• Do not keep outdated medicine or medicine no longer needed. Flush the contents of the container down the toilet, unless otherwise directed.

Precautions While Using This Medicine

Do not drink large amounts of caffeine-containing coffee, tea, or colas while you are taking this medicine. To do so may cause unwanted effects.

For patients taking this medicine for nasal congestion:

• **If symptoms do not improve within 7 days or if you also have a high fever, check with your doctor.** These signs may mean that you have other medical problems.

Side Effects of This Medicine

Along with its needed effects, a medicine may cause some unwanted effects. Although not all of these side effects appear very often, when they do occur they may require medical attention. Check with your doctor as soon as possible if any of the following side effects occur:

Rare
Painful or difficult urination
Tightness in chest
Unusually fast, pounding, or irregular heartbeat (especially with high doses)

Early signs of overdose
Abdominal or stomach pain
Headache (severe)
Nausea and vomiting (severe)
Nervousness (severe)
Restlessness (severe)
Unusually fast, pounding, or irregular heartbeat
Unusual sweating not associated with exercise

Late signs of overdose
Confusion
Convulsions (seizures)
Hallucinations (seeing, hearing, or feeling things that are not there)
Hostile behavior
Muscle trembling
Rapid breathing
Rapid and irregular pulse

Other side effects may occur which usually do not require medical attention. These side effects may go away during treatment as your body adjusts to the medicine. However, check with your doctor if

any of the following side effects continue or are bothersome:

Less common—more common with high doses

    Dizziness
    Dryness of nose or mouth
    Headache (mild)
    Nausea (mild)
    Nervousness (mild)
    Restlessness (mild)
    Trouble in sleeping
    Unusual feeling of well-being

The above side effects are more likely to occur in elderly patients, who are usually more sensitive to the effects of phenylpropanolamine.

Other side effects not listed above may also occur in some patients. If you notice any other effects, check with your doctor.

PILOCARPINE (Ophthalmic)

Some commonly used brand names are:

Adsorbocarpine	Ocusert Pilo
Akarpine	Pilocar
Almocarpine	Pilokair
Isopto Carpine	Pilopine HS
Miocarpine*	P. V. Carpine
Ocu-Carpine	Liquifilm

Generic name product may also be available.

---

*Not available in the United States.

Pilocarpine (pye-loe-KAR-peen) is used in the eye to treat glaucoma and other eye conditions.

This medicine is available only with your doctor's prescription.

Before Using This Medicine

In order to decide on the best treatment for your medical problem, your doctor should be told:

—if you have ever had any unusual or allergic reaction to pilocarpine.

—if you are allergic to any substance, such as certain preservatives. Most medicines contain more than their active ingredient. Your doctor or pharmacist can help you avoid products that may cause a problem.

—if you are pregnant or if you intend to become pregnant while using this medicine, since ophthalmic pilocarpine may be absorbed into the body. Studies on birth defects have not been done in either animals or humans.

—if you are breast-feeding an infant, since ophthalmic pilocarpine may be absorbed into the body. Although it is not known whether pilocarpine passes into the breast milk and this medicine has not been shown to cause problems in humans, the chance always exists.

—if you have asthma.

—if you are now using any of the following medicines in the eye:

    Atropine
    Cyclopentolate
    Homatropine
    Scopolamine

Proper Use of This Medicine

Use this medicine only as directed. Do not use more of it and do not use it more often than your doctor ordered. To do so may increase the chance of too much medicine being absorbed into the body and the chance of side effects.

For patients using the eye drop form of pilocarpine:

• How to apply this medicine: First, wash hands. With middle finger, apply pressure to the inside corner of the eye (and continue to apply pressure for 1 or 2 minutes after the medicine has been placed in the eye). Tilt head back and with the index finger of the same hand, pull lower eyelid away from eye to form a pouch. Drop the medicine into the pouch and gently close eyes. Do not blink. Keep eyes closed for 1 or 2 minutes to allow the medicine to be absorbed.

• To prevent contamination of the eye drops, do not touch the applicator tip to any surface (including the eye) and keep the container tightly closed.

• If you miss a dose of this medicine, apply it as soon as possible. However, if it is almost time for your next dose, skip the missed dose and apply your next dose at the regularly scheduled time. Then continue with your regular dosing schedule.

For patients using the eye gel form of pilocarpine:

• How to apply this medicine: First, wash hands. Pull lower eyelid away from eye to form a pouch. Squeeze a thin strip of gel into the pouch. A 1½-cm (approximately ½-inch) strip of gel is usually enough unless otherwise directed by your doctor. Gently close eyes and keep them closed for 1 or 2 minutes to allow the medicine to be absorbed.

• To prevent contamination of the eye gel, do not touch the applicator tip to any surface (including the eye), wipe the tip of the gel tube with a clean tissue, and keep the tube tightly closed.

• If you miss a dose of this medicine, apply it as soon as possible. However, if you do not remember the missed dose until the next day, skip it and apply your next dose at the regularly scheduled time. Then continue with your regular dosing schedule.

For patients using the eye system form of pilocarpine:

• This medicine usually comes with patient directions. Read them carefully before using this medicine.

• If you think this medicine unit may be damaged, do not use it. If you have any questions about this, check with your doctor or pharmacist.

• If the unit seems to be releasing too much medicine into your eye, remove it and replace with a new unit. If you have any questions about this, check with your doctor.

How to store this medicine:

• Store away from heat and direct light.

• **Keep out of the reach of children.**

• Store the eye system form of this medicine in the refrigerator.

• Store the gel form of this medicine in the refrigerator or at room temperature. If stored at room temperature, discard any unused medicine after 8 weeks.

• Do not store in the bathroom medicine cabinet because the heat or moisture may cause the medicine to break down.

• Keep the gel or solution form of this medicine from freezing.

• Do not keep outdated medicine or medicine no longer needed. Flush the gel or solution form of this medicine down the toilet, unless otherwise directed.

Precautions While Using This Medicine

Your doctor should check your eye pressure at regular visits.

For patients using the eye drop or gel form of this medicine:

• For a short time after you apply this medicine, your vision may be blurred or there may be a change in your near or distant vision. **Make sure your vision is clear before you drive or do other jobs that require you to see well.**

For patients using the eye system form of this medicine:

• For the first several hours after inserting this unit in the eye, your vision may be blurred or there may be a change in your near or distant vision. Therefore, insert this unit in the eye at bedtime, unless otherwise directed by your doctor. If this unit is inserted in the eye at any other time of the day, **make sure your vision is clear before you drive or do other jobs that require you to see well.**

Side Effects of This Medicine

Along with its needed effects, a medicine may cause some unwanted effects. Although not all of these side effects appear very often, when they do occur they may require medical attention. Check with your doctor as soon as possible if any of the following side effects occur:

Possible signs of too much medicine being absorbed into the body

    Muscle tremors
    Nausea, vomiting, or diarrhea
    Troubled breathing or wheezing
    Unusual increase in sweating
    Unusual watering of mouth

Other side effects may occur which usually do not require medical attention. These side effects may go away during treatment as your body adjusts to the medicine. However, check with your doctor if any of the following side effects continue or are bothersome:

More common

    Blurred vision or change in near or distant vision
    Eye pain

Less common

    Browache
    Headache
    Irritation of eyes

Other side effects not listed above may also occur in some patients. If you notice any other effects, check with your doctor.

POTASSIUM SUPPLEMENTS
(Systemic)

This information applies to the following medicines:

Potassium Acetate
Potassium Bicarbonate
Potassium Bicarbonate and Potassium Chloride
Potassium Bicarbonate and Potassium Citrate
Potassium Chloride
Potassium Chloride, Potassium Bicarbonate, and Potassium Citrate
Potassium Gluconate
Potassium Gluconate and Potassium Chloride
Potassium Gluconate and Potassium Citrate
Potassium Gluconate, Potassium Citrate, and Ammonium Chloride
Trikates

This information does *not* apply to:

Potassium Citrate
Potassium Iodide
Potassium Permanganate
Potassium Phosphates

Some commonly used brand names and other names are:	Generic names:
	Potassium Acetate†
	Potassium Bicarbonate†
Klorvess K-Lyte/Cl K-Lyte-Cl 50	Potassium Bicarbonate and Potassium Chloride
K-Lyte K-Lyte DS	Potassium Bicarbonate and Potassium Citrate
Cena-K EM-K-10% Kaochlor Kaochlor S-F Kaon-Cl Kaon-Cl 10 Kaon-Cl 20% Kato Kay Ciel K-Lor Klor-10% Klor-Con Klor-Con 20% Klor-Con/25 Klorvess 10% Klotrix K-Tab Micro-K Micro-K 10	Potassium Chloride†

Potachlor Potage Potasalan Potassine Rum-K SK-Potassium Chloride Slow-K	Potassium Chloride†
Kaochlor-Eff	Potassium Chloride, Potassium Bicarbonate, and Potassium Citrate
Bayon Kaon Kao-Nor Kaylixir K-G Elixir	Potassium Gluconate†
Kolyum	Potassium Gluconate and Potassium Chloride
Bi-K Twin-K	Potassium Gluconate and Potassium Citrate
Twin-K-Cl	Potassium Gluconate, Potassium Citrate, and Ammonium Chloride
Potassium Triplex Tri-K	Trikates

†Generic name product available.

Potassium (poe-TASS-ee-um) is needed to maintain good health. Potassium supplements may be needed by patients who do not have enough potassium in their regular diet and by those who have lost too much potassium because of illness or treatment with certain medicines.

Since too much potassium may also cause health problems, most potassium supplements are available only with your doctor's prescription.

Before Using This Medicine

In order to decide on the best treatment for your medical problem, your doctor should be told:

—if you have ever had any unusual reaction to potassium preparations.

—if you are on a low-salt, low-sugar, or any other special diet, or if you are allergic to any substance, such as sulfites or other preservatives or dyes. Most medicines contain more than their active ingredient, and many liquid medicines contain alcohol. Your doctor or pharmacist can help you avoid products that may cause a problem.

—if you are pregnant or if you intend to become pregnant while using this medicine. Although potassium supplements have not been shown to cause problems in humans, the chance always exists.

—if you are breast-feeding an infant. Although this medicine has not been shown to cause problems in humans, the chance always exists since potassium supplements pass into breast milk.

—if you have any of the following medical problems:
Addison's disease (underactive adrenal glands)
Diarrhea
Heart disease
Intestinal blockage
Kidney disease
Stomach ulcer

—if you are now taking any of the following medicines or types of medicine:
Adrenocorticoids (cortisone-like medicine)
Amiloride
Antimuscarinics (medicine for stomach spasms or cramps)
Calcium-containing medicines
Captopril
Corticotropin (ACTH)
Heart medicine such as digitoxin or digoxin
Laxatives
Potassium-containing medicines, other
Quinidine

Sodium polystyrene sulfonate
Spironolactone
Triamterene
Vitamin B$_{12}$

—if you are now using salt substitutes or drinking low-salt milk.

Proper Use of This Medicine

For patients taking the liquid form of this medicine:

• This medicine must be diluted in at least ½ glass (4 ounces) of cold water or juice to reduce possible stomach irritation or laxative effect.

For patients taking the soluble granule, soluble powder, or soluble tablet form of this medicine:

• This medicine must be completely dissolved in at least ½ glass (4 ounces) of cold water or juice to reduce possible stomach irritation or laxative effect.

• Allow any "fizzing" to stop before taking the dissolved medicine.

For patients taking the extended-release tablet form of this medicine:

• Swallow the tablets whole. Do not crush, chew, or suck on the tablet.

• If you have trouble swallowing tablets or if they seem to stick in your throat, check with your doctor. When this medicine is not properly released, it can cause irritation which may lead to ulcers.

For patients using juices to dilute or dissolve this medicine:

• If you are on a salt (sodium)-restricted diet, check with your doctor before using tomato juice to dilute your medicine. Tomato juice has a high salt (sodium) content.

Take this medicine immediately after meals or with food to lessen possible stomach upset or laxative action.

Take this medicine only as directed by your doctor. Do not take more of it, do not take it more often, and do not take it for a longer period of time than your doctor ordered. **This is especially important if you are also taking both diuretics (water pills) and digitalis medicines for your heart.**

If you miss a dose of this medicine and remember within 2 hours, take the missed dose right away with food or liquids. Then go back to your regular dosing schedule. However, if you do not remember until later, skip the missed dose and go back to your regular dosing schedule. Do not double doses.

How to store this medicine:

• Store away from heat and direct light.

• **Keep out of the reach of children.**

• Do not store in the bathroom medicine cabinet because the heat or moisture may cause the medicine to break down.

• Keep the liquid from freezing.

• Do not keep outdated medicine or medicine no longer needed. Flush the contents of the container down the toilet, unless otherwise directed.

Precautions While Using This Medicine

Your doctor should check your progress at regular visits.

Since salt substitutes and low-salt milk may contain potassium, do not use them unless told to do so by your doctor.

Check with your doctor at once if you notice blackish stools or other signs of stomach or intestinal bleeding. This medicine may cause such a condition to become worse, especially when taken in tablet form.

Side Effects of This Medicine

Along with its needed effects, a medicine may cause some unwanted effects. Although not all of these side effects appear very often, when they do occur they may require medical attention. **Stop taking this medicine and check with your doctor immediately if any of the following side effects occur:**

Rare
Confusion
Irregular heartbeat
Numbness or tingling in hands, feet, or lips
Shortness of breath or difficult breathing
Unexplained anxiety
Unusual tiredness or weakness
Weakness or heaviness of legs

Other side effects may occur which usually do not require medical attention. These side effects may go away during treatment as your body adjusts to the medicine. However, check with your doctor if any of the following side effects continue or are bothersome:

Less common
Diarrhea
Nausea
Stomach pain or discomfort
Vomiting

Other side effects not listed above may also occur in some patients. If you notice any other effects, check with your doctor.

PRAZOSIN (Systemic)

A commonly used brand name is Minipress.

Prazosin (PRA-zoe-sin) belongs to the general class of medicines called antihypertensives. It is taken by mouth to treat high blood pressure.

High blood pressure adds to the workload of the heart and arteries. If it continues for a long time, they may not function properly. This can damage the blood vessels of the brain, heart, and kidneys resulting in a stroke, heart attack, or kidney failure. These problems may be avoided if blood pressure is controlled.

Prazosin works by relaxing blood vessels so that blood passes through them more easily. This helps to lower blood pressure.

Prazosin may also be used for other conditions as determined by your doctor.

Prazosin is available only with your doctor's prescription.

Before Using This Medicine

In order to decide on the best treatment for your medical problem, your doctor should be told:

—if you have ever had any unusual or allergic reaction to prazosin.

—if you are on a low-salt, low-sugar, or any other special diet, or if you are allergic to any substance, such as sulfites or other preservatives or dyes. Most medicines contain more than their active ingredient. Your doctor or pharmacist can help you avoid products that may cause a problem.

—if you are pregnant or if you intend to become pregnant while taking this medicine. Prazosin has not been shown to cause birth defects or other problems in animals; however, studies have not been done in humans.

—if you are breast-feeding an infant. Although prazosin has not been shown to cause problems in humans, the chance always exists.

—if you have any of the following medical problems:
Angina (chest pain)
Heart disease
Kidney disease

—if you are now taking any of the following medicines or types of medicine:
Diuretics (water pills)
Inflammation medicine, especially indomethacin

Other antihypertensives (high blood pressure medicine)

Proper Use of This Medicine

Importance of diet—When prescribing medicine for your condition, your doctor may also prescribe a personal diet for you. Such a diet may be low in sodium (salt). Most people eat much more sodium than they need and too much sodium in the diet may increase blood pressure. Some foods that contain large amounts of sodium include canned soup, pickles, ketchup, green and ripe olives, relish, frankfurters, soy sauce, and carbonated beverages. Your doctor may want you to limit the amounts of these and other high-sodium foods in your diet. Medicine is usually more effective when such a diet is properly followed.

Also, it may be very important for you to go on a reducing diet. However, check with your doctor before going on any diet.

Many patients who have high blood pressure will not notice any signs of the problem. In fact, many may feel normal. It is very important that you take your medicine exactly as directed and that you keep your doctor's appointments even if you feel well.

Remember that prazosin will not cure your high blood pressure but it does help control it. Therefore, you must continue to take it as directed if you expect to lower your blood pressure and keep it down. **You may have to take medicine for the rest of your life.** If high blood pressure is not treated, it can cause serious problems such as heart failure, blood vessel disease, stroke, or kidney disease.

In order to help remember to take your medicine, try to get into the habit of taking it at the same time each day.

If you miss a dose of this medicine, take it as soon as possible. However, if it is almost time for your next dose, skip the missed dose and go back to your regular dosing schedule. Do not double doses.

How to store this medicine:

• Store away from heat and direct light.

• **Keep out of the reach of children.**

• Do not store in the bathroom medicine cabinet because the heat or moisture may cause the medicine to break down.

• Do not keep outdated medicine or medicine no longer needed. Flush the contents of the container down the toilet, unless otherwise directed.

Precautions While Using This Medicine

It is important that your doctor check your progress at regular visits in order to make sure that this medicine is working properly.

Do not take other medicines unless they have been discussed with your doctor. This especially includes over-the-counter (nonprescription) medicines for appetite control, asthma, colds, cough, hay fever, or sinus problems, since they may tend to increase your blood pressure.

Dizziness or drowsiness may occur after the first dose of this medicine. Taking the first dose at bedtime may prevent problems. **Avoid driving or performing hazardous tasks for the first 24 hours after you start taking this medicine or when the dose is increased. Make sure you know how you react to this medicine before you drive, use machines, or do other jobs that require you to be alert.**

Dizziness, lightheadedness, or fainting may occur, especially when you get up from a lying or sitting position. Getting up slowly may help lessen this problem. **If you begin to feel dizzy, lie down so that you** do not faint. Then sit for a few moments before standing to prevent the dizziness from returning.

The dizziness, lightheadedness, or fainting is also more likely to occur if you drink alcohol, stand for long periods of time, exercise, or if the weather is hot. **While you are taking this medicine, be careful in the amount of alcohol you drink. Also, use extra care during exercise or hot weather or if you must stand for long periods of time.**

Side Effects of This Medicine

Along with its needed effects, a medicine may cause some unwanted effects. Although not all of these side effects appear very often, when they do occur they may require medical attention. Check with your doctor as soon as possible if any of the following side effects occur:

More common

Dizziness or lightheadedness, especially when getting up from a lying or sitting position

Less common

Chest pain
Fainting (sudden)
Irregular heartbeat
Shortness of breath
Swelling of feet or lower legs
Weight gain

Rare

Inability to control urination
Numbness or tingling of hands or feet

Other side effects may occur which usually do not require medical attention. These side effects may go away during treatment as your body adjusts to the medicine. However, check with your doctor if any of the following side effects continue or are bothersome:

Less common

Drowsiness
Headache
Lack of energy
Nausea and vomiting

Dizziness, lightheadedness, or fainting may be more likely to occur in the elderly, who are more sensitive to the effects of prazosin.

Other side effects not listed above may also occur in some patients. If you notice any other effects, check with your doctor.

PRAZOSIN AND POLYTHIAZIDE (Systemic)

A commonly used brand name is Minizide.

Prazosin (PRA-zoe-sin) and polythiazide (pol-i-THYE-a-zide) combination is used in the treatment of high blood pressure.

High blood pressure adds to the workload of the heart and arteries. If it continues for a long time, they may not function properly. This can damage the blood vessels of the brain, heart, and kidneys resulting in a stroke, heart attack, or kidney failure. These problems may be avoided if blood pressure is controlled.

Prazosin works by relaxing blood vessels so that blood passes through them more easily. The polythiazide in this combination helps to reduce the amount of water in the body by increasing the flow of urine. Both of these actions help to lower blood pressure.

This medicine is available only with your doctor's prescription.

For information about the precautions and side effects of the medicines in this combination, see:

Prazosin (Systemic)
Diuretics, Thiazide (Systemic)

Combination products are designed for specific uses. These uses may not be the same as the uses of the individual ingredients. Therefore, some of the information provided in the individual listings may not be relevant to the combination product. If questions arise, check with your doctor, nurse, or pharmacist.

PROBENECID (Systemic)

Some commonly used brand names are Benemid, Benuryl*, and SK-Probenecid.

Generic name product may also be available.

---

*Not available in the United States.

Probenecid (proe-BEN-e-sid) is used in the treatment of chronic gout or gouty arthritis. These conditions are caused by too much uric acid in the blood. The medicine works by removing the extra uric acid from the body. Probenecid does not cure gout, but after you have been taking it for a few months it will help prevent gout attacks. This medicine will help prevent gout attacks only as long as you continue to take it.

Probenecid is also used to prevent or treat other medical problems that may occur if too much uric acid is present in the body.

Probenecid is sometimes used with certain kinds of antibiotics to make them more effective in the treatment of infections.

Probenecid is available only with your doctor's prescription.

Before Using This Medicine

In order to decide on the best treatment for your medical problem, your doctor should be told:

—if you have ever had any unusual or allergic reaction to probenecid.

—if you are on a low-salt, low-sugar, or any other special diet, or if you are allergic to any substance, such as sulfites or other preservatives or dyes. Most medicines contain more than their active ingredient. Your doctor or pharmacist can help you avoid products that may cause a problem.

—if you are pregnant or if you intend to become pregnant while taking this medicine. Although probenecid has not been shown to cause problems in humans, the chance always exists.

—if you are breast-feeding an infant. Although probenecid has not been shown to cause problems in humans, the chance always exists.

—if you have any of the following medical problems:
 Blood disease
 Kidney disease or stones (or history of)
 Stomach ulcer (history of)

—if you are now taking any of the following medicines or types of medicine:
 Antidiabetics, oral (diabetes medicine you take by mouth)
 Anti-inflammatory analgesics, such as diflunisal, fenoprofen, ibuprofen, indomethacin, meclofenamate, mefenamic acid, naproxen, oxyphenbutazone, phenylbutazone, piroxicam, sulindac, and tolmetin
 Antineoplastics (medicine for cancer)
 Aspirin or other salicylates
 Clofibrate
 Diazoxide
 Diuretics (water pills)
 Dyphylline
 Heparin
 Mecamylamine
 Medicine for infection, including tuberculosis or virus infection
 Nitrofurantoin
 Other gout medicine
 Riboflavin (vitamin B_2)

Proper Use of This Medicine

If probenecid upsets your stomach, it may be taken with food. If this does not work, an antacid may be taken. If stomach upset (nausea, vomiting, or loss of appetite) continues, check with your doctor.

For patients taking probenecid for gout:
 • After you begin to take probenecid, gout attacks may continue to occur for a

while. However, if you take this medicine regularly as directed by your doctor, the attacks will gradually become less frequent and less painful than before. After you have been taking probenecid for several months, they may stop completely.

• This medicine will help prevent gout attacks but it will not relieve an attack that has already started. **Even if you take another medicine for gout attacks, continue to take this medicine also.** If you have any questions about this, check with your doctor.

For patients taking probenecid for gout or to help remove uric acid from the body:

• When you first begin taking probenecid, the amount of uric acid in the kidneys is greatly increased. This may cause kidney stones in some people. To help prevent this, your doctor may want you to drink at least 10 to 12 full glasses (8 ounces each) of fluids each day, or to take another medicine to make your urine less acid. It is important that you follow your doctor's instructions very carefully.

If you are taking probenecid regularly and you miss a dose, take the missed dose as soon as possible. However, if you do not remember until it is almost time for the next dose, skip the missed dose and go back to your regular dosing schedule. Do not double doses.

How to store this medicine:

• Store away from heat and direct light.

• **Keep out of the reach of children.**

• Do not store in the bathroom medicine cabinet because the heat or moisture may cause the medicine to break down.

• Do not keep outdated medicine or medicine no longer needed. Flush the contents of the container down the toilet, unless otherwise directed.

Precautions While Using This Medicine

If you will be taking probenecid for more than a few weeks, your doctor should check your progress at regular visits.

For diabetics: Probenecid may cause false test results with copper sulfate urine sugar tests (Clinitest®), but not with glucose enzymatic urine sugar tests (Clinistix®). If you have any questions about this, check with your doctor or pharmacist.

For patients taking probenecid for gout or to help remove uric acid from the body:

• Taking aspirin or other salicylates will lessen the effects of probenecid. Also, drinking too much alcohol may increase the amount of uric acid in the blood and lessen the effects of this medicine. Therefore, **do not take aspirin or other salicylates or drink alcoholic beverages while taking this medicine,** unless you have first checked with your doctor.

Side Effects of This Medicine

Along with its needed effects, a medicine may cause some unwanted effects. Although not all of these side effects appear very often, when they do occur they may require medical attention. Check with your doctor as soon as possible if any of the following side effects occur:

Less common
    Bloody urine
    Lower back pain
    Painful urination
Rare
    Difficulty in breathing
    Fever
    Skin rash or itching
    Sore throat and fever
    Sudden decrease in amount of urine
    Swelling of feet, lower legs, or face
    Unusual bleeding or bruising
    Unusual tiredness or weakness
    Unusual weight gain
    Yellowing of eyes or skin

Signs of overdose
   Convulsions (seizures)
   Vomiting (severe and continuing)

Other side effects may occur which usually do not require medical attention. These side effects may go away during treatment as your body adjusts to the medicine. However, check with your doctor if any of the following side effects continue or are bothersome:

More common
   Headache
   Loss of appetite
   Nausea or vomiting (mild)

Less common
   Dizziness
   Flushing or redness of face
   Frequent urge to urinate
   Sore gums

Other side effects not listed above may also occur in some patients. If you notice any other effects, check with your doctor.

PROCAINAMIDE (Systemic)

Some commonly used brand names are Procan SR, Promine, Pronestyl, and Pronestyl-SR.

Generic name product may also be available.

Procainamide (proe-KANE-a-mide) is used to correct irregular heartbeats to a normal rhythm and to slow an overactive heart. This allows the heart to work more efficiently. It produces its beneficial effects by slowing nerve impulses in the heart and reducing sensitivity of heart tissues.

Procainamide is taken by mouth in capsules, tablets, or extended-release (long-acting) tablets. It is also given by injection in emergencies or when a rapid effect is needed.

Procainamide is available only with your doctor's prescription.

Before Using This Medicine

In order to decide on the best treatment for your medical problem, your doctor should be told:

—if you have ever had any unusual or allergic reaction to procainamide, procaine, or any "caine-type" medicine.

—if you are on a low-salt, low-sugar, or any other special diet, or if you are allergic to any substance, such as sulfites or other preservatives or dyes. Most medicines contain more than their active ingredient. Your doctor or pharmacist can help you avoid products that may cause a problem.

—if you are pregnant or if you intend to become pregnant while taking this medicine. Although procainamide has not been shown to cause problems in humans, the chance always exists since it is known to pass from the mother to the fetus.

—if you are breast-feeding an infant. Although procainamide has not been shown to cause problems in humans, the chance always exists since it passes into breast milk.

—if you have any of the following medical problems:
   Asthma
   Kidney disease
   Liver disease
   Lupus erythematosus (history of)
   Myasthenia gravis

—if you are now taking any of the following medicines or types of medicine:
   Antidyskinetics (medicine for Parkinson's disease)
   Antihistamines or medicine for hay fever, other allergies, or colds
   Antihypertensives (high blood pressure medicine)
   Antimuscarinics (medicine for abdominal or stomach spasms or cramps)
   Bethanechol
   Medicine for myasthenia gravis
   Other heart medicine

Proper Use of This Medicine

Take procainamide exactly as directed by your doctor, even though you may feel well. Do not take more medicine than ordered.

Procainamide should be taken with a glass of water on an empty stomach 1 hour before or 2 hours after meals so that it will be absorbed more quickly. However, to lessen stomach upset, your doctor may want you to take the medicine with food or milk.

For patients taking the extended-release tablets:
• Swallow the tablet whole without breaking, crushing, or chewing it.

This medicine works best when there is a constant amount in the blood. **To help keep this amount constant, do not miss any doses. Also, it is best to take each dose at evenly spaced times day and night.** For example, if you are to take 6 doses a day, each dose should be spaced about 4 hours apart. If this interferes with your sleep or other daily activities, or if you need help in planning the best times to take your medicine, check with your doctor, nurse, or pharmacist.

If you do miss a dose of this medicine and remember within 2 hours (4 hours if you are taking the long-acting tablets), take it as soon as possible. However, if you do not remember until later, skip the missed dose and go back to your regular dosing schedule. Do not double doses.

How to store this medicine:
• Store away from heat and direct light.
• **Keep out of the reach of children.**
• Do not store in the bathroom medicine cabinet or refrigerator because the moisture usually present in these areas may cause the medicine to break down. Keep the container tightly closed and store in a dry place.

• Do not keep outdated medicine or medicine no longer needed. Flush the contents of the container down the toilet, unless otherwise directed.

Precautions While Using This Medicine

It is important that your doctor check your progress at regular visits to make sure the medicine is working properly. This will allow necessary changes in the amount of medicine you are taking, which also may help reduce side effects.

Do not stop taking this medicine without first checking with your doctor. Stopping it suddenly may cause a serious change in the activity of your heart. Your doctor may want you to reduce gradually the amount you are taking before stopping completely.

Before having any kind of surgery (including dental surgery) or emergency treatment, tell the physician or dentist in charge that you are taking this medicine.

Your doctor may want you to carry a medical identification card or bracelet stating that you are taking this medicine.

Dizziness or lightheadedness may occur, especially in elderly patients and when large doses are used. **Elderly patients should use extra care to avoid falling. Make sure you know how you react to this medicine before you drive, use machines, or do other jobs that require you to be alert.**

Side Effects of This Medicine

Along with its needed effects, a medicine may cause some unwanted effects. Although not all of these side effects appear very often, when they do occur they may require medical attention. Check with your doctor as soon as possible if any of the following side effects occur:

Less common
　Fever and chills
　Joint pain or swelling

Pains with breathing
Skin rash or itching

Rare

Confusion
Fever or sore mouth, gums, or throat
Hallucinations (seeing, hearing, or feeling things that are not there)
Mental depression
Unusual bleeding or bruising
Unusual tiredness or weakness

Possible signs of overdose

Confusion
Dizziness (severe) or fainting
Drowsiness
Nausea and vomiting
Unusual decrease in urination
Unusually fast or irregular heartbeat

Other side effects may occur which usually do not require medical attention. These side effects may go away during treatment as your body adjusts to the medicine. However, check with your doctor if any of the following side effects continue or are bothersome:

More common

Diarrhea
Loss of appetite

Less common

Dizziness or lightheadedness

Dizziness or lightheadedness are more likely to occur in the elderly who are usually more sensitive to the effects of this medicine.

The medicine in the extended-release tablets is contained in a special wax form (matrix). The medicine is slowly released, after which the wax matrix passes out of the body. Sometimes it may be seen in the stool. This is normal and is no cause for concern.

Other side effects not listed above may also occur in some patients. If you notice any other effects, check with your doctor.

QUINIDINE (Systemic)

Some commonly used brand names are:

Cardioquin	Quinidex
Cin-Quin	Extentabs
Duraquin	Quinora
Quinaglute	SK-Quinidine
Duratabs	Sulfate

Generic name product may also be available.

Quinidine (KWIN-i-deen) is most often used to correct certain irregular heartbeats to a normal rhythm and to slow an overactive heart.

Quinidine acts directly on the heart tissues to make them less responsive. It also slows impulses along special nerve networks to the heart. This allows the heart to work more efficiently.

Do not confuse this medicine with *quinine*, which, although related, has different medical uses.

Quinidine is available only with your doctor's prescription.

Before Using This Medicine

In order to decide on the best treatment for your medical problem, your doctor should be told:

—if you have ever had any unusual or allergic reaction to quinidine or quinine.

—if you are on a low-salt, low-sugar, or any other special diet, or if you are allergic to any substance, such as sulfites or other preservatives or dyes. Most medicines contain more than their active ingredient. Your doctor or pharmacist can help you avoid products that may cause a problem.

—if you are pregnant or if you intend to become pregnant while taking this medicine. Although studies have not been done in either humans or animals, a closely related medicine, quinine, has been shown to cause birth defects of the nervous system, fingers, and toes and decreased hearing in the infant. Quinine also may cause contractions of the uterus.

—if you are breast-feeding an infant. Although quinidine has not been reported to cause problems in humans, the chance always exists since it has been shown to pass into the breast milk.

—if you have any of the following medical problems:

Asthma or emphysema
Blood disease
Infection
Kidney disease
Liver disease
Myasthenia gravis
Overactive thyroid
Psoriasis

—if you are now taking or have taken within the past 2 weeks any of the following medicines or types of medicine:

Acetazolamide
Antacids (when used frequently)
Anticoagulants, oral (blood thinners you take by mouth)
Anticonvulsants, hydantoin (seizure medicine)
Barbiturates
Bethanechol
Calcium carbonate
Carbamazepine
Cimetidine
Dichlorphenamide
Methazolamide
Medicine for myasthenia gravis
Other heart medicine (especially digoxin)
Phenothiazines
Potassium supplements
Primidone
Quinine
Reserpine
Rifampin
Sodium bicarbonate (baking soda)

Proper Use of This Medicine

Take quinidine with a full glass (8 ounces) of water on an empty stomach 1 hour before or 2 hours after meals so that it will be absorbed more quickly. However, to lessen stomach upset, your doctor may want you to take the medicine with food or milk.

For patients taking the extended-release tablet form of this medicine:

• These tablets are to be swallowed whole.

• Do not break, crush, or chew before swallowing.

Take quinidine exactly as directed by your doctor even though you may feel well. Do not take more medicine than ordered and do not miss any doses.

If you do miss a dose of this medicine and remember within 2 hours of the missed dose, take it as soon as possible. However, if you do not remember until later, skip the missed dose and go back to your regular dosing schedule. Do not double doses.

How to store this medicine:

• Store away from heat and direct light.

• **Keep out of the reach of children.**

• Do not store in the bathroom medicine cabinet because the heat or moisture may cause the medicine to break down.

• Do not keep outdated medicine or medicine no longer needed. Flush the contents of the container down the toilet, unless otherwise directed.

Precautions While Using This Medicine

It is very important that your doctor check your progress at regular visits to make sure the quinidine is working properly and does not cause unwanted effects.

Do not stop taking this medicine without first checking with your doctor, in order to avoid possible worsening of your condition.

Before having any kind of surgery (including dental surgery) or emergency treatment, tell the physician or dentist in charge that you are taking this medicine.

Your doctor may want you to carry a medical identification card or bracelet stating that you are using this medicine.

Some people who are unusually sensitive to this medicine may have side effects after the first dose or first few doses. Check with your doctor right away if the following side effects occur: breathing difficulty, changes in vision, dizziness, fever, headache, ringing in ears, or skin rash.

Side Effects of This Medicine

Along with its needed effects, a medicine may cause some unwanted effects. Although not all of these side effects appear very often, when they do occur they may require medical attention. **Check with your doctor immediately** if any of the following side effects occur:

Less common
   Blurred vision or any change in vision
   Dizziness, lightheadedness, or fainting
   Fever
   Headache (severe)
   Ringing or buzzing in the ears or any loss of hearing
   Skin rash, hives, or itching
   Wheezing, shortness of breath, or troubled breathing

Rare
   Unusual bleeding or bruising
   Unusually fast heartbeat
   Unusual tiredness or weakness

Other side effects may occur which usually do not require medical attention. These side effects may go away during treatment as your body adjusts to the medicine. However, check with your doctor if any of the following side effects continue or are bothersome:

More common
   Bitter taste
   Diarrhea
   Flushing of skin with itching
   Loss of appetite
   Nausea or vomiting
   Stomach pain or cramping

Less common
   Confusion

Other side effects not listed above may also occur in some patients. If you notice any other effects, check with your doctor.

RANITIDINE (Systemic)
A commonly used brand name is Zantac.

Ranitidine (ra-NIT-te-deen) is a medicine used to treat duodenal and gastric ulcers. It is also used in some conditions in which the stomach produces too much acid, such as in Zollinger-Ellison disease. Ranitidine may also be used for other conditions as determined by your doctor.

Ranitidine works by decreasing the amount of acid produced by the stomach.

Ranitidine is available only with your doctor's prescription.

Before Using This Medicine

In order to decide on the best treatment for your medical problem, your doctor should be told:

   —if you have ever had any unusual or allergic reaction to ranitidine or cimetidine.

   —if you are on a low-salt, low-sugar, any other special diet, or if you are allergic to any substance, such as sulfites or other preservatives or dyes. Most medicines contain more than their active ingredient. Your doctor or pharmacist can help you avoid products that may cause a problem.

   —if you are pregnant or if you intend to become pregnant while using this medicine. Studies have not been done in humans; however, ranitidine has not been shown to cause birth defects or other problems in animal studies.

—if you are breast-feeding an infant. Although ranitidine has not been shown to cause problems in humans, the chance always exists since this medicine passes into the breast milk.

—if you have any of the following medical problems:

Kidney disease
Liver disease

—if you are now taking any other medicine, especially the following medicines or types of medicine:

Antacids
Ketoconazole

Proper Use of This Medicine

It may take several days for ranitidine to begin to relieve stomach pain. Antacids may be taken with ranitidine, but not at the same time, to help relieve pain, unless your doctor has told you not to use them. However, one hour should pass between taking the antacid and the ranitidine.

Take this medicine for the full time of treatment, even if you begin to feel better. Also, it is important that you keep your doctor's appointments for check-ups so that your doctor will be better able to tell you when to stop taking ranitidine.

If you miss a dose of this medicine, take it as soon as possible. However, if it is almost time for your next dose, skip the missed dose and go back to your regular dosing schedule. Do not double doses.

How to store this medicine:

• Store away from heat and direct light.

• **Keep out of the reach of children.**

• Do not store in the bathroom medicine cabinet because the heat or moisture may cause the medicine to break down.

• Do not keep outdated medicine or medicine no longer needed. Flush the contents of the container down the toilet, unless otherwise directed.

Precautions While Using This Medicine

Before you have any skin tests for allergies, tell the doctor in charge that you are taking ranitidine. The results of the test may be affected by this medicine.

Remember that certain medicines, such as aspirin, and certain foods and drinks that irritate the stomach may make your problem worse.

Cigarette smoking tends to decrease the effect of ranitidine. This is more likely to affect the stomach's nighttime production of acid. While taking ranitidine, stop smoking completely, or at least do not smoke after taking the last dose of the day.

Follow your doctor's orders and check with him or her if your ulcer pain continues or gets worse.

Side Effects of This Medicine

Along with its needed effects, a medicine may cause some unwanted effects. Although not all of these side effects appear very often, when they do occur they may require medical attention. Check with your doctor as soon as possible if any of the following side effects occur:

Rare

Confusion (especially in very ill elderly patients)
Sore throat and fever
Unusual bleeding or bruising
Unusually slow, fast, or irregular heartbeat
Unusual tiredness or weakness

Other side effects may occur which usually do not require medical attention. These side effects may go away during treatment as your body adjusts to the medicine. However, check with your doctor if any of the following side effects continue or are bothersome:

Less common or rare

Constipation
Dizziness or headache

Nausea
Skin rash
Stomach pain

The above side effects are more likely to occur in elderly patients with kidney and/or liver disease, who are usually more sensitive to the effects of ranitidine.

Other side effects not listed above may also occur in some patients. If you notice any other effects, check with your doctor.

RAUWOLFIA ALKALOIDS
(Systemic)

This information applies to the following medicines:

Alseroxylon (al-ser-OX-i-lon)
Deserpidine (de-SER-pi-deen)
Rauwolfia Serpentina (rah-WOOL-fee-a serpen-TEE-na)
Reserpine (re-SER-peen)

Some commonly used brand names are:	Generic names:
Rauwiloid	Alseroxylon
Harmonyl	Deserpidine
Raudixin Rauverid Wolfina	Rauwolfia Serpentina†
Releserp-5 Sandril Serpasil SK-Reserpine	Reserpine†

†Generic name product may also be available.

Rauwolfia alkaloids belong to the general class of medicines called antihypertensives. They are taken by mouth to treat high blood pressure.

High blood pressure adds to the workload of the heart and arteries. If it continues for a long time, they may not function properly. This can damage the blood vessels of the brain, heart, and kidneys, resulting in a stroke, heart attack, or kidney failure. These problems may be avoided if blood pressure is controlled.

Rauwolfia alkaloids work by controlling nerve impulses along certain nerve pathways. As a result, they act on the heart and blood vessels to lower blood pressure.

Rauwolfia alkaloids may also be used to treat other conditions as determined by your doctor.

These medicines are available only with your doctor's prescription.

Before Using This Medicine

In order to decide on the best treatment for your medical problem, your doctor should be told:

—if you have ever had any unusual or allergic reaction to rauwolfia alkaloids.

—if you are on a low-salt, low-sugar, or any other special diet, or if you are allergic to any substance, such as sulfites or other preservatives or dyes. Most medicines contain more than their active ingredient. Your doctor or pharmacist can help you avoid products that may cause a problem.

—if you are pregnant or if you intend to become pregnant while using this medicine. Too much use of rauwolfia alkaloids during pregnancy may cause unwanted effects (difficult breathing, low temperature, loss of appetite) in the baby. In rats, use of rauwolfia alkaloids during pregnancy decreases survival of the newborn. Be sure you have discussed this with your doctor before taking this medicine.

—if you are breast-feeding an infant. Rauwolfia alkaloids pass into the breast milk and may cause unwanted effects (difficult breathing, low temperature, loss of appetite) in infants of mothers taking large doses of this medicine. Be sure you have discussed this with your doctor before taking this medicine.

—if you have any of the following medical problems:

Allergies or other breathing problems
Asthma
Epilepsy
Gallstones
Heart disease
Kidney disease
Mental depression (or history of)
Parkinson's disease
Pheochromocytoma (PCC)
Stomach ulcer
Ulcerative colitis

—if you are now using any of the following medicines or types of medicine:

Acebutolol
Antimuscarinics (medicine for abdominal or stomach spasms or cramps)
Atenolol
Digitalis glycosides (heart medicine)
Diuretics (water pills) or other antihypertensives (blood pressure medicine)
Inflammation medicines, especially indomethacin
Labetalol
Levodopa
Metoprolol
Nadolol
Oxprenolol
Pindolol
Propranolol
Quinidine
Sotalol
Timolol

—if you are now taking central nervous system (CNS) depressants, such as:

Anticonvulsants (seizure medicine)
Antihistamines or medicine for hay fever, other allergies, or colds
Barbiturates
Muscle relaxants
Narcotics
Prescription pain medicine
Sedatives, tranquilizers, or sleeping medicine

—if you are now taking or have taken within the past 2 weeks monoamine oxidase (MAO) inhibitors, such as:

Furazolidone
Isocarboxazid
Pargyline
Phenelzine
Procarbazine
Tranylcypromine

Proper Use of This Medicine

Importance of diet—When prescribing medicine for your condition, your doctor may also prescribe a personal diet for you. Such a diet may be low in sodium (salt). Most people eat much more sodium than they need and too much sodium in the diet may increase blood pressure. Some foods that contain large amounts of sodium include canned soup, pickles, ketchup, green and ripe olives, relish, frankfurters, soy sauce, and carbonated beverages. Your doctor may want you to limit the amounts of these and other high-sodium foods in your diet. Medicine is usually more effective when such a diet is properly followed.

Also, it may be very important for you to go on a reducing diet. However, check with your doctor before going on any diet.

Many patients who have high blood pressure will not notice any signs of the problem. In fact, many may feel normal. It is very important that you take your medicine exactly as directed and that you keep your doctor's appointments even if you feel well.

Remember that this medicine will not cure your high blood pressure but it does control it. Therefore, you must continue to take it as directed if you expect to lower your blood pressure and keep it down. **You may have to take medicine for the rest of your life.** If high blood pressure is not treated, it can cause serious problems such as heart failure, blood vessel disease, stroke, or kidney disease.

In order to help remember to take your medicine, try to get into the habit of taking it at the same time each day.

This medicine is sometimes given together with certain other medicines. If you are using a combination of drugs, make sure that you take each medicine at the proper time and do not mix them. Ask your doctor, nurse, or pharmacist to help you plan a way to remember to take your medicines at the right time.

If this medicine upsets your stomach, it may be taken with meals or milk. If stomach upset (nausea, vomiting, stomach cramps or pain) continues or gets worse, check with your doctor.

If you miss a dose of this medicine, do not take the missed dose at all and do not double the next one. Instead, go back to your regular dosing schedule.

How to store this medicine:

- Store away from heat and direct light.
- **Keep out of the reach of children.**
- Do not store in the bathroom medicine cabinet because the heat or moisture may cause the medicine to break down.
- Do not keep outdated medicine or medicine no longer needed. Flush the contents of the container down the toilet, unless otherwise directed.

Precautions While Using This Medicine

It is important that your doctor check your progress at regular visits in order to make sure that this medicine is working properly.

In some patients, this medicine may cause mental depression. **Tell your doctor right away:**

—if you or anyone else notices unusual changes in your mood.

—if you start having early-morning sleeplessness or unusually vivid dreams or nightmares.

This medicine will add to the effects of alcohol and other CNS depressants (medicines that slow down the nervous system, possibly causing drowsiness). Some examples of CNS depressants are antihistamines or medicine for hay fever, other allergies, or colds; sedatives, tranquilizers, or sleeping medicine; prescription pain medicine or narcotics; barbiturates; medicine for seizures; muscle relaxants; or anesthetics, including some dental anesthetics. **Check with your doctor before taking any of the above while you are using this medicine.**

This medicine may cause some people to become drowsy or less alert than they are normally. This is more likely to happen when you begin to take it or when you increase the amount of medicine you are taking. **Make sure you know how you react to this medicine before you drive, use machines, or do other jobs that require you to be alert.**

Your mouth, nose, and throat may feel very dry while you are taking this medicine. To help relieve mouth dryness, chew sugarless gum or dissolve bits of ice in your mouth.

Before having any kind of surgery (including dental surgery) or emergency treatment, **tell the physician or dentist in charge that you are taking this medicine.**

This medicine often causes stuffiness in the nose. However, do not use nasal decongestant medicines without first checking with your doctor or pharmacist.

Do not take other medicines unless they have been discussed with your doctor. This especially includes over-the-counter (nonprescription) medicines for appetite control, asthma, colds, cough, hay fever, or sinus problems, since they may tend to increase your blood pressure.

Side Effects of This Medicine

Suggestions that rauwolfia alkaloids may increase the risk of breast cancer occurring later have not been proven. However, rats and mice given 100 to 300 times the human dose had an increased risk of tumors.

Along with its needed effects, a medicine may cause some unwanted effects. Although not all of these side effects appear very often, when they do occur they may require medical attention. **Check with your doctor immediately** if any of the following side effects occur:

Less common
  Drowsiness or faintness
  Impotence or decreased sexual interest
  Lack of energy or weakness
  Mental depression or inability to
    concentrate
  Nervousness or anxiety
  Vivid dreams or nightmares or early-
    morning sleeplessness

Check with your doctor as soon as possible if any of the following side effects occur:

Less common
  Black tarry stools
  Bloody vomit
  Chest pain
  Headache
  Irregular or slow heartbeat
  Shortness of breath
  Stomach cramps or pain

Rare
  Painful or difficult urination
  Skin rash or itching
  Stiffness
  Trembling and shaking of hands and
    fingers
  Unusual bleeding or bruising

Possible signs of overdose
  Dizziness or drowsiness (severe)
  Flushing of skin

Pinpoint pupils of eyes
Slow pulse

Other side effects may occur which usually do not require medical attention. These side effects may go away during treatment as your body adjusts to the medicine. However, check with your doctor if any of the following side effects continue or are bothersome:

More common
  Diarrhea
  Dizziness
  Dry mouth
  Loss of appetite
  Nausea and vomiting
  Stuffy nose

Less common
  Swelling of feet and lower legs

Dizziness may be more likely to occur in the elderly, who are more sensitive to the effects of rauwolfia alkaloids.

After you stop using this medicine, it may still produce some side effects that need attention. During this period of time **check with your doctor immediately** if you notice any of the following side effects:

  Drowsiness or faintness
  Impotence or decreased sexual interest
  Irregular or slow heartbeat
  Lack of energy or weakness
  Mental depression or inability to
    concentrate
  Nervousness or anxiety
  Vivid dreams or nightmares or early-
    morning sleeplessness

Other side effects not listed above may also occur in some patients. If you notice any other effects, check with your doctor.

RAUWOLFIA ALKALOIDS AND THIAZIDE DIURETICS (Systemic)

This information applies to the following medicines:

Deserpidine (de-SER-pi-deen) and Hydrochlorothiazide (hye-droe-klor-oh-THYE-a-zide)

Deserpidine and Methyclothiazide (meth-i-kloe-THYE-a-zide)

Rauwolfia Serpentina (rah-WOOL-fee-a serpen-TEE-na) and Bendroflumethiazide (bendroe-floo-meth-EYE-a-zide)

Reserpine (re-SER-peen) and Chlorothiazide (klor-oh-THYE-a-zide)

Reserpine and Chlorthalidone (klor-THAL-idone)

Reserpine and Hydrochlorothiazide (hye-droe-klor-oh-THYE-a-zide)

Reserpine and Hydroflumethiazide (hye-droe-floo-meth-EYE-a-zide)

Reserpine and Methyclothiazide (meth-i-kloe-THYE-a-zide)

Reserpine and Polythiazide (pol-i-THYE-a-zide)

Reserpine and Quinethazone (kwin-ETH-a-zone)

Reserpine and Trichlormethiazide (trye-klor-meth-EYE-a-zide)

Some commonly used brand names are:	Generic names:
Oreticyl Oreticyl Forte	Deserpidine and Hydrochlorothiazide
Enduronyl	Deserpidine and Methyclothiazide†
Rauzide	Rauwolfia Serpentina and Bendroflumethiazide
Diupres	Reserpine and Chlorothiazide†
Demi-Regroton Regroton	Reserpine and Chlorthalidone
Hydropres Serpasil-Esidrix	Reserpine and Hydrochlorothiazide†
Salutensin Salutensin-Demi	Reserpine and Hydroflumethiazide†
Diutensen-R	Reserpine and Methyclothiazide
Renese-R	Reserpine and Polythiazide
Hydromox-R	Reserpine and Quinethazone
Metatensin Naquival	Reserpine and Trichlormethiazide†

†Generic name product may also be available.

Rauwolfia alkaloid and thiazide diuretic combinations are used in the treatment of high blood pressure.

High blood pressure adds to the workload of the heart and arteries. If it continues for a long time, they may not function properly. This can damage the blood vessels of the brain, heart, and kidneys, resulting in a stroke, heart attack, or kidney failure. These problems may be avoided if blood pressure is controlled.

Rauwolfia alkaloids work by controlling nerve impulses along certain nerve pathways. As a result, they act on the heart and blood vessels to lower blood pressure. Thiazide diuretics help to reduce the amount of water in the body by increasing the flow of urine. This also helps to lower blood pressure.

These medicines are available only with your doctor's prescription.

For information about the precautions and side effects of the medicines in this combination, see:

Rauwolfia Alkaloids (Systemic)
Diuretics, Thiazide (Systemic)

Combination products are designed for specific uses. These uses may not be the same as the uses of the individual ingredients. Therefore, some of the information provided in the individual listings may not be relevant to the combination product. If questions arise, check with your doctor, nurse, or pharmacist.

RESERPINE AND HYDRALAZINE
(Systemic)

A commonly used brand name is Serpasil-Apresoline.

The reserpine (re-SER-peen) and hydralazine (hye-DRAL-a-zeen) combination is taken by mouth to treat high blood pressure.

High blood pressure adds to the workload of the heart and arteries. If it continues for a long time, they may not function properly. This can damage the blood vessels of the brain, heart, and kidneys, resulting in a stroke, heart attack, or kidney failure. These problems may be avoided if blood pressure is controlled.

Reserpine works by controlling nerve impulses along certain nerve pathways. As a result, it acts on the heart and blood vessels to lower blood pressure. Hydralazine works by relaxing blood vessels and increasing the supply of blood and oxygen to the heart while reducing its work load.

Reserpine and hydralazine combination is available only with your doctor's prescription.

For information about the precautions and side effects of the medicines in this combination, see:

Rauwolfia Alkaloids (Systemic)
Hydralazine (Systemic)

Combination products are designed for specific uses. These uses may not be the same as the uses of the individual ingredients. Therefore, some of the information provided in the individual listings may not be relevant to the combination product. If questions arise, check with your doctor, nurse, or pharmacist.

RESERPINE, HYDRALAZINE, AND HYDROCHLOROTHIAZIDE
(Systemic)

Some commonly used brand names are:

Hydrap-Es	Ser-Ap-Es
Hyserp	Tri-Hydroserpine
R-HCTZ-H	Unipres

Generic name product may also be available.

Reserpine (re-SER-peen), hydralazine (hye-DRAL-a-zeen), and hydrochlorothiazide (hye-droe-KLOR-oh-THYE-a-zide) combinations are taken by mouth to treat high blood pressure.

High blood pressure adds to the workload of the heart and arteries. If it continues for a long time, they may not function properly. This can damage the blood vessels of the brain, heart, and kidneys, resulting in a stroke, heart attack, or kidney failure. These problems may be avoided if blood pressure is controlled.

Reserpine works by controlling nerve impulses along certain nerve pathways. As a result, it acts on the heart and blood vessels to lower blood pressure. Hydralazine works by relaxing blood vessels and increasing the supply of blood to the heart while reducing its work load. Hydrochlorothiazide helps to reduce the amount of water in the body by increasing the flow of urine. This also helps to lower blood pressure.

This medicine is available only with your doctor's prescription.

For information about the precautions and side effects of the medicines in this combination, see:

Rauwolfia Alkaloids (Systemic)
Hydralazine (Systemic)
Diuretics, Thiazide (Systemic)

Combination products are designed for specific uses. These uses may not be the same as the uses of the individual ingredients. Therefore, some of the information provided in the individual listings may not be relevant to the combination product. If questions arise, check with your doctor, nurse, or pharmacist.

SALICYLATES (Systemic)

This information applies to the following medicines:

Aspirin (AS-pir-in)
Buffered Aspirin
Choline Salicylate (KOE-leen sa-LI-si-late)
Choline and Magnesium (mag-NEE-zhum) Salicylates
Magnesium Salicylate
Salicylamide (sal-i-SILL-a-mide)
Salsalate (SAL-sa-late)
Sodium Salicylate

Some commonly used brand names and other names are:

For Aspirin†‡

Acetylsalicylic Acid	Ecotrin
Apo-Asen*	Empirin
Arthritis Bayer Timed-Release	Encaprin
	Entrophen*
ASA	Hiprin
A.S.A.	Measurin
A.S.A. Enseals	Novasen*
Aspergum	Riphen-10*
Astrin*	Sal-Adult*
Bayer Aspirin	Sal-Infant*
Bayer Timed-Release Arthritic Pain Formula*	St. Joseph Aspirin for Children
Coryphen*	Supasa*
Cosprin	Triaphen-10*
Easprin	Zorprin

For Aspirin and Caffeine

Accurate*	Major-cin
Acotin*	Neo-Tigol*
Alsidol*	Nervine*
Anacin	P-A-C Revised
Asafen*	Formula
CP-2	Paradol*
C2*	Synalgos
812*	T-R-C Regular
Instantine*	217*

For Buffered Aspirin†

Alka-Seltzer Effervescent Pain Reliever and Antacid	Buff-A
	Buffaprin
	Bufferin
Arthritic Pain Formula*	Buffinol
	Buf-Tabs
Arthritis Pain Formula	Cama Arthritis Reliever
Ascriptin	
Ascriptin A/D	Wesprin Buffered
Asperbuf	

For Choline Salicylate
Arthropan

For Choline and Magnesium Salicylates

Choline Magnesium Trisalicylate	Trilisate

For Magnesium Salicylate

Doan's Pills§	Magan
Durasal	Mobidin
Efficin	MS-650

For Salicylamide†
Uromide

For Salsalate

Artha-G	Mono-Gesic
Disalcid	Salicylsalicylic Acid

For Sodium Salicylate†
Uracel

*Not available in the United States.
†Generic name product may also be available.
‡In Canada, *Aspirin* is also a brand name. Acetylsalicylic acid is the generic name in Canada.
§In Canada, *Doan's Pills* brand does not contain magnesium salicylate. It contains other pain relievers.

Salicylates are medicines used to relieve pain and reduce fever. Most salicylates are also used to relieve some symptoms caused by arthritis or rheumatism, such as swelling, stiffness, and joint pain. However, they do not cure arthritis and will help you only as long as you continue to take them. Aspirin may also be used, under the advice of a doctor, to lessen the chance of heart attack in patients with certain heart problems and to lessen the chance of stroke in some men.

There have been reports suggesting that use of aspirin in children with fever due to a viral infection (especially flu or chicken pox) may cause a serious illness called Reye's syndrome. Therefore, do not give aspirin or other salicylates to a child with flu or chicken pox without first discussing this with your child's doctor.

The caffeine present in some of these products may provide additional relief of headache pain or faster pain relief.

Some salicylates are available only with your physician's or dentist's prescription. Others are available without a prescription; however, your physician or dentist may have special instructions on the proper dose of these medicines for your medical condition.

Before Using This Medicine

Before you take a salicylate, check with your doctor or pharmacist:

—if you have ever had any unusual or allergic reaction to aspirin or other salicylates including diflunisal or methyl salicylate (oil of wintergreen), or to any of the following medicines:

    Fenoprofen
    Ibuprofen
    Indomethacin
    Meclofenamate
    Mefenamic acid
    Naproxen
    Oxyphenbutazone
    Phenylbutazone
    Piroxicam
    Sulindac
    Tolmetin
    Zomepirac

—if you are on a low-salt, low-sugar, or any other special diet, or if you are allergic to any substance, such as sulfites or other preservatives or dyes. Most medicines contain more than their active ingredient, and many liquid medicines contain alcohol. Your doctor or pharmacist can help you avoid products that may cause a problem.

—if you are pregnant or if you intend to become pregnant while using this medicine. Salicylates have not been shown to cause birth defects in humans. Studies on birth defects in humans have been done with aspirin but not with other salicylates. However, studies in animals have shown that salicylates cause birth defects.

Some reports have suggested that too much use of aspirin late in pregnancy may cause a decrease in the newborn's weight and possible death of the fetus or newborn infant. However, the mothers in these reports had been taking much larger amounts of aspirin than are usually recommended. Studies of mothers taking aspirin in the doses that are usually recommended did not show these unwanted effects. However, there is a chance that regular use of salicylates late in pregnancy may cause unwanted effects on the heart or blood flow in the fetus or in the newborn infant.

Use of salicylates, especially aspirin, during the last 2 weeks of pregnancy may cause bleeding problems in the fetus before or during delivery or in the newborn infant. Also, too much use of salicylates during the last 3 months of pregnancy may increase the length of pregnancy, prolong labor, cause other problems during delivery, or cause severe bleeding in the mother before, during, or after delivery.

Studies in humans have not shown that caffeine causes birth defects. However, studies in animals have shown that caffeine causes birth defects when given in very large doses (amounts equal to the amount of caffeine present in 12 to 24 cups of coffee a day).

—if you are breast-feeding an infant. Salicylates have not been shown to cause problems in humans. However, the chance always exists, especially if large amounts are taken regularly, as for arthritis or rheumatism. Salicylates pass into the breast milk.

Caffeine passes into the breast milk in small amounts.

—if you have any of the following medical problems:

Anemia
Asthma, allergies, and nasal polyps (history of)
Glucose-6-phosphate dehydrogenase (G6PD) deficiency
Gout
Heart disease
Hemophilia or other bleeding problems
High blood pressure (for buffered aspirin effervescent tablets and sodium salicylate only)
Kidney disease
Liver disease
Overactive thyroid
Stomach ulcer or other stomach problems

—if you are taking aspirin or buffered aspirin and are also taking any of the following medicines or types of medicine:

Ascorbic acid (vitamin C)
Dipyridamole
Divalproex
Valproic acid

—if you are taking any of the salicylates and are also taking any of the following medicines or types of medicine:

Acetazolamide
Adrenocorticoids (cortisone-like medicine)
Aminoglycoside antibiotics
Anticoagulants (blood thinners)
Antidiabetics, oral (medicine for sugar diabetes you take by mouth)
Antiemetics (medicine for nausea or vomiting or motion sickness)
Anti-inflammatory analgesics, such as diflunisal, fenoprofen, ibuprofen, indomethacin, meclofenamate, mefenamic acid, naproxen, oxyphenbutazone, phenylbutazone, piroxicam, sulindac, or tolmetin
Bumetanide
Capreomycin
Cisplatin
Corticotropin (ACTH)
Dichlorphenamide
Ethacrynic acid
Furosemide

Heparin
Insulin
Laxatives containing cellulose
Methazolamide
Methotrexate
Nifedipine
Probenecid
Sulfinpyrazone
Urine acidifiers (medicine to make your urine more acid)
Urine alkalizers (medicine to make your urine less acid)
Vancomycin
Verapamil
Vitamin K

—if you regularly take large amounts of acetaminophen or antacids.

—if you are taking buffered aspirin, choline and magnesium salicylates, or magnesium salicylate and are also taking tetracycline.

—if you are taking one of the products containing caffeine and are also taking any of the following medicines or types of medicine:

Amantadine
Aminophylline
Amphetamines
Appetite suppressants (diet pills)
Chlophedianol
Dyphylline
Epinephrine
Lithium
Medicine for hay fever or other allergies (including nose drops or sprays)
Medicine for asthma or breathing problems (including oral inhalations)
Methylphenidate
Oxtriphylline
Pemoline
Theophylline

Proper Use of This Medicine

Unless otherwise directed by your physician or dentist:

• Do not take more of this medicine than recommended on the label in order to lessen the chance of side effects.

• Children up to 12 years of age should not take this medicine more than 5 times a day or for more than 5 days in a row.

• Adults should not take this medicine for more than 10 days in a row.

• Aspirin chewing gum tablets should not be used for more than 2 days in a row if they are being used to relieve a sore throat.

When used for arthritis or rheumatism, this medicine must be taken regularly as ordered by your doctor in order for it to help you. Up to 2 to 3 weeks or longer may pass before you feel the full effects of this medicine.

Take this medicine after meals or with food (except for aspirin suppositories) to lessen stomach irritation.

Take tablet or capsule forms of this medicine with a full glass (8 ounces) of water. Also, do not lie down for about 15 to 30 minutes after swallowing the medicine. This helps to prevent irritation that may lead to trouble in swallowing.

For patients taking aspirin or buffered aspirin:

• **Do not use aspirin or buffered aspirin if it has a strong, vinegar-like odor,** since this means the medicine is breaking down. If you have any questions about this, check with your doctor or pharmacist.

• If you have just had your tonsils removed, a tooth pulled, or other dental or mouth surgery and you are to take aspirin or buffered aspirin during the next 7 days, be sure to swallow the aspirin whole. Do not chew aspirin during this time.

• Do not place aspirin or buffered aspirin tablets directly on a tooth or gum surface. This may cause a burn.

• There are several different forms of aspirin or buffered aspirin. If you are using:

—*chewable aspirin tablets,* they may be chewed, dissolved in liquid, crushed, or swallowed whole.

—*effervescent buffered aspirin tablets,* they must be dissolved in water (between ⅓ and ½ cup of water for each tablet) just before taking. Drink all of the liquid in order to be sure you are taking the full amount of medicine. It is best to add more water to the glass and drink that also, to make sure that you are taking all of the medicine.

—*enteric-coated aspirin tablets,* they are to be swallowed whole. Do not crush them or break them up before taking.

—*extended-release (long-acting) aspirin tablets,* check with your pharmacist as to how they should be taken. Some may be gently broken up before swallowing if you cannot swallow them whole. Others should not be broken up and must be swallowed whole.

—*aspirin suppositories,* first remove the foil wrapper and moisten the suppository with water. Lie down on your side and push the suppository well up into the rectum with your finger.

For patients taking the liquid form of choline and magnesium salicylates:

• The liquid may be mixed with fruit juice just before taking.

• Drink a full glass (8 ounces) of water after taking the medicine.

For patients taking enteric-coated sodium salicylate tablets:

• The tablets must be swallowed whole. Do not crush them or break them up before taking.

If your physician or dentist has ordered you to take this medicine according to a regular schedule and you miss a dose, take it as soon as you remember. However, if it is almost time for your next dose, skip the missed dose and go back to your regular dosing schedule. Do not double doses.

How to store this medicine:

• Store away from heat and direct light.

• **Keep out of the reach of children** because overdose is very dangerous in young children.

• Do not store in the bathroom medicine cabinet because the heat or moisture may cause the medicine to break down.

• Keep liquid forms of this medicine from freezing.

• Store aspirin suppositories in a cool place. It is usually best to keep them in the refrigerator, but keep them from freezing.

• Do not keep outdated medicine or medicine no longer needed. Flush the contents of the container down the toilet, unless otherwise directed.

Precautions While Using This Medicine

Check the labels of all over-the-counter (OTC), nonprescription, and prescription medicines you now take. If any contain aspirin or other salicylates, including bismuth subsalicylate, be especially careful. Also, be especially careful if you regularly use a shampoo or other medicine for your skin that contains salicylic acid. Using them while taking this medicine may lead to overdose. If you have any questions about this, check with your doctor or pharmacist.

If you will be taking salicylates for a long time (more than 5 days in a row for children or 10 days in a row for adults) or in large amounts, your doctor should check your progress at regular visits.

Check with your doctor:
—if your symptoms do not improve or if they become worse.

—if you are taking this medicine to bring down a fever, and the fever lasts for more than 3 days or returns.

—if you are taking this medicine regularly, as for arthritis or rheumatism, and you notice a ringing or buzzing in the ear or severe or continuing headaches. These are often the first signs that too much salicylate is being taken. Your doctor may want to change the amount of medicine you are taking every day.

Do not regularly take acetaminophen, ibuprofen, or other anti-inflammatory analgesics such as diflunisal, fenoprofen, indomethacin, meclofenamate, mefenamic acid, naproxen, oxyphenbutazone, phenylbutazone, piroxicam, sulindac, or tolmetin, while you are taking a salicylate unless your physician or dentist directs you to do so. This is especially important if you are taking large amounts of salicylates, or if you must take them for a long time (as for arthritis or rheumatism). Taking these medicines with a salicylate may increase the chance of unwanted effects.

For diabetics—False urine sugar test results may occur if you are regularly taking large amounts of salicylates, such as:

—Aspirin: 8 or more 325-mg (5-grain), or 4 or more 500-mg or 650-mg (10-grain), or 3 or more 800-mg (or higher strength), doses a day.

—Buffered aspirin or
—Sodium salicylate: 8 or more 325-mg (5-grain), or 4 or more 500-mg or 650-mg (10-grain), doses a day.

—Choline salicylate: 4 or more teaspoonfuls (each teaspoonful containing 870 mg) a day.

—Choline and magnesium salicylates: 5 or more 500-mg tablets or teaspoonfuls, or 4 or more 750-mg tablets, a day.

—Magnesium salicylate: 7 or more 325-mg, or 4 or more 480-mg (or higher strength), tablets a day.

—Salsalate: 6 or more 325-mg doses, or 4 or more 500-mg doses, a day.

Smaller doses or occasional use of salicylates usually will not affect urine sugar tests. However, check with your doctor, nurse, or pharmacist (especially if your diabetes is not well-controlled) if:

—you are not sure how much salicylate you are taking every day.

—you notice any change in your urine sugar test results.

—you have any other questions about this possible problem.

Do not take aspirin for 5 days before any surgery, including dental surgery, unless otherwise directed by your physician or dentist. Taking aspirin during this time may cause bleeding problems.

For patients taking buffered aspirin, choline and magnesium salicylates, or magnesium salicylate:

• If you are also taking a tetracycline antibiotic, do not take the two medicines within 1 hour of each other. Taking them too close together may prevent the tetracycline from being absorbed by your body. If you have any questions about this, check with your doctor or pharmacist.

If you are taking a laxative containing cellulose, take the salicylate at least 2 hours before or after you take the laxative. Taking these medicines too close together may lessen the effects of the salicylate.

For patients on a sodium-restricted (low-salt) diet—Buffered aspirin effervescent tablets and sodium salicylate contain a large amount of sodium. Do not take these medicines without first checking with your doctor or pharmacist.

For patients taking this medicine by mouth:

• Stomach problems may be more likely to occur if you drink alcoholic beverages while being treated with this medicine, especially if you are taking it in high doses or for a long time. Check with your doctor if you have any questions about this.

For patients using aspirin suppositories:

• Too much use of aspirin suppositories may cause irritation of the rectum. Check with your doctor if this occurs.

If you think that you or anyone else may have taken an overdose, get emergency help at once. Taking an overdose of these medicines may cause unconsciousness or death. Signs of overdose include convulsions (seizures), hearing loss, mental confusion, ringing or buzzing in the ear, severe drowsiness or tiredness, severe excitement or nervousness, and unusually fast or deep breathing.

Side Effects of This Medicine

Along with its needed effects, a medicine may cause some unwanted effects. Although not all of these side effects appear very often, when they do occur they may require medical attention. When this medicine is used for short periods of time at low doses, side effects usually are rare. However, **get emergency help immediately** if any of the following signs of overdose occur:

Any loss of hearing
Bloody urine
Confusion
Convulsions (seizures)
Diarrhea
Dizziness or lightheadedness
Drowsiness (severe)
Excitement or nervousness (severe)
Hallucinations (seeing, hearing, or feeling things that are not there)
Nausea or vomiting (severe or continuing)
Shortness of breath or troubled breathing (for salicylamide only)

Stomach pain (severe or continuing)
Unexplained fever
Unusual increase in sweating
Unusually fast or deep breathing
Unusual thirst
Unusual or uncontrollable flapping movements of the hands, especially in elderly patients
Vision problems

Signs of overdose in children
Changes in behavior
Drowsiness or tiredness (severe)
Unusually fast or deep breathing

Also, check with your doctor as soon as possible if any of the following side effects occur:

More common
Nausea or vomiting
Stomach pain

Less common or rare
Bloody or black tarry stools
Headache (severe or continuing)
Ringing or buzzing in ear (continuing)
Shortness of breath, troubled breathing, tightness in chest, or wheezing
Skin rash, hives, or itching
Unusual tiredness or weakness
Vomiting of blood or material that looks like coffee grounds

The above side effects are more likely to occur in children, especially those with fever or who are dehydrated (those who have lost large amounts of body fluid because of vomiting, diarrhea, or sweating), and in elderly patients (60 years of age or older). These patients are usually more sensitive to the effects of salicylates.

Other side effects may occur which usually do not require medical attention. These side effects may go away during treatment as your body adjusts to the medicine. However, check with your doctor or pharmacist if any of the following side effects continue or are bothersome:
Drowsiness (for salicylamide only)
Heartburn or indigestion
Sleeplessness, nervousness, or jitters (for products containing caffeine only)

Other side effects not listed above may also occur in some patients. If you notice any other effects, check with your doctor.

SKELETAL MUSCLE RELAXANTS (Systemic)

This information applies to the following medicines:
Carisoprodol (kar-eye-soe-PROE-dole)
Chlorphenesin (klor-FEN-e-sin)
Chlorzoxazone (klor-ZOX-a-zone)
Metaxalone (me-TAX-a-lone)
Methocarbamol (meth-oh-KAR-ba-mole)

This information does *not* apply to the following medicines: Baclofen, cyclobenzaprine, dantrolene, diazepam, and orphenadrine.

Some commonly used brand names are:	Generic names
Rela Soma Soprodol	Carisoprodol†
Maolate Mycil*	Chlorphenesin
Paraflex	Chlorzoxazone†
Skelaxin	Metaxalone
Delaxin Marbaxin Robaxin	Methocarbamol†

*Not available in the United States.
†Generic name product may also be available.

Skeletal muscle relaxants are medicines used to relax certain muscles in your body and relieve the pain and discomfort caused by strains, sprains, or other injury to your muscles. However, these medicines do not take the place of rest, exercise or physical therapy, or other treatment that your doctor may recommend for your medical problem.

Methocarbamol is also used to relieve some of the muscle problems caused by tetanus.

Skeletal muscle relaxants act in the central nervous system (CNS) to produce their muscle relaxant effects. Their actions in the CNS may also produce some of their side effects.

In the United States, these medicines are available only with your doctor's prescription. In Canada, some of these medicines are available without a prescription.

Before Using This Medicine

In order to decide on the best treatment for your medical problem, your doctor should be told:

—if you have ever had any unusual or allergic reaction to this medicine.

—if you are taking carisoprodol and have ever had any unusual or allergic reaction to carbromal, mebutamate, meprobamate, or tybamate.

—if you are on a low-salt, low-sugar, or any other special diet, or if you are allergic to any substance, such as sulfites or other preservatives or dyes. Most medicines contain more than their active ingredient. Your doctor or pharmacist can help you avoid products that may cause a problem.

—if you are taking metaxalone and any other medicine you have taken has ever caused an allergy or reaction that affected your blood.

—if you are pregnant or if you intend to become pregnant while using this medicine. Although skeletal muscle relaxants have not been shown to cause birth defects or other problems, the chance always exists. Studies on birth defects have not been done in humans. Studies in animals with metaxalone have not shown that it causes birth defects.

—if you are breast-feeding an infant. Carisoprodol passes into the breast milk and may cause drowsiness or stomach upset in infants of nursing mothers taking the medicine. Although chlorphenesin, chlorzoxazone, metaxalone, and methocarbamol have not been shown to cause problems, the chance always exists.

—if you have either of the following medical problems:
Kidney disease
Liver disease

—if you are taking carisoprodol and have porphyria.

—if you are taking chlorzoxazone and have a history of allergies.

—if you are receiving methocarbamol by injection and have epilepsy.

—if you are now using central nervous system (CNS) depressants, such as:
Anticonvulsants (seizure medicine)
Antihistamines or medicine for hay fever, other allergies, or colds
Barbiturates
Narcotics
Other muscle relaxants
Prescription pain medicine
Sedatives, tranquilizers, or sleeping medicine
Tricyclic antidepressants (medicine for depression)

—if you are now taking or have taken within the past 2 weeks monoamine oxidase (MAO) inhibitors, such as:
Furazolidone
Isocarboxazid
Pargyline
Phenelzine
Procarbazine
Tranylcypromine

Proper Use of This Medicine

Chlorzoxazone, metaxalone, or methocarbamol tablets may be crushed and mixed with a little food or liquid if needed to make the tablets easier to swallow.

If you miss a dose of this medicine and remember within an hour or so of the missed dose, take it right away. But if you do not remember until later, skip the missed dose and go back to your regular dosing schedule. Do not double doses.

How to store this medicine:

• Store away from heat and direct light.

• **Keep out of the reach of children.**

• Do not store in the bathroom medicine cabinet because the heat or moisture may cause the medicine to break down.

• Do not keep outdated medicine or medicine no longer needed. Flush the contents of the container down the toilet, unless otherwise directed.

Precautions While Using This Medicine

If you will be taking this medicine for a long period of time (for example, more than a few weeks), your doctor should check your progress at regular visits.

This medicine will add to the effects of alcohol and other CNS depressants (medicines that slow down the nervous system, possibly causing drowsiness). Some examples of CNS depressants are antihistamines or medicine for hay fever, other allergies, or colds; sedatives, tranquilizers, or sleeping medicine; prescription pain medicine or narcotics; barbiturates; medicine for seizures; tricyclic antidepressants (medicine for depression); other muscle relaxants; or anesthetics, including some dental anesthetics. **Check with your doctor before taking any of the above while you are using this medicine.**

Skeletal muscle relaxants may cause blurred vision or clumsiness or unsteadiness in some people. They may also cause some people to feel drowsy, dizzy, lightheaded, faint, or less alert than they are normally. **Make sure you know how you react to this medicine before you drive, use machines, or do other jobs that require you to be alert, well-coordinated, and able to see well.**

For diabetics taking metaxalone—Metaxalone may cause false test results with one type of test for sugar in your urine. If your urine sugar test shows an unusually large amount of sugar, or if you have any questions about this, check with your doctor, nurse, or pharmacist. This is especially important if your diabetes is not well controlled.

Side Effects of This Medicine

Along with its needed effects, a medicine may cause some unwanted effects. Although not all of these side effects appear very often, when they do occur they may require medical attention. Check with your doctor as soon as possible if any of the following side effects occur:

Less common

Fainting
Fever
Mental depression
Skin rash, hives, itching, or redness
Stinging or burning of eyes
Stuffy nose and red or bloodshot eyes
Swelling of face, lips, or tongue
Unusually fast, slow, or pounding heartbeat
Wheezing, shortness of breath, or troubled breathing

Rare

Bloody or black tarry stools
Convulsions or seizures (methocarbamol injection only)
Sore throat and fever
Unusual bruising or bleeding
Unusual tiredness or weakness
Yellowing of eyes or skin

Other side effects may occur which usually do not require medical attention. These side effects may go away during treatment as your body adjusts to the medicine. However, check with your doctor if any of the following side effects continue or are bothersome:

More common

Blurred or double vision or any change in vision
Dizziness or lightheadedness
Drowsiness

Less common or rare
Abdominal or stomach cramps or pain
Clumsiness or unsteadiness
Confusion
Constipation
Diarrhea
Flushing or redness of face
Headache
Heartburn
Hiccups
Nausea or vomiting
Pain or peeling of skin at place of
     injection (methocarbamol only)
Trembling
Trouble in sleeping
Uncontrolled movements of eyes (metho-
     carbamol injection only)
Unusual excitement, nervousness, rest-
     lessness, or irritability
Unusual muscle weakness

Although not all of the side effects listed above have been reported for all of these medicines, they have been reported for at least one of them. However, since all of these skeletal muscle relaxants have similar effects, it is possible that any of the above side effects may occur with any of these medicines.

In addition to the other side effects listed above, chlorzoxazone may cause your urine to turn orange or reddish purple. Methocarbamol may cause your urine to turn black, brown, or green. This effect is harmless and will go away when you stop taking the medicine. However, if you have any questions about this, check with your doctor.

Other side effects not listed above may also occur in some patients. If you notice any other effects, check with your doctor.

SUCRALFATE (Oral)

Some commonly used brand names are Carafate and Sulcrate*.

---

*Not available in the United States.

Sucralfate (soo-KRAL-fate) is taken by mouth to treat duodenal ulcer. This medicine may also be used for other conditions as determined by your doctor.

Sucralfate is available only with your doctor's prescription.

Before Using This Medicine

In order to decide on the best treatment for your medical problem, your doctor should be told:

—if you have ever had any unusual or allergic reaction to sucralfate.

—if you are on a low-salt, low-sugar, or any other special diet, or if you are allergic to any substance, such as sulfites or other preservatives or dyes. Most medicines contain more than their active ingredient. Your doctor or pharmacist can help you avoid products that may cause a problem.

—if you are pregnant or if you intend to become pregnant while taking this medicine. Studies have not been done in humans. However, sucralfate has not been shown to cause birth defects or other problems in animal studies.

—if you are breast-feeding an infant. Although sucralfate has not been shown to cause problems in humans, the chance always exists.

—if you are now taking any of the following medicines or types of medicine:
Antacids
Cimetidine
Phenytoin
Tetracyclines
Vitamins A, D, E, or K

Proper Use of This Medicine

This medicine is best taken with water on an empty stomach 1 hour before meals and at bedtime, unless otherwise directed by your doctor. For best results, do not chew the tablets.

Take this medicine for the full time of treatment, even if you begin to feel better. Also, it is important that you keep your doctor's appointments for check-ups so that your doctor will be better able to tell you when to stop taking this medicine.

Do not take this medicine for more than 8 weeks unless your doctor has prescribed or ordered a special schedule for you.

If you miss a dose of this medicine, take it as soon as possible. However, if it is almost time for your next dose, skip the missed dose and go back to your regular dosing schedule. Do not double doses.

How to store this medicine:

• Store away from heat and direct light.

• **Keep out of the reach of children.**

• Do not store in the bathroom medicine cabinet because the heat or moisture may cause the medicine to break down.

• Do not keep outdated medicine or medicine no longer needed. Flush the contents of the container down the toilet, unless otherwise directed.

Precautions While Using This Medicine

Antacids may be taken with sucralfate to help relieve any stomach pain, unless your doctor has told you not to use them. **However, antacids should not be taken within ½ hour before or 1 hour after sucralfate.** Taking these medicines too close together may keep sucralfate from working as well.

Side Effects of This Medicine

Along with its needed effects, a medicine may cause some unwanted effects. Some side effects may occur which usually do not require medical attention. These side effects may go away during treatment as your body adjusts to the medicine. However, check with your

doctor as soon as possible if any of the following side effects continue or are bothersome:

More common
  Constipation

Less common or rare
  Backache
  Diarrhea
  Dizziness or lightheadedness
  Drowsiness
  Dryness of mouth
  Indigestion
  Nausea
  Skin rash, hives, or itching
  Stomach cramps or pain

Other side effects not listed above may also occur in some patients. If you notice any other effects, check with your doctor.

SULFONAMIDES (Systemic)

This information applies to the following medicines:

Sulfacytine (sul-fa-SYE-teen)
Sulfamethoxazole (sul-fa-meth-OX-a-zole)
Sulfamethoxazole and Trimethoprim (sul-fa-meth-OX-a-zole and trye-METH-oh-prim)
Sulfisoxazole (sul-fi-SOX-a-zole)

Some commonly used brand names or other names are:	Generic names:
Renoquid	Sulfacytine
Gantanol Methoxanol	Sulfamethoxa-zole†
Apo-Sulfatrim* Bactrim Cotrim Co-trimoxazole Novotrimel* Protrin* Roubac* Septra SMZ-TMP Sulfamethoprim	Sulfamethoxazole and Trimethoprim†

Gantrisin
Lipo Gantrisin
Novosoxazole*   Sulfisoxazole†
SK-Soxazole
Sulfafurazole

---

*Not available in the United States.
†Generic name product may also be available.

Sulfonamides (sul-FON-a-mides) or sulfa medicines belong to the general family of medicines called anti-infectives. They are taken by mouth or given by injection to help the body overcome infections. They will not work for colds, flu, or other virus infections.

Sulfonamides are available only with your doctor's prescription.

Before Using This Medicine

In order to decide on the best treatment for your medical problem, your doctor should be told:

—if you have ever had any unusual or allergic reaction to any of the sulfonamides, furosemide or thiazide diuretics (water pills), oral antidiabetic agents (diabetes medicine you take by mouth), or glaucoma medicine you take by mouth (for example, acetazolamide, dichlorphenamide, methazolamide).

—if you are on a low-salt, low-sugar, or any other special diet, or if you are allergic to any substance, such as sulfites or other preservatives or dyes. Most medicines contain more than their active ingredient, and many liquid medicines contain alcohol. Your doctor or pharmacist can help you avoid products that may cause a problem.

—if you are pregnant or if you intend to become pregnant while taking this medicine, although sulfonamides have not been shown to cause birth defects in humans. Liver problems, although possible, do not usually occur.

—if you are breast-feeding an infant. Sulfonamides pass into the breast milk in small amounts and may cause unwanted effects in the infant with glucose-6-phosphate dehydrogenase (G6PD) deficiency.

—if you have any of the following medical problems:
Glucose-6-phosphate dehydrogenase (G6PD) deficiency
Kidney disease
Liver disease
Porphyria

—if you are now taking any of the following medicines or types of medicine:
Acetaminophen
Aminobenzoic acid (PABA)
Anthralin
Anticoagulants, coumarin- or indandione-type (blood thinners)
Anticonvulsants (seizure medicine)
Antidiabetic agents, oral (diabetes medicine you take by mouth)
Antithyroid agents (medicine for overactive thyroid)
Bone marrow depressants, such as: antineoplastics (cancer medicine), azathioprine, chloramphenicol, colchicine, flucytosine, gold compounds, oxyphenbutazone, penicillamine, phenylbutazone, plicamycin, primaquine, pyrimethamine, trimethoprim
Carmustine
Chloroquine
Coal tar
Dantrolene
Dapsone
Daunorubicin
Dipyrone
Diuretics (water pills or high blood pressure medicine)
Doxorubicin
Estrogens (female hormones)
Furazolidone
Hydroxychloroquine
Ketoconazole
Mercaptopurine
Methenamine
Methotrexate
Methoxsalen
Nalidixic acid
Nitrofurantoin
Oral contraceptives (birth control pills)

Penicillins
Phenothiazines (tranquilizers)
Probenecid
Sulfinpyrazone
Sulfoxone
Tetracyclines
Trioxsalen
Valproic acid
Vitamin K

Proper Use of This Medicine

Do not give sulfonamides to infants under 1 month of age unless otherwise directed by your doctor. However, sulfacytine should not be given to children under 14 years of age.

Sulfonamides are best taken with a full glass (8 ounces) of water on an empty stomach (either 1 hour before or 2 hours after meals). **Several additional glasses of water should be taken every day,** unless otherwise directed by your doctor. Drinking extra water will help to prevent unwanted side effects of sulfonamides.

For patients taking the oral liquid form of this medicine:

• Use a specially marked measuring spoon or other device to measure each dose accurately since the average household teaspoon may not hold the right amount of liquid.

To help clear up your infection completely, **keep taking this medicine for the full time of treatment** even if you begin to feel better after a few days. If you stop taking this medicine too soon, your symptoms may return.

This medicine works best when there is a constant amount in the blood or urine. **To help keep this amount constant, do not miss any doses. Also, it is best to take each dose at evenly spaced times day and night.** For example, if you are to take 4 doses a day, each dose should be spaced about 6 hours apart. If this interferes with your sleep or other daily activities,

or if you need help in planning the best times to take your medicine, check with your doctor, nurse, or pharmacist.

If you do miss a dose of this medicine, take it as soon as possible. This will help to keep a constant amount of medicine in the blood or urine. However, if it is almost time for your next dose and your dosing schedule is:

• 2 doses a day—Space the missed dose and the next dose 5 to 6 hours apart.

• 3 or more doses a day—Space the missed dose and the next dose 2 to 4 hours apart or double your next dose.

Then go back to your regular dosing schedule.

How to store this medicine:

• Store away from heat and direct light.

• **Keep out of the reach of children.**

• Do not store in the bathroom medicine cabinet because the heat or moisture may cause the medicine to break down.

• Keep the oral liquid forms of this medicine from freezing.

• Do not keep outdated medicine or medicine no longer needed. Flush the contents of the container down the toilet, unless otherwise directed.

Precautions While Using This Medicine

It is important that your doctor check your progress at regular visits if you will be taking this medicine for a long time.

If your symptoms do not improve within a few days or if they become worse, check with your doctor.

Some people who take sulfonamides may become more sensitive to sunlight than they are normally. When you begin to take this medicine, avoid too much sun or too much use of a sunlamp until you see how you react, especially if you tend to burn easily. You may still be more sensitive to sunlight or sunlamps for many months after you stop taking this medicine. If you have a severe reaction, check with your doctor.

Before having any kind of surgery (including dental surgery) with a general anesthetic, tell the physician or dentist in charge that you are taking a sulfonamide.

Side Effects of This Medicine

Along with its needed effects, a medicine may cause some unwanted effects. Although not all of these side effects appear very often, when they do occur they may require medical attention. **Stop taking this medicine and check with your doctor immediately if any of the following side effects occur:**

More common
Itching
Skin rash

Less common
Aching of joints and muscles
Difficulty in swallowing
Pale skin
Redness, blistering, peeling, or loosening of skin
Sore throat and fever
Unusual bleeding or bruising
Unusual tiredness or weakness
Yellowing of eyes or skin

Rare
Blood in urine
Lower back pain
Pain or burning while urinating
Swelling of front part of neck

Also, check with your doctor as soon as possible if the following side effect occurs:

More common
Increased sensitivity of skin to sunlight

Other side effects may occur which usually do not require medical attention. These

side effects may go away during treatment as your body adjusts to the medicine. However, check with your doctor if any of the following side effects continue or are bothersome:

More common
Diarrhea
Dizziness
Headache
Loss of appetite
Nausea or vomiting

Other side effects not listed above may also occur in some patients. If you notice any other effects, check with your doctor.

SULFONAMIDES AND PHENAZOPYRIDINE (Systemic)

This information applies to the following medicines:

Sulfamethoxazole (sul-fa-meth-OX-a-zole) and Phenazopyridine (fen-az-oh-PEER-i-deen)
Sulfisoxazole (sul-fi-SOX-a-zole) and Phenazopyridine

Some commonly used brand names or other names are:	Generic names:
Azo Gantanol Azo Sulfamethoxazole	Sulfamethoxazole and Phenazopyridine†
Azo Gantrisin Azo-Soxazole Azo-Sulfisoxazole Suldiazo Sulfafurazole and Phenazopyridine	Sulfisoxazole and Phenazopyridine†

†Generic name product may also be available.

Sulfonamides and phenazopyridine, combination products containing a sulfa medicine and a urinary pain reliever, belong to the general family of medicines called anti-infectives. They are taken by mouth to help the body overcome infections of the urinary tract and to help relieve the pain, burning, and irritation of these infections.

Sulfonamides and phenazopyridine combinations are available only with your doctor's prescription.

For information about the precautions and side effects of the medicines in this combination, see:

Sulfonamides (Systemic)
Phenazopyridine (Systemic)

Combination products are designed for specific uses. These uses may not be the same as the uses of the individual ingredients. Therefore, some of the information provided in the individual listings may not be relevant to the combination product. If questions arise, check with your doctor, nurse, or pharmacist.

TERBUTALINE (Systemic)

Some commonly used brand names are Brethaire, Brethine, and Bricanyl.

Terbutaline (ter-BYOO-ta-leen) is taken by inhalation or mouth or given by injection to treat bronchial asthma, bronchitis, and emphysema. It relieves wheezing, shortness of breath, and troubled breathing. Terbutaline may be used for other conditions as determined by your doctor.

This medicine is available only with your doctor's prescription.

Before Using This Medicine

In order to decide on the best treatment for your medical problem, your doctor should be told:

—if you have ever had any unusual or allergic reaction to medicines like terbutaline, such as amphetamines, ephedrine, epinephrine, isoproterenol, metaproterenol, norepinephrine, phenylephrine, phenylpropanolamine, or pseudoephedrine.

—if you are on a low-salt, low-sugar, or any other special diet, or if you are allergic to any substance, such as sulfites or other preservatives or dyes. Most medicines contain more than their active ingredient. Your doctor or pharmacist can help you avoid products that may cause a problem.

—if you are pregnant or if you intend to become pregnant while taking this medicine. Studies on birth defects have not been done in humans. However, terbutaline has not been shown to cause birth defects in animal studies when given in doses many times the human dose. Terbutaline given by injection during pregnancy has been reported to cause an unusually fast heartbeat in the fetus. Also, terbutaline may delay labor.

—if you are breast-feeding an infant. Although this medicine has not been shown to cause problems in humans, the chance always exists since terbutaline passes into the breast milk.

—if you have any of the following medical problems:

Convulsions (seizures) (history of)
Diabetes mellitus (sugar diabetes)
Heart disease
High blood pressure
Overactive thyroid

—if you are now taking any of the following medicines or types of medicine:

Acebutolol
Amantadine
Amphetamines
Antihypertensives (high blood pressure medicine)
Appetite suppressants (diet pills)
Atenolol
Caffeine
Chlophedianol
Digitalis glycosides (heart medicine)
Labetalol
Levodopa
Medicine for colds, hay fever, or other allergies (including nose drops or sprays)
Methylphenidate
Metoprolol

Nadolol
Nitrates (medicine for angina)
Other medicine (including oral inhalations) for asthma or breathing problems
Pemoline
Pindolol
Propranolol
Thyroid hormones
Timolol

Proper Use of This Medicine

Take terbutaline only as directed. Do not take more of it and do not take it more often than your doctor ordered. To do so may increase the chance of serious side effects. Inhalation aerosol medicines similar to terbutaline have been reported to cause death when too much of the medicine was used.

For patients using the inhalation aerosol form of terbutaline:

• This medicine usually comes with patient directions. Read them carefully before using this medicine.

• Keep spray away from the eyes.

If you miss a dose of this medicine and remember within an hour or so of the missed dose, use it right away. However, if you do not remember until later, skip the missed dose and go back to your regular dosing schedule. Do not double doses.

How to store this medicine:

• Store away from heat.

• **Keep out of the reach of children.**

• Store the tablet form of this medicine away from direct light and the inhalation aerosol form of this medicine away from direct sunlight.

• Do not store in the bathroom medicine cabinet because the heat or moisture may cause the medicine to break down.

• Keep the inhalation aerosol form of this medicine from freezing.

• Do not puncture, break, or burn the inhalation aerosol container, even if it is empty.

• Do not keep outdated medicine or medicine no longer needed. Flush the tablet form of this medicine down the toilet, unless otherwise directed.

Precautions While Using This Medicine

If you still have trouble breathing after taking this medicine, or if your condition gets worse, check with your doctor at once.

For patients using the inhalation aerosol form of terbutaline:

• If you are also using the inhalation aerosol form of an adrenocorticoid (cortisone-like medicine, such as beclomethasone, dexamethasone, flunisolide, or triamcinolone), **allow 15 minutes between using the terbutaline and an adrenocorticoid,** unless otherwise directed by your doctor. This will help to reduce the possibility of side effects.

Side Effects of This Medicine

Along with its needed effects, a medicine may cause some unwanted effects. Although not all of these side effects appear very often, when they do occur they may require medical attention. Check with your doctor as soon as possible if any of the following side effects occur:

Possible signs of overdose
   Dizziness (severe)
   Drowsiness (severe)
   Headache (continuing or severe)
   Increase in blood pressure (severe)
   Muscle cramps (severe)
   Nausea or vomiting (continuing)
   Unusually fast or pounding heartbeat (continuing)
   Unusual nervousness or restlessness
   Weakness (severe)

Other side effects may occur which usually do not require medical attention. These side effects may go away during treatment as your body adjusts to the medicine. However, check with your doctor if

any of the following side effects continue or are bothersome:

More common

Nervousness
Restlessness
Trembling

Less common

Dizziness or lightheadedness
Drowsiness
Headache
Increase in blood pressure
Muscle cramps or twitching
Nausea or vomiting
Unusual increase in sweating
Unusually fast or pounding heartbeat
Weakness

The above side effects are more likely to occur in elderly patients, who are usually more sensitive to the effects of terbutaline.

Other side effects not listed above may also occur in some patients. If you notice any other effects, check with your doctor.

TERPIN HYDRATE (Systemic)

Terpin hydrate (TER-pin HYE-drate) is taken by mouth to relieve coughs due to colds and mild bronchial irritations. It may also loosen mucus or phlegm (pronounced flem) in the lungs.

This medicine is usually not used for the chronic cough that occurs with smoking, asthma, or emphysema or when there is an unusually large amount of mucus or phlegm with the cough.

Terpin hydrate elixir has a very high alcohol content. Do not give this medicine to children up to 12 years of age without first checking with your doctor.

Terpin hydrate is available without a prescription; however, your doctor may have special instructions on the proper dose of this medicine for your medical condition.

Before Using This Medicine

Before you use this medicine, check with your doctor or pharmacist:

—if you have ever had any unusual or allergic reaction to terpin hydrate.

—if you are on a low-salt, low-sugar, or any other special diet, or if you are allergic to any substance, such as sulfites or other preservatives or dyes. Most medicines contain more than their active ingredient, and many liquid medicines contain alcohol. Your doctor or pharmacist can help you avoid products that may cause a problem.

—if you are pregnant or if you intend to become pregnant while using this medicine. This medicine contains 42.5% of alcohol. Too much use of alcohol during pregnancy may cause birth defects. In addition, although terpin hydrate has not been shown to cause birth defects or other problems in humans, the chance always exists.

—if you are breast-feeding an infant. The alcohol in this medicine passes into the breast milk. Although the amount of alcohol in recommended doses of this medicine does not usually cause problems in humans, the chance always exists.

—if you are now taking any central nervous system (CNS) depressants, such as:

Anticonvulsants (seizure medicine)
Antihistamines or medicine for hay fever, other allergies, or colds
Barbiturates
Muscle relaxants
Narcotics
Prescription pain medicine
Sedatives, tranquilizers, or sleeping medicine

—if you are now taking tricyclic antidepressants, such as:

Amitriptyline
Amoxapine
Clomipramine
Desipramine

Doxepin
Imipramine
Nortriptyline
Protriptyline
Trimipramine

Proper Use of This Medicine

Take this medicine only as directed. Do not take more of it and do not take it more often than recommended on the label, unless otherwise directed by your doctor. If too much is taken, it may become habit-forming since this medicine contains a large amount of alcohol.

To help loosen mucus or phlegm (flem) in the lungs, **drink a glass of water after each dose of this medicine,** unless otherwise directed by your doctor.

If you must take this medicine regularly and you miss a dose, take it as soon as possible. However, if it is almost time for your next dose, skip the missed dose and go back to your regular dosing schedule. Do not double doses.

How to store this medicine:

• Store away from heat and direct light.

• **Keep out of the reach of children.**

• Do not store in the bathroom medicine cabinet because the heat or moisture may cause the medicine to break down.

• Keep this medicine from freezing.

• Do not keep outdated medicine or medicine no longer needed. Flush the contents of the container down the toilet, unless otherwise directed.

Precautions While Using This Medicine

If your cough has not improved after 7 days or if you have a high fever, skin rash, continuing headache, or sore throat with the cough, check with your doctor. These signs may mean that you have other medical problems.

If crystals form in this solution, dissolve them by warming the closed container of solution in warm water and then gently shaking it.

The alcohol in this medicine will add to the effects of other alcohol and CNS depressants (medicines that slow down the nervous system, possibly causing drowsiness). Some examples of CNS depressants are antihistamines or medicine for hay fever, other allergies, or colds; sedatives, tranquilizers, or sleeping medicine; prescription pain medicine or narcotics; barbiturates; medicine for seizures; muscle relaxants; or anesthetics, including some dental anesthetics. **Check with your doctor before taking any of the above while you are using this medicine.**

Side Effects of This Medicine

Along with its needed effects, a medicine may cause some unwanted effects. Although no serious side effects have been reported for terpin hydrate, the following side effects may be noticed by some patients. Check with your doctor if any of these effects continue or are bothersome:

Less common or rare
    Nausea
    Stomach pain
    Vomiting

Other side effects not listed above may also occur in some patients. If you notice any other effects, check with your doctor.

TETRACYCLINES (Systemic)

This information applies to the following medicines:

Demeclocycline (dem-e-kloe-SYE-kleen)
Doxycycline (dox-i-SYE-kleen)

Methacycline (meth-a-SYE-kleen)
Minocycline (mi-noe-SYE-kleen)
Oxytetracycline (ox-i-te-tra-SYE-kleen)
Tetracycline (te-tra-SYE-kleen)

Some commonly used brand names are:	Generic names:
Declomycin	Demeclocycline
Doxy Doxy-Caps Doxychel Doxy-Tabs Vibramycin Vibra-Tabs	Doxycycline†
Rondomycin	Methacycline
Minocin	Minocycline
Terramycin	Oxytetracycline†
Achromycin Achromycin V Bristacycline Cefracycline* Cyclopar Kesso-Tetra Medicycline* Neo-Tetrine* Novotetra* Panmycin Retet-S Robitet SK-Tetracycline Sumycin Tetracyn Tetralean* Tetrex Tetrex-S	Tetracycline†

*Not available in the United States.
†Generic name product may also be available.

Tetracyclines belong to the general family of medicines called antibiotics. They are taken by mouth or given by injection to help the body overcome infections. They are also taken by mouth to help control acne. Demeclocycline and doxycycline may also be used for other problems as determined by your doctor. Tetracyclines will not work for colds, flu, or other virus infections.

Tetracyclines are available only with your doctor's prescription.

Before Using This Medicine

In order to decide on the best treatment for your medical problem, your doctor should be told:

—if you have ever had any unusual or allergic reaction to any of the tetracyclines or combination medicines containing a tetracycline.

—if you have ever had any unusual or allergic reaction to lidocaine, procaine, or other "caine-type" anesthetics (medicines which cause numbing) (applies only to oxytetracycline and tetracycline given by injection into the muscle).

—if you are pregnant or if you intend to become pregnant while taking this medicine. Use is not recommended during the last half of pregnancy. Tetracyclines may cause the unborn infant's teeth to become discolored and may slow down the growth of the infant's teeth and bones if they are taken during that time. In addition, liver problems may occur in pregnant women, especially those receiving high doses by injection into a vein.

—if you are breast-feeding an infant. Use is not recommended since tetracyclines pass into the breast milk. They may cause the infant's teeth to become discolored and may slow down the growth of the infant's teeth and bones. They may also cause increased sensitivity of the infant's skin to sunlight and fungal infections of the mouth and vagina. In addition, minocycline may cause dizziness, lightheadedness, or unsteadiness in the infant.

—if you have either of the following medical problems:
> Kidney disease (does not apply to
>   doxycycline or minocycline)
> Liver disease

—if you have diabetes insipidus (water diabetes) and you are taking demeclocycline.

—if you are now taking any of the tetracyclines and are also taking any of the following medicines or types of medicine:

Aminosalicylate calcium
Antacids
Calcium supplements such as calcium gluconate, calcium lactate, or dicalcium phosphate
Choline and magnesium salicylates
Colestipol
Iron supplements
Laxatives (magnesium-containing)
Magnesium salicylate
Penicillins
Sodium bicarbonate (baking soda)

—if you are now taking demeclocycline and are also taking desmopressin.

—if you are now taking doxycycline and are also taking any of the following medicines or types of medicine:

Barbiturates
Carbamazepine
Phenytoin

Proper Use of This Medicine

To help clear up your infection completely, **keep taking this medicine for the full time of treatment** even if you begin to feel better after a few days. If you stop taking this medicine too soon, your symptoms may return.

This medicine works best when there is a constant amount in the blood or urine. **To help keep this amount constant, do not miss any doses. Also, it is best to take each dose at evenly spaced times day and night.** For example, if you are to take 4 doses a day, each dose should be spaced about 6 hours apart. If this interferes with your sleep or other daily activities, or if you need help in planning the best times to take your medicine, check with your doctor, nurse, or pharmacist.

If you do miss a dose of this medicine, take it as soon as possible. This will help to keep a constant amount of medicine in the blood or urine. However, if it is almost time for your next dose and your dosing schedule is:

• 1 dose a day (for example, for acne)— Space the missed dose and the next dose 10 to 12 hours apart.

• 2 doses a day—Space the missed dose and the next dose 5 to 6 hours apart.

• 3 or more doses a day—Space the missed dose and the next dose 2 to 4 hours apart or double your next dose.

Then go back to your regular dosing schedule.

Do not give tetracyclines to infants or children under 8 years of age unless directed by your doctor since they may cause permanently discolored teeth and other problems.

Tetracyclines should be taken with a full glass (8 ounces) of water to prevent irritation of the esophagus (tube between the throat and stomach) or stomach. In addition, most tetracyclines (except doxycycline and minocycline) are best taken on an empty stomach (either 1 hour before or 2 hours after meals). However, if this medicine still upsets your stomach, your doctor may want you to take it with food.

Do not take milk, milk formulas, or other dairy products within 1 to 2 hours of the time you take tetracyclines (except doxycycline and minocycline) by mouth since they may keep this medicine from working as well.

If this medicine has changed color, taste, or looks different, has become outdated (old), has been stored incorrectly (too warm or too damp), or otherwise appears to have broken down, do not use it. To do so may cause serious side effects. Discard by flushing it down the toilet. If you have any questions about this, check with your doctor or pharmacist.

For patients taking the oral liquid form of this medicine:

• Use a specially marked measuring spoon or other device to measure each dose accurately, since the average household teaspoon may not hold the right amount of liquid.

• Do not use after the expiration date on the label since the medicine may not work as well. Check with your pharmacist if you have any questions about this.

For patients taking doxycycline or minocycline:

• These medicines may be taken with food or milk if they upset your stomach.

How to store this medicine:

• Store away from heat and direct light, out of the reach of children.

• Do not store in the bathroom medicine cabinet because the heat or moisture may cause the medicine to break down.

• Keep the the oral liquid forms of this medicine from freezing.

• Do not keep outdated medicine or medicine no longer needed. Flush it down the toilet.

Precautions While Using This Medicine

If your symptoms do not improve within a few days (or a few weeks or months for acne patients) or if they become worse, check with your doctor.

Do not take aminosalicylate calcium; antacids; calcium supplements such as calcium gluconate, calcium lactate, or dicalcium phosphate; choline and magnesium salicylates combination; magnesium salicylate; magnesium-containing laxatives such as Epsom salt; or sodium bicarbonate (baking soda) within 1 to 2 hours of the time you take any of the tetracyclines by mouth. In addition, do not take iron preparations (included also in some vitamin preparations) within 2 to 3 hours of the time you take tetracyclines by mouth. To do so may keep this medicine from working as well.

Before having surgery (including dental surgery) with a general anesthetic, tell the physician or dentist in charge that you are taking a tetracycline. This does not apply to doxycycline, however.

Some people who take tetracyclines may become more sensitive to sunlight than they are normally. **When you first begin taking this medicine, avoid too much sun or too much use of a sunlamp until you see how you react,** especially if you tend to burn easily. You may still be more sensitive to sunlight or sunlamps for 2 weeks to several months or more after stopping this medicine. **If you have a severe reaction, check with your doctor.**

For patients taking minocycline:

• In addition to the precautions mentioned above, minocycline may cause some people to become dizzy, lightheaded, or unsteady. **Make sure you know how you react to this medicine before you drive, use machines, or do other jobs that require you to be alert.** If these reactions are especially bothersome, check with your doctor.

Side Effects of This Medicine

Along with its needed effects, a medicine may cause some unwanted effects. In some infants and children, tetracyclines may cause the teeth to become discolored. Even though this may not happen right away, check with your doctor as soon as possible if you notice this effect or if you have any questions about it.

Also, check with your doctor as soon as possible if the following side effects occur:

Less common with demeclocycline
   Greatly increased frequency of urination or amount of urine
   Unusual thirst
   Unusual tiredness or weakness
Less common with minocycline
   Pigmentation (darker color or discoloration) of skin and mucous membranes

Other side effects may occur which usually do not require medical attention. These side effects may go away during treatment as your body adjusts to the medicine. However, check with your doctor if any of the following side effects continue or are bothersome:

More common with all tetracyclines
   Cramps or burning of the stomach
   Diarrhea
   Increased sensitivity of skin to sunlight (rare with minocycline)
   Itching of the rectal or genital (sex organ) areas
   Nausea or vomiting
   Sore mouth or tongue
More common with minocycline
   Dizziness, lightheadedness, or unsteadiness

In some patients tetracyclines may cause the tongue to become darkened or discolored. This is only temporary and will go away when you stop taking this medicine.

Other side effects not listed above may also occur in some patients. If you notice any other effects, check with your doctor.

THEOPHYLLINE AND GUAIFENESIN (Systemic)

Some commonly used brand names are:

Asbron G	Glyceryl T
Inlay-Tabs	Lanophyllin-GG
Bronchial	Quibron
Elixophyllin-GG	Slo-Phyllin GG
Synophylate-GG	Theolair-Plus
Theocolate	Theolate

Generic name product may also be available.

Theophylline (thee-OFF-i-lin) and guaifenesin (gwye-FEN-e-sin) combination is taken by mouth to treat the symptoms of bronchial asthma, chronic bronchitis, emphysema, and other lung diseases. This medicine relieves cough, wheezing, shortness of breath, and troubled breathing. It works by opening up the bronchial tubes or air passages of the lungs and increasing the flow of air through them.

This medicine is available only with your doctor's prescription.

For information about the precautions and side effects of the medicines in this combination, see:

   Xanthine-derivative Bronchodilators (Systemic)
   Guaifenesin (Systemic)

Combination products are designed for specific uses. These uses may not be the same as the uses of the individual ingredients. Therefore, some of the information provided in the individual listings may not be relevant to the combination product. If questions arise, check with your doctor, nurse, or pharmacist.

THIOXANTHENES (Systemic)

This information applies to the following medicines:

Chlorprothixene (klor-proe-THIX-een)
Thiothixene (thye-oh-THIX-een)

Some commonly used brand names are:	Generic names:
Taractan	
Tarasan*	Chlorprothixene

Navane	Thiothixene

*Not available in the United States.

This medicine belongs to the general family of medicines known as thioxanthenes. It is used in the treatment of nervous, mental, and emotional conditions. Improvement in such conditions is thought to result from the effect of the medicine on nerve pathways in specific areas of the brain. The thioxanthene medicines are usually taken by mouth, but may be given by injection when necessary.

Thioxanthene medicines are available only with your doctor's prescription.

Before Using This Medicine

In order to decide on the best treatment for your medical problem, your doctor should be told:

—if you have ever had any unusual or allergic reaction to other thioxanthene or phenothiazine medicines.

—if you are on a low-salt, low-sugar, or any other special diet, or if you are allergic to any substance, such as sulfites or other preservatives or dyes. Most medicines contain more than their active ingredient, and many liquid medicines contain alcohol. Your doctor or pharmacist can help you avoid products that may cause a problem.

—if you are pregnant or if you intend to become pregnant while taking this medicine. Studies have not been done in humans. Although animal studies have not shown thioxanthenes to cause birth defects, the studies have shown that they caused a decrease in fertility and a reduced number of successful pregnancies.

—if you are breast-feeding an infant. Although thioxanthenes have not been shown to cause problems in humans, the chance always exists. It is not known if thioxanthenes pass into the breast milk.

—if you have any of the following medical problems:

Alcoholism
Blood disease
Enlarged prostate
Glaucoma
Heart or blood vessel disease
Liver disease
Lung disease
Parkinson's disease
Reye's syndrome
Stomach ulcers
Urination problems

—if you are now taking any of the following medicines or types of medicine:

Amphetamines
Antacids
Anticonvulsants (seizure medicine)
Antimuscarinics (medicine for abdominal or stomach spasms or cramps)
Aspirin or other salicylates
Bromocriptine
Bumetanide
Capreomycin
Cisplatin
Diarrhea medicine
Epinephrine
Ethacrynic acid
Furosemide
High blood pressure medicine
Levodopa
Papaverine
Paromomycin
Phenothiazines
Quinine
Stomach ulcer medicine
Vancomycin

—if you are now taking central nervous system (CNS) depressants, such as:

Alcohol
Antihistamines or medicine for hay fever, other allergies, or colds
Barbiturates
Muscle relaxants
Narcotics
Prescription pain medicine
Sedatives, tranquilizers, or sleeping medicine

—if you are now taking tricyclic antidepressants (medicine for depression), such as:

Amitriptyline
Amoxapine

Clomipramine
Desipramine
Doxepin
Imipramine
Nortriptyline
Protriptyline
Trimipramine

—if you are now taking or have taken within the past 2 weeks monoamine oxidase (MAO) inhibitors, such as:

Furazolidone
Isocarboxazid
Pargyline
Phenelzine
Procarbazine
Tranylcypromine

—if you are now taking aminoglycosides by injection (medicine for serious infection), such as:

Amikacin
Gentamicin
Kanamycin
Neomycin
Netilmicin
Streptomycin
Tobramycin

Proper Use of This Medicine

This medicine may be taken with food or a full glass (8 ounces) of water or milk to reduce stomach irritation. Liquid forms of this medicine may be taken undiluted or mixed with milk, water, fruit juice, or carbonated beverages.

Do not take more of this medicine or take it more often than your doctor ordered. This is particularly important when it is given to children, since they may react very strongly to the effects of the medicine.

Sometimes this medicine must be taken for several weeks before its full effect is reached in the treatment of certain mental and emotional conditions.

If you miss a dose of this medicine, take it as soon as possible. However, if it is within 2 hours of your next dose, skip the missed dose and go back to your regular dosing schedule. Do not double doses.

How to store this medicine:

• Store away from heat and direct light.

• **Keep out of the reach of children.**

• Do not store in the bathroom medicine cabinet because the heat or moisture may cause the medicine to break down.

• Keep the liquid from freezing.

• Do not keep outdated medicine or medicine no longer needed. Flush the contents of the container down the toilet, unless otherwise directed.

Precautions While Using This Medicine

Your doctor should check your progress at regular visits. This will allow the dosage of the medicine to be adjusted when necessary and also reduce the possibility of side effects.

Do not stop taking this medicine without first checking with your doctor. If you suddenly stop taking this medicine you may have side effects and your medical condition may become worse. Your doctor may want you to gradually reduce the amount you are taking before stopping completely.

This medicine will add to the effects of alcohol and other CNS depressants (medicines that slow down the nervous system, possibly causing drowsiness). Some examples of CNS depressants are antihistamines or medicine for hay fever, other allergies, or colds; sedatives, tranquilizers, or sleeping medicine; prescription pain medicine or narcotics; barbiturates; medicine for seizures; muscle relaxants; or anesthetics, including some dental anesthetics. **Check with your doctor before taking any such depressants while you are using this medicine.**

Do not take this medicine within an hour of taking antacids or medicine for diarrhea. Taking them too close together may make this medicine less effective.

This medicine may cause some people to become drowsy or less alert than they are normally, especially during the first few weeks the medicine is being taken. Even if you take this medicine only at bedtime, you may feel drowsy or less alert on arising. **Make sure you know how you react to this medicine before you drive, use machines, or do other jobs that require you to be alert.**

Dizziness, lightheadedness, or fainting may occur, especially when you get up from a lying or sitting position. Getting up slowly may help. If the problem continues or gets worse, check with your doctor.

Sometimes, patients may show signs of restlessness and excitement after taking this medicine. If this occurs, stop taking the medicine and check with your doctor.

This medicine will often make you sweat less, allowing your body temperature to increase. **Use extra care not to become overheated during exercise or hot weather while you are taking this medicine,** since overheating could possibly result in heat stroke. Also, hot baths or saunas may make you feel dizzy or faint while you are taking this medicine.

A few people who take this medicine may become more sensitive to sunlight than they are normally. When you first begin taking this medicine, avoid too much sun or too much use of a sunlamp until you see how you react. If you have a severe reaction, check with your doctor.

Your mouth may feel very dry while you are taking this medicine. To keep your mouth comfortably moist, chew sugarless gum, melt bits of ice in your mouth, or use a saliva substitute as often as necessary.

Try to avoid getting liquid forms of this medicine on the skin or clothing. Skin rash and irritation have been caused by similar medicines.

Side Effects of This Medicine

Along with its needed effects, a medicine may cause some unwanted effects. Although not all of these side effects appear very often, when they do occur they may require medical attention. **Stop taking this medicine and get emergency help immediately** if any of the following side effects occur:

Rare
    Convulsions (seizures)
    Difficulty in breathing
    Fever
    High or low (irregular) blood pressure
    Increased sweating
    Loss of bladder control
    Muscle stiffness (severe)
    Unusual feeling of tiredness
    Unusually fast heartbeat
    Unusually pale skin

Also, check with your doctor as soon as possible if any of the following side effects occur:

More common
    Blurred vision or other eye problems
    Difficulty in talking or swallowing
    Fainting
    Loss of balance control
    Mask-like face
    Muscle spasms, especially of neck and
        back
    Restlessness or desire to keep moving
    Shuffling walk
    Stiffness of arms and legs
    Trembling and shaking of hands and
        fingers
    Unusual fixation of eyes
    Unusual twisting movements of body

Less common
    Chewing movements
    Difficult urination
    Lip smacking or puckering

Puffing of cheeks
Rapid or worm-like movements of tongue
Skin discoloration
Skin rash
Unusual, uncontrolled movements of
arms and legs
Rare
Sore throat and fever
Yellowing of eyes and skin
Signs of overdose
Dizziness (severe)
Drowsiness (severe)
Muscle trembling, jerking, stiffness, or
uncontrolled movements (severe)
Unusual excitement
Unusually small pupils
Unusual tiredness or weakness (severe)

Other side effects may occur which usually
do not require medical attention. These
side effects may go away during treatment as your body adjusts to the medicine. However, check with your doctor if
any of the following side effects continue or are bothersome:

More common
Constipation
Decreased sweating
Dizziness, lightheadedness, or fainting
Drowsiness (mild)
Dry mouth
Increased sensitivity of skin to sunlight
Nasal congestion
Less common
Changes in menstrual period
Decreased sexual ability
Swelling of breasts

After you stop taking this medicine your
body may need time to adjust, especially
if you took this medicine in high doses or
for a long period of time. If you stop
taking it too quickly, the following withdrawal effects may occur and should be
reported to your doctor:

*Possible effects of stopping medicine
too quickly*
Dizziness
Nausea and vomiting
Trembling of fingers and hands

Stomach pain
Uncontrolled, continuing movements of
mouth, tongue, or jaw

Although not all of the side effects listed
above have been reported for both chlorprothixene and thiothixene, they have
been reported for at least one of them.
However, since chlorprothixene and
thiothixene are very similar, any of the
above side effects may occur with either
of these medicines.

The above side effects, especially constipation, dizziness or fainting, drowsiness,
dry mouth, uncontrolled movements of
the mouth and tongue, and trembling of
fingers and hands are more likely to occur in the elderly, who are usually more
sensitive to the effects of thioxanthenes.

Other side effects not listed above may also
occur in some patients. If you notice any
other effects, check with your doctor.

THYROID HORMONES (Systemic)

This information applies to the following medicines:

Levothyroxine (lee-voe-thye-ROX-een)
Liothyronine (lye-oh-THYE-roe-neen)
Liotrix (LYE-oh-trix)
Thyroglobulin (thye-roe-GLOB-yoo-lin)
Thyroid (THYE-roid)

This information does not apply to Thyrotropin.

Some commonly used brand names are:	Generic names:
Levothroid Noroxine Synthroid	Levothyroxine
Cytomel	Liothyronine
Euthroid Thyrolar	Liotrix

Proloid	Thyroglobulin
	Thyroid†

†Generic name product may also be available.

Thyroid medicines belong to the general group of medicines called hormones. They are used when the thyroid gland does not produce enough hormone.

These medicines are available only with your doctor's prescription.

Before Using This Medicine

In order to decide on the best treatment for your medical problem, your doctor should be told:

—if you have ever had any unusual or allergic reaction to thyroid medicine.

—if you are on a low-salt, low-sugar, or any other special diet, or if you are allergic to any substance, such as sulfites or other preservatives or dyes. Most medicines contain more than their active ingredient. Your doctor or pharmacist can help you avoid products that may cause a problem.

—if you are pregnant or if you intend to become pregnant while you are using this medicine. It is essential that your baby receives the right amount of thyroid for normal development. Although use of thyroid hormones has not been shown to cause problems, you may need to take different amounts while you are pregnant. In addition, you may respond differently than usual to some tests. Your doctor should check your progress at regular visits while you are pregnant.

—if you are breast-feeding an infant. Although thyroid hormones have not been shown to cause problems in humans, the chance always exists.

—if you have any of the following medical problems:

Diabetes mellitus (sugar diabetes)
Hardening of the arteries
Heart disease
High blood pressure
History of overactive thyroid
Kidney disease
Underactive adrenal gland
Underactive pituitary gland

—if you are now taking or have recently taken any other medicines, including:

Acebutolol
Adrenocorticoids (cortisone-like medicine)
Anticoagulants, oral (blood thinners you take by mouth)
Antidiabetics, oral (diabetes medicine you take by mouth)
Atenolol
Barbiturates
Carbamazepine
Cholestyramine
Colestipol
Cough syrup or cold medicine
Estrogens
Insulin
Labetalol
Metoprolol
Nadolol
Oral contraceptives (birth control pills)
Oxprenolol
Phenytoin
Pindolol
Primidone
Propranolol
Rifampin
Sotalol
Timolol
Tricyclic antidepressants (medicine for depression)

Proper Use of This Medicine

Use this medicine only as directed by your doctor. Do not use more or less of it, and do not use it more often than your doctor ordered. Your doctor has prescribed the exact amount your body needs and if you take different amounts, you may experience symptoms of an overactive or underactive thyroid. Take it at the same time each day to make sure it always has the same effect.

If your condition is due to a lack of thyroid hormone, you may have to take this medicine for the rest of your life. It is very important that you **do not stop taking this medicine without first checking with your doctor.**

If you miss a dose of this medicine, take it as soon as possible. However, if it is almost time for your next dose, skip the missed dose and go back to your regular dosing schedule. Do not double doses. If you miss more than 2 or 3 doses or if you have any questions about this, check with your doctor.

How to store this medicine:

• Store away from heat and direct light.

• **Keep out of the reach of children.**

• Do not store in the bathroom medicine cabinet because the heat or moisture may cause the medicine to break down.

• Do not keep outdated medicine or medicine no longer needed. Flush the contents of the container down the toilet, unless otherwise directed.

Precautions While Using This Medicine

It is very important that your doctor check your progress at regular visits, in order to make sure that this medicine is working properly.

If you have some kinds of heart disease, this medicine may cause chest pain or shortness of breath when you exert yourself. Do not overdo exercise or physical work. If you have any questions about this, check with your doctor.

Before having any kind of surgery (including dental surgery) or emergency treatment, **tell the doctor or dentist in charge that you are taking this medicine.**

Do not take any other medicine unless prescribed by your doctor. Some medicines may increase or decrease the effects of thyroid on your body and cause problems in controlling your condition. Also,

thyroid may change the effects of other medicines.

Side Effects of This Medicine

Along with its needed effects, a medicine may cause some unwanted effects. Although not all of these side effects appear very often, when they do occur they may require medical attention. Check with your doctor as soon as possible if any of the following side effects occur since they may indicate an overdose or an allergic reaction:

Rare
    Headache (severe) in children
    Hives
    Skin rash

Possible signs of overdose
    Chest pain
    Rapid or irregular heartbeat
    Shortness of breath

This medicine may take a few days or weeks to have a noticeable effect on your condition. Until it begins to work, you may experience no change in your symptoms. Check with your doctor if the following symptoms continue:
    Clumsiness
    Coldness
    Constipation
    Dry, puffy skin
    Listlessness
    Muscle aches
    Sleepiness
    Tiredness
    Unusual weight gain
    Weakness

Other effects may occur if the dose of the medicine is not exactly right. These side effects will go away when the dose is corrected. Check with your doctor if any of the following symptoms occur:
    Changes in appetite
    Changes in menstrual periods
    Diarrhea
    Fever
    Hand tremors
    Headache

Irritability
Leg cramps
Nervousness
Sensitivity to heat
Sleeplessness
Unusual sweating
Vomiting
Weight loss

Other side effects not listed above may also occur in some patients. If you notice any other effects, check with your doctor.

TIMOLOL (Ophthalmic)

A commonly used brand name is Timoptic.

Timolol (TYE-moe-lole) is used in the eye to treat certain types of glaucoma. It works by lowering the pressure in the eye.

This medicine is available only with your doctor's prescription.

Before Using This Medicine

In order to decide on the best treatment for your medical problem, your doctor should be told:

—if you have ever had any unusual or allergic reaction to timolol.

—if you are allergic to any substance, such as certain preservatives. Most medicines contain more than their active ingredient. Your doctor or pharmacist can help you avoid products that may cause a problem.

—if you are pregnant or if you intend to become pregnant while using this medicine, since ophthalmic timolol may be absorbed into the body. Studies on birth defects have not been done in humans. However, studies in animals have not shown that timolol causes birth defects. Studies in animals have shown that timolol delays the formation of bone and increases the chance of death in the animal fetus when given in doses many times the maximum recommended human oral dose.

—if you are breast-feeding an infant, since this medicine may be absorbed into the body. Although ophthalmic timolol has not been shown to cause problems in humans, the chance always exists.

—if you have any of the following medical problems:

Asthma, chronic bronchitis, or emphysema
Diabetes mellitus (sugar diabetes)
Heart disease
Myasthenia gravis
Overactive thyroid

—if you are now using any of the following medicines or types of medicine:

Acebutolol
Antidiabetic agents, oral (diabetes medicine you take by mouth)
Antihypertensives (high blood pressure medicine)
Atenolol
Diazoxide
Digitalis glycosides (heart medicine)
Insulin
Labetalol
Lidocaine
Medicine for asthma or other breathing problems
Medicine for colds, hay fever, or other allergies (including nose drops or sprays)
Metoprolol
Nadolol
Phenothiazines (tranquilizers)
Pindolol
Propranolol
Timolol taken by mouth
Verapamil

Proper Use of This Medicine

Use this medicine only as directed. Do not use more of it and do not use it more often than your doctor ordered. To do so may increase the chance of too much medicine being absorbed into the body and the chance of side effects.

How to apply this medicine: First, wash hands. With middle finger, apply pressure to the inside corner of the eye (and continue to apply pressure for 1 or 2 minutes after the medicine has been placed in the eye). Tilt head back and with the index finger of the same hand, pull the lower eyelid away from eye to form a pouch. Drop the medicine into the pouch and gently close eyes. Do not blink. Keep eyes closed for 1 or 2 minutes to allow the medicine to be absorbed.

To prevent contamination of the eye drops, do not touch the applicator tip to any surface (including the eye) and keep the container tightly closed.

If you miss a dose of this medicine and your dosing schedule is one dose to be applied:

Once a day—
Apply the missed dose as soon as possible. However, if you do not remember the missed dose until the next day, skip it and apply your regularly scheduled dose.

More than once a day—
Apply the missed dose as soon as possible. However, if it is almost time for your next dose, skip the missed dose and apply your next dose at the regularly scheduled time. Then continue with your regular dosing schedule.

How to store this medicine:

• Store away from heat and direct light.

• **Keep out of the reach of children.**

• Do not store in the bathroom medicine cabinet because the heat or moisture may cause the medicine to break down.

• Keep the medicine from freezing.

• Do not keep outdated medicine or medicine no longer needed. Flush the contents of the container down the toilet, unless otherwise directed.

Precautions While Using This Medicine

Your doctor should check your eye pressure at regular visits in order to make certain that your glaucoma is being controlled.

Before having any kind of surgery (including dental surgery) or emergency treatment, tell the physician or dentist in charge that you are using this medicine.

Diabetics—**This medicine may cause your blood sugar levels to fall. Also, this medicine may cover up signs of hypoglycemia (low blood sugar),** such as change in pulse rate or increased blood pressure. If you have any questions about this, check with your doctor.

Side Effects of This Medicine

Along with its needed effects, a medicine may cause some unwanted effects. Although not all of these side effects appear very often, when they do occur they may require medical attention. Check with your doctor as soon as possible if any of the following side effects occur:

Irritation of eye or changes in vision
Skin rash or hives

Signs of too much medicine being absorbed into the body

Confusion or mental depression
Headache or dizziness
Irregular heartbeat
Nausea or feeling faint
Unusually slow or pounding heartbeat
Unusual tiredness or weakness
Wheezing or troubled breathing

Other side effects not listed above may also occur in some patients. If you notice any other effects, check with your doctor.

TOCAINIDE (Systemic)
A commonly used brand name is Tonocard.

Tocainide (toe-KAY-nide) belongs to the group of medicines known as antiarrhythmics. It is taken by mouth to correct irregular heartbeats to a normal rhythm.

Tocainide produces its helpful effects by slowing nerve impulses in the heart and making the heart tissue less sensitive.

Tocainide is available only with your doctor's prescription.

Before Using This Medicine

In order to decide on the best treatment for your medical problem, your doctor should be told:

—if you have ever had any unusual or allergic reaction to tocainide or anesthetics.

—if you are on a low-salt, low-sugar, or any other special diet, or if you are allergic to any substance, such as sulfites or other preservatives or dyes. Most medicines contain more than their active ingredient. Your doctor or pharmacist can help you avoid products that may cause a problem.

—if you are pregnant or if you intend to become pregnant while using this medicine. Although tocainide has not been shown to cause birth defects or other problems in humans, the chance always exists. Studies in animals have shown that high doses of tocainide may increase the possibility of death in the animal fetus, although it has not been shown to cause birth defects.

—if you are breast-feeding an infant. Although it is not known whether tocainide passes into breast milk and it has not been shown to cause problems in humans, the chance always exists.

—if you have either of the following medical problems:
Kidney disease
Liver disease

—if you are now taking any of the following medicines or types of medicine:
Antineoplastics (cancer medicine)
Azathioprine
Beta-adrenergic blocking agents (acebutolol, atenolol, labetalol, metoprolol, nadolol, oxprenolol, pindolol, propranolol, sotalol, or timolol)
Chloramphenicol
Colchicine
Flucytosine
Other heart medicine
Oxyphenbutazone
Penicillamine
Phenylbutazone
Primaquine
Pyrimethamine
Trimethoprim

Proper Use of This Medicine

Take tocainide exactly as directed by your doctor, even though you may feel well. Do not take more medicine than ordered.

If tocainide upsets your stomach, your doctor may advise you to take it with food or milk.

This medicine works best when there is a constant amount in the blood. **To help keep this amount constant, do not miss any doses. Also, it is best to take each dose at evenly spaced times day and night.** For example, if you are to take 3 doses a day, the doses should be spaced about 8 hours apart. If this interferes with your sleep or other daily activities, or if you need help in planning the best times to take your medicine, check with your doctor, nurse, or pharmacist.

If you miss a dose of tocainide and remember within 4 hours, take it as soon as possible. Then go back to your regular dosing schedule. However, if you do not remember until later, skip the missed dose and go back to your regular dosing schedule. Do not double doses.

How to store this medicine:

- Store away from heat and direct light.
- **Keep out of the reach of children.**
- Do not store in the bathroom medicine cabinet because the heat or moisture may cause the medicine to break down.
- Do not keep outdated medicine or medicine no longer needed. Flush the contents of the container down the toilet, unless otherwise directed.

Precautions While Using This Medicine

It is important that your doctor check your progress at regular visits to make sure the medicine is working properly. This will allow for changes to be made in the amount of medicine you are taking, if necessary.

Your doctor may want you to carry a medical identification card or bracelet stating that you are using this medicine.

Tocainide may cause some people to become dizzy, lightheaded, or less alert than they are normally. **Make sure you know how you react to this medicine before you drive, use machines, or do other jobs that require you to be alert.**

Before having any kind of surgery (including dental surgery) or emergency treatment, tell the physician or dentist in charge that you are taking this medicine.

Side Effects of This Medicine

Along with its needed effects, a medicine may cause some unwanted effects. Although not all of these side effects appear very often, when they do occur they may require medical attention. Check with your doctor as soon as possible if any of the following side effects occur:

Less common
  Trembling or shaking

Rare
  Cough or shortness of breath
  Fever, chills, or sore throat

Irregular heartbeats
Unusual bleeding or bruising

Other side effects may occur which usually do not require medical attention. These side effects may go away during treatment as your body adjusts to the medicine. However, check with your doctor if any of the following side effects continue or are bothersome:

More common
  Dizziness or lightheadedness
  Loss of appetite
  Nausea

Less common
  Blurred vision
  Confusion
  Headache
  Nervousness
  Numbness or tingling of fingers and toes
  Skin rash
  Sweating
  Vomiting

Dizziness or lightheadedness is more likely to occur in the elderly, who are usually more sensitive to the effects of tocainide.

Other side effects not listed above may also occur in some patients. If you notice any other effects, check with your doctor.

TRAZODONE (Systemic)
A commonly used brand name is Desyrel.

Trazodone (TRAZ-oh-done) belongs to the group of medicines known as antidepressants or "mood elevators." It is taken by mouth to relieve mental depression and depression that sometimes occurs with anxiety.

Trazodone is available only with your doctor's prescription.

Before Using This Medicine

In order to decide on the best treatment for your medical problem, your doctor should be told:

—if you have ever had any unusual or allergic reaction to trazodone.

—if you are on a low-salt, low-sugar, or any other special diet, or if you are allergic to any substance, such as sulfites or other preservatives or dyes. Most medicines contain more than their active ingredient. Your doctor or pharmacist can help you avoid products that may cause a problem.

—if you are pregnant or if you intend to become pregnant while using this medicine. Studies have not been done in humans. However, studies in animals have shown that trazodone causes birth defects and fetal death when given in doses up to 50 times the largest recommended human dose.

—if you are breast-feeding an infant. Although it is not known whether trazodone passes into breast milk and this medicine has not been shown to cause problems in humans, the chance always exists. Trazodone has been found in the milk of test animals.

—if you have any of the following medical problems:

   Alcoholism
   Heart disease
   Kidney disease
   Liver disease

—if you are now taking high blood pressure medicine, such as:

   Clonidine
   Guanabenz
   Methyldopa
   Metyrosine
   Pargyline
   Rauwolfia alkaloids

—if you are now taking other central nervous system (CNS) depressants, such as:

   Anticonvulsants (seizure medicine)
   Antihistamines or medicine for hay fever, other allergies, or colds
   Barbiturates
   Muscle relaxants
   Narcotics
   Prescription pain medicine
   Sedatives, tranquilizers, or sleeping medicine

Proper Use of This Medicine

To lessen stomach upset, take this medicine with food, even for a daily bedtime dose, unless your doctor has told you to take it on an empty stomach.

Take trazodone only as directed by your doctor, to benefit your condition as much as possible.

Sometimes trazodone must be taken for up to 4 weeks before you begin to feel better, although most people notice improvement within 2 weeks.

If you miss a dose of this medicine, take it as soon as possible. However, if it is within 4 hours of your next dose, skip the missed dose and go back to your regular dosing schedule. Do not double doses.

How to store this medicine:

• Store away from heat and direct light.

• **Keep out of the reach of children.**

• Do not store in the bathroom medicine cabinet because the heat or moisture may cause the medicine to break down.

• Do not keep outdated medicine or medicine no longer needed. Flush the contents of the container down the toilet, unless otherwise directed.

Precautions While Using This Medicine

It is very important that your doctor check your progress at regular visits. This will allow your doctor to check the medicine's effects and to change the dose if needed.

Do not stop taking this medicine without first checking with your doctor. Your doctor may want you to reduce gradually the amount you are using before stopping completely, in order to prevent a possible return of your medical problem.

Before having any kind of surgery (including dental surgery) or emergency treatment, tell the doctor or dentist in charge that you are using this medicine.

This medicine will add to the effects of alcohol and other CNS depressants (medicines that slow down the nervous system, possibly causing drowsiness). Some examples of CNS depressants are antihistamines or medicine for hay fever, other allergies, or colds; sedatives, tranquilizers, or sleeping medicine; prescription pain medicine or narcotics; barbiturates; medicine for seizures; muscle relaxants; or anesthetics, including some dental anesthetics. **Check with your doctor before taking any of the above while you are using this medicine.**

This medicine may cause some people to become drowsy or less alert than they are normally. **Make sure you know how you react to this medicine before you drive, use machines, or do other jobs that require you to be alert.**

Dizziness, lightheadedness, or fainting may occur, especially when you get up from a lying or sitting position. Getting up slowly may help. If this problem continues or gets worse, check with your doctor.

Your mouth may feel very dry while you are taking trazodone. To keep your mouth comfortably moist, chew sugarless gum, melt bits of ice in your mouth, or use a saliva substitute as often as necessary.

Side Effects of This Medicine

Along with its needed effects, a medicine may cause some unwanted effects. Although not all of these side effects appear very often, when they do occur they may require medical attention. **Stop taking this medicine and check with your doctor immediately** if the following side effect occurs:

Rare
Prolonged, painful, inappropriate penile erection

Also, check with your doctor as soon as possible if any of the following side effects occur:

Less common
Confusion
Muscle tremors

Rare
Skin rash
Unusually fast or slow heartbeat

Other side effects may occur which usually do not require medical attention. These side effects may go away during treatment as your body adjusts to the medicine. However, check with your doctor if any of the following side effects continue or are bothersome:

More common
Blurred vision
Dizziness or lightheadedness
Drowsiness
Dry mouth
Headache
Nausea and vomiting

Less common
Constipation
Diarrhea
Muscle aches or pains
Unusual tiredness or weakness

The above side effects, especially drowsiness, dizziness, confusion, vision problems, dry mouth, and constipation, are more likely to occur in elderly patients, who are usually more sensitive to the effects of trazodone.

Other side effects not listed above may also occur in some patients. If you notice any other effects, check with your doctor.

TRIMETHOBENZAMIDE
(Systemic)

Some commonly used brand names are:

Tegamide	Tigan
Ticon	Tiject-20

Trimethobenzamide (trye-meth-oh-BEN-za-mide) is a medicine used to treat nausea and vomiting.

Trimethobenzamide is available only with your doctor's prescription.

Before Using This Medicine

In order to decide on the best treatment for your medical problem, your doctor should be told:

—if you have ever had any unusual or allergic reaction to trimethobenzamide.

—if you are allergic or sensitive to benzocaine or other local anesthetics (the suppository form of this medicine contains benzocaine), or if you are allergic to any substance, such as sulfites or other preservatives or dyes. Most medicines contain more than their active ingredient. Your doctor or pharmacist can help you avoid products that may cause a problem.

—if you are pregnant or if you intend to become pregnant while using this medicine. Studies have not been done in humans. However, although studies in animals have not shown that trimethobenzamide causes birth defects, it has been shown to increase the chance of a miscarriage.

—if you are breast-feeding an infant. Although trimethobenzamide has not been shown to cause problems in humans, the chance always exists.

—if you have either of the following medical problems:

High fever
Intestinal infection

—if you are now taking any other medicine, especially the following medicines or types of medicine:

Aspirin or other salicylates
Cisplatin
Clonidine
Guanabenz
Methyldopa
Metyrosine
Paromomycin
Vancomycin

—if you are now taking any central nervous system (CNS) depressants, such as:

Anticonvulsants (seizure medicine)
Antihistamines or medicine for hay fever, other allergies, or colds
Barbiturates
Narcotics
Phenothiazines
Prescription pain medicine
Sedatives, tranquilizers, or sleeping medicine

—if you are now taking tricyclic antidepressants (medicine for depression), such as:

Amitriptyline
Amoxapine
Clomipramine
Desipramine
Doxepin
Imipramine
Nortriptyline
Protriptyline
Trimipramine

Proper Use of This Medicine

Do not use this medicine to treat nausea and vomiting in children unless otherwise directed by your doctor. If you are giving this medicine to a child, be especially careful not to give more than is prescribed since side effects may be more serious in children.

Trimethobenzamide is used only to relieve or prevent nausea and vomiting. Use it only as directed. Do not use more of it and do not use it more often than your doctor ordered. To do so may increase the chance of side effects.

For patients using the rectal suppository dosage form of this medicine:

- How to insert suppository: First, remove foil wrapper and moisten the suppository with water. Lie down on side and push the suppository well up into the rectum with finger. If the suppository is too soft to insert because of storage in a warm place, before removing the foil wrapper chill the suppository in the refrigerator for 30 minutes or run cold water over it.

If you must use this medicine regularly and you miss a dose, use it as soon as possible. However, if it is almost time for your next dose, skip the missed dose and go back to your regular dosing schedule. Do not double doses.

How to store this medicine:

- Store away from heat and direct light.
- **Keep out of the reach of children.**
- Do not store in the bathroom medicine cabinet because the heat or moisture may cause the medicine to break down.
- Do not keep outdated medicine or medicine no longer needed. Flush the contents of the container down the toilet, unless otherwise directed.

Precautions While Using This Medicine

Trimethobenzamide will add to the effects of alcohol and other CNS depressants (medicines that slow down the nervous system, possibly causing drowsiness). Some examples of CNS depressants are antihistamines or medicine for hay fever, other allergies, or colds; sedatives, tranquilizers, or sleeping medicine; prescription pain medicine or narcotics; barbiturates; medicine for seizures; muscle relaxants; or anesthetics, including some dental anesthetics. **Check with your doctor before taking any of the above while you are using this medicine.**

This medicine may cause some people to become dizzy, lightheaded, drowsy, or less alert than they are normally. **Make sure you know how you react to this medicine before you drive, use machines, or do other jobs that require you to be alert.**

When using trimethobenzamide on a regular basis, make sure your doctor knows if you are taking large amounts of aspirin at the same time (as in arthritis or rheumatism). Effects of too much aspirin, such as ringing in the ears, may be covered up by this medicine.

Side Effects of This Medicine

Along with its needed effects, a medicine may cause some unwanted effects. Although not all of these side effects appear very often, when they do occur they may require medical attention. Check with your doctor as soon as possible if any of the following side effects occur:

Rare
 Back pain
 Convulsions (seizures)
 Mental depression
 Shakiness or tremors
 Sore throat and fever
 Unusual feeling of tiredness
 Vomiting (severe or continuing)
 Yellowing of eyes and skin

Other side effects may occur which usually do not require medical attention. These side effects may go away during treatment as your body adjusts to the medicine. However, check with your doctor if any of the following side effects continue or are bothersome:

More common
 Drowsiness

Less common
 Blurred vision
 Diarrhea
 Dizziness
 Headache
 Muscle cramps

Other side effects not listed above may also occur in some patients. If you notice any other effects, check with your doctor.

XANTHINE-DERIVATIVE BRONCHODILATORS (Systemic)

This information applies to the following medicines:

Aminophylline (am-in-OFF-i-lin)
Dyphylline (DYE-fi-lin)
Oxtriphylline (ox-TRYE-fi-lin)
Theophylline (thee-OFF-i-lin)

Some commonly used brand names are:	Generic names:
Aminophyllin	
Amoline	
Corophyllin*	
Lixaminol	
Palaron*	Aminophylline†
Phyllocontin	
Somophyllin	
Somophyllin-DF	
Truphylline	

Asminyl	
Dilin	
Dilor	
Droxine	
Droxine L.A.	
Droxine S.F.	
Dyflex	Dyphylline†
Dylline	
Dy-Phyl-Lin	
Lufyllin	
Neothylline	
Oxystat	
Protophylline*	

Apo-Oxtriphylline*	
Choledyl	
Choledyl SA	Oxtriphylline†
Novotriphyl*	

Accurbron	
Aerolate	
Aquaphyllin	Theophylline†
Asmalix	
Bronkodyl	

Bronkodyl S-R	
Constant-T	
Duraphyl	
Elixicon	
Elixomin	
Elixophyllin	
Elixophyllin SR	
LaBID	
Lanophyllin	
Liquophylline	
Lixolin	
Lodrane	
PMS Theophylline*	
Pulmophylline*	
Quibron-T Dividose	
Quibron-T/SR Dividose	
Respbid	
Slo-bid Gyrocaps	
Slo-Phyllin	
Slo-Phyllin Gyrocaps	
Somophyllin-12*	
Somophyllin-CRT	Theophylline†
Somophyllin-T	
Sustaire	
Theo-24	
Theobid Duracaps	
Theobid Jr. Duracaps	
Theobron SR	
Theoclear	
Theoclear L.A. Cenules	
Theo-Dur	
Theo-Dur Sprinkle	
Theolair	
Theolair-SR	
Theo-Lix	
Theolixir	
Theon	
Theophyl	
Theophyl-SR	
Theospan SR	
Theostat	
Theo-Time	
Theovent	
Uniphyl	

Synophylate	Theophylline Sodium Glycinate

*Not available in the United States.
†Generic name product may also be available.

Xanthine-derivative bronchodilators are used to treat the symptoms of bronchial asthma, chronic bronchitis, and emphysema. These medicines relieve cough, wheezing, shortness of breath, and troubled breathing. They work by opening up the bronchial tubes or air passages of the lungs and increasing the flow of air through them.

Aminophylline and theophylline may also be used for other conditions as determined by your doctor.

Xanthine-derivative bronchodilators are taken by mouth, given by injection, or used rectally. The oral liquid, uncoated or chewable tablet, capsule, and rectal enema dosage forms may be used for treatment of the acute attack and for chronic (long-term) treatment. If rectal enemas are used, they should not be used for longer than 48 hours because they may cause rectal irritation. The enteric-coated tablet and extended-release dosage forms are usually used only for chronic treatment. Sometimes, aminophylline rectal suppositories may be used but they generally are not recommended because of poor absorption.

These medicines are available only with your doctor's prescription.

Before Using This Medicine

In order to decide on the best treatment for your medical problem, your doctor should be told:

—if you have ever had any unusual or allergic reaction to aminophylline, caffeine, dyphylline, ethylenediamine (contained in aminophylline), oxtriphylline, theobromine, or theophylline.

—if you are on a low-salt, low-sugar, or any other special diet, or if you are allergic to any substance, such as sulfites or other preservatives or dyes. Most medicines contain more than their active ingredient, and many liquid medicines contain alcohol. Your doctor or pharmacist can help you avoid products that may cause a problem.

—if you are pregnant or if you intend to become pregnant while using this medicine. Studies on birth defects have not been done in humans. However, some studies in animals have shown that theophylline (includes aminophylline and oxtriphylline) causes birth defects when given in doses many times the human dose. Also, use of aminophylline, oxtriphylline, or theophylline during pregnancy may cause unwanted effects such as unusually fast heartbeat, jitteriness, irritability, gagging, vomiting, and breathing problems in the newborn infant. Studies with dyphylline on birth defects have not been done in either humans or animals.

—if you are breast-feeding an infant. Theophylline passes into the breast milk and may cause irritability, fretfulness, or trouble in sleeping in infants of mothers taking either aminophylline, oxtriphylline, or theophylline. Although dyphylline has not been shown to cause problems in humans, the chance always exists since it passes into the breast milk.

—if you are using any of the xanthines and have any of the following medical problems:

Diarrhea
Enlarged prostate
Fibrocystic breast disease
Heart disease
Stomach ulcer (or history of) or other stomach problems

—if you are using aminophylline, oxtriphylline, or theophylline and have any of the following medical problems:

Fever
Liver disease
Overactive thyroid
Respiratory infections, such as influenza (flu)

—if you are using the aminophylline rectal enema and have irritation or infection of the rectum or lower colon.

—if you are using dyphylline and have kidney disease.

—if you are using any of the xanthines and are also taking any of the following medicines or types of medicine:

Acebutolol
Amantadine
Amphetamines
Appetite suppressants (diet pills)
Atenolol
Caffeine
Chlophedianol
Diarrhea medicine
Labetalol
Lithium
Methylphenidate
Metoprolol
Nadolol
Other medicine for asthma or breathing problems
Pemoline
Pindolol
Propranolol
Timolol

—if you are using any of the xanthines and are also taking any other prescription or nonprescription medicines, especially medicines for colds or allergies.

—if you are using aminophylline, oxtriphylline, or theophylline and are also taking any of the following medicines or types of medicine:

Allopurinol
Barbiturates
Carbamazepine
Cimetidine
Erythromycin
Nicotine chewing gum or other medicine to help you stop smoking
Phenytoin
Primidone
Rifampin
Troleandomycin

—if you are using aminophylline, oxtriphylline, or theophylline and:

• you are also going to receive an influenza (flu) vaccine.
• you also smoke or have smoked (tobacco or marijuana) regularly within the last 2 years. The amount of medicine you need may vary, depending on how much and how recently you have smoked.

• you are also on a low-protein, high-carbohydrate or high-protein, low-carbohydrate diet.

—if you are using dyphylline and are also taking probenecid.

Proper Use of This Medicine

Use this medicine only as directed by your doctor. Do not use more of it, do not use it more often, and do not use it for a longer period of time than your doctor ordered. To do so may increase the chance of serious side effects.

In order for this medicine to help your medical problem, it must be taken every day in regularly spaced doses as ordered by your doctor. This is necessary to keep a constant amount of this medicine in the blood. To help keep this amount constant, do not miss any doses.

If you do miss a dose of this medicine, take it as soon as possible. However, if it is almost time for your next dose, skip the missed dose and go back to your regular dosing schedule. Do not double doses.

For patients taking this medicine by mouth:

• If you are taking the capsule, tablet, liquid, or extended-release (not including the once-a-day capsule or tablet) form of this medicine, **it works best when taken with a glass of water on an empty stomach** (either 30 minutes to 1 hour before meals or 2 hours after meals). That way the medicine will get into the blood sooner. However, in some cases your doctor may want you to take this medicine with meals or right after meals to lessen stomach upset. If you have any questions about how you should be taking this medicine, check with your doctor.

• If you are taking the once-a-day capsule or tablet form of this medicine, **take one dose each morning after fasting**

overnight and about 2 hours before eating. Try to take the medicine about the
same time each day.

• There are several different forms of
xanthines capsules and tablets. If you
are taking:

—chewable tablets, chew the tablets before swallowing.

—enteric-coated tablets, swallow the
tablets whole. Do not crush, break, or
chew before swallowing.

—extended-release capsules, swallow
the capsule whole. Do not crush, break,
or chew before swallowing.

—extended-release tablets, swallow the
tablets whole. Do not break (unless tablet is scored for breaking), crush, or
chew before swallowing.

For patients using the aminophylline
enema:

• This medicine usually comes with patient directions. Read them carefully before using this medicine.

• If crystals form in the solution, dissolve
them by placing the closed container of
solution in warm water. If the crystals do
not dissolve, do not use the medicine.

How to store this medicine:

• Store away from heat and direct light.

• **Keep out of the reach of children.**

• Do not store in the bathroom medicine
cabinet because the heat or moisture
may cause the medicine to break down.

• Keep the liquid form of this medicine
from freezing.

• Do not keep outdated medicine or medicine no longer needed. Flush the capsule, tablet, or liquid form of this medicine down the toilet, unless otherwise directed.

Precautions While Using This Medicine

Your doctor should check your progress at
regular visits, especially for the first few
weeks after you begin using this medicine. A blood test may be taken to help
your doctor decide whether the dose of
this medicine should be changed.

**Do not change brands or dosage forms of
this medicine without first checking with
your doctor.** Different products may not
work the same way. If you refill your
medicine and it looks different, check
with your pharmacist.

This medicine may add to the central nervous system stimulant effects of caffeine-containing foods or beverages
such as chocolate, cocoa, tea, coffee,
and cola drinks. **Avoid eating or drinking
large amounts of these foods or beverages while using this medicine.** If you
have any questions about this, check
with your doctor.

For patients using aminophylline, oxtriphylline, or theophylline:

• Do not eat charcoal-broiled foods every
day while using this medicine since
these foods may keep the medicine from
working as well.

• **Check with your doctor at once if you
develop symptoms of influenza (flu) or a
fever** since either of these may increase
the chance of side effects with this
medicine.

• Also, **check with your doctor if diarrhea
occurs** because the dose of this medicine
may need to be changed.

For patients using the aminophylline
enema:

• If burning or other irritation of the
rectal area occurs after you use this
medicine and it continues or becomes
worse, check with your doctor.

Side Effects of This Medicine

Along with its needed effects, a medicine may cause some unwanted effects. Although not all of these side effects appear very often, when they do occur they may require medical attention. Check with your doctor as soon as possible if any of the following side effects occur:

Less common

Heartburn and/or vomiting

Rare

Skin rash or hives (with aminophylline only)

Possible signs of overdose

Bloody or black tarry stools
Confusion or change in behavior
Convulsions (seizures)
Diarrhea
Dizziness or lightheadedness
Flushing or redness of face
Headache
Increased urination
Irritability
Loss of appetite
Muscle twitching
Nausea (continuing or severe) or vomiting
Stomach cramps or pain
Trembling
Trouble in sleeping
Unusually fast breathing
Unusually fast, pounding, or irregular heartbeat
Unusual tiredness or weakness
Vomiting blood or material that looks like coffee grounds

Other side effects may occur which usually do not require medical attention. These side effects may go away during treatment as your body adjusts to the medicine. However, check with your doctor if any of the following side effects continue or are bothersome:

More common

Nausea
Nervousness or restlessness

Less common

Burning or irritation of rectum (for rectal enema only)

The above side effects are more likely to occur in elderly patients and newborn infants, who are usually more sensitive to the effects of these medicines.

Other side effects not listed above may also occur in some patients. If you notice any other effects, check with your doctor.

Appendix I:
General Information About Use of Medicines

For your own safety, health, and well-being, it is important that you learn about the proper use of your medicines. The information that follows is general in nature and applies to the use of any medicine. This information must be supplemented with the drug-specific information which is found in the individual listings of this book.

It is a good idea for you to learn both the generic and brand names of your medicine and even to write them down and keep them for future use.

Many prescriptions may not be refilled unless your pharmacist has first checked with your doctor. To save time, do not wait until you have run out of medicine before requesting a refill. This is especially important if you must take your medicine every day.

If you want more information about your medicines, ask your doctor, nurse, or pharmacist. Do not be embarrassed to ask questions about any medicine you are taking. To help you remember, it may be helpful to write down any questions you have and bring these questions with you on your next visit to your doctor or pharmacist.

Before Using Your Medicine

Before you use any medicine, your doctor, nurse, and pharmacist should be told:

—if you have ever had an allergic or unusual reaction to any medicine, food, or other substance.

—if you are on a low-salt, low-sugar, or any other special diet, or if you are allergic to any substance, such as yellow dye or sulfites. Most medicines contain more than their active ingredient, and many liquid medicines contain alcohol.

—if you are pregnant or if you plan to become pregnant. Certain medicines may cause birth defects or other problems in the unborn child. For other medicines, safe use during pregnancy has not been established. The use of any medicine during pregnancy must be carefully considered.

—if you are breast-feeding a baby. Some medicines may pass into the breast milk and cause unwanted effects in the infant.

—if you have any medical problems.

—if you have taken any medicines in the past few weeks. Don't forget over-the-counter (nonprescription) medicines such as aspirin, laxatives, and antacids.

Proper Use of Your Medicine

Take any medicine exactly as directed, at the right time, and for the full length of time prescribed by your doctor. If you are using an over-the-counter (nonprescription) medicine, follow the directions on the label, unless otherwise directed by your doctor. If you feel that your medicine is not working for you, check with your doctor.

To avoid mistakes, do not take medicine in the dark. Always read the label before taking, noting especially the expiration date, if any, of the contents.

Child-proof caps on most prescription medicines for oral use are required by law. However, if there are no children in your home, and you find it hard to open such caps, you may ask your pharmacist for a regular, easier-to-open cap. He or she is authorized by law to furnish you with a regular cap if you request it.

Different medicines should never be mixed in one container. Always keep your medicine tightly capped in its original container, when not in use. Do not remove the label since directions for use and other special information appear there.

How to store your medicine:

• Store away from heat and direct sunlight.

• **Keep out of the reach of children.**

• Do not store in the bathroom medicine cabinet because the heat or moisture may cause the medicine to break down.

• Keep liquid medicines from freezing.

• Do not keep outdated medicine or medicine no longer needed. Flush the contents of the container down the toilet, unless otherwise directed.

Precautions While Using Your Medicine

Never give your medicine to anyone else. It has been prescribed for your personal medical problem and may not be the correct treatment for another person.

Before having any kind of surgery (including dental surgery) or emergency treatment, tell the physician or dentist in charge about any medicine you are taking.

If you think you have taken an overdose of any medicine or if a child has taken a medicine by accident: Call your poison control center or your doctor or pharmacist, at once. Keep those telephone numbers handy. Also, keep a bottle of Ipecac Syrup safely stored in your home in case you are told to cause vomiting. Read the directions on the label of Ipecac Syrup before using.

Side Effects of Your Medicine

Along with its needed effects, a medicine may cause some unwanted effects. Some of these side effects may need medical attention, while others may not. It is important for you to know what side effects may occur and what you should do if you notice signs of them.

If you notice any other unusual reactions or side effects, check with your doctor, nurse, or pharmacist.

Appendix II
Members of the United States Pharmacopeial Convention and the Institutions and Organizations Represented

Howard University, College of Medicine: Robert E. Taylor, M.D., Ph.D.
Howard University, College of Pharmacy & Pharmacal Sciences: Wendell T. Hill, Jr., Pharm.D.
Medical Society of the District of Columbia: Michael D. Abramowitz, M.D.

FLORIDA

Florida A & M University, College of Pharmacy and Pharmaceutical Sciences: Henry Lewis, III, Pharm.D.
University of Florida, College of Medicine: Thomas F. Muther, Ph.D.
University of Florida, College of Pharmacy: Michael A. Schwartz, Ph.D.
University of South Florida, College of Medicine: Joseph J. Krzanowski, Jr., Ph.D.
Florida Pharmacy Association: George Browning

GEORGIA

Medical College of Georgia, School of Medicine: Merle W. Riley, Ph.D.
Mercer University, Southern School of Pharmacy: A. Vincent Lopez, Ph.D.
Morehouse School of Medicine: Ralph W. Trottier, Ph.D.
University of Georgia, College of Pharmacy: Howard C. Ansel, Ph.D.
Georgia Pharmaceutical Association: Charles L. Braucher, Ph.D.
Medical Association of Georgia: E.D. Bransome, Jr., M.D.

IDAHO

Idaho State University, College of Pharmacy: Eugene I. Isaacson, Ph.D.

ILLINOIS

Chicago Medical School/University of Health Sciences: Seymour Ehrenpreis, Ph.D.
Southern Illinois University, School of Medicine: Ronald A. Browning, Ph.D.
University of Illinois, College of Medicine: Marten M. Kernis, Ph.D.
University of Illinois, College of Pharmacy: Martin I. Blake, Ph.D.
Illinois Pharmacists Association: Ronald W. Gottrich
Illinois State Medical Society: Vincent A. Costanzo, Jr., M.D.

INDIANA

Butler University, College of Pharmacy: Margaret A. Shaw, Ph.D.
Indiana University, School of Medicine: George R. Aronoff, M.D.
Purdue University, School of Pharmacy and Pharmacal Sciences: Adelbert M. Knevel, Ph.D.

IOWA

Drake University, College of Pharmacy: Wendell Southard, Ph.D.
University of Iowa, College of Pharmacy: Robert A. Wiley, Ph.D.
Iowa Pharmacists Association: Robert Osterhaus

KANSAS

University of Kansas, School of Medicine: Edward J. Walaszek, Ph.D.
University of Kansas, School of Pharmacy: Siegfried Lindenbaum, Ph.D.
Kansas Pharmacists Association: John Owen

KENTUCKY

University of Kentucky, College of Pharmacy: Patrick P. DeLuca, Ph.D.
University of Louisville, School of Medicine: Peter P. Rowell, Ph.D.

Kentucky Medical Association: Ellsworth C. Seeley, M.D.
Kentucky Pharmacists Association: Chester L. Parker, Pharm.D.

LOUISIANA

Northeast Louisiana University, School of Pharmacy: Robert D. Kee, Ph.D.
Tulane University, School of Medicine: Floyd R. Domer, Ph.D.
Xavier University of Louisiana, College of Pharmacy: Josephine Daigle, Ph.D.
Louisiana Pharmacists Association: William G. Day
Louisiana State Medical Society: John Adriani, M.D.

MARYLAND

Johns Hopkins University, School of Medicine: E. Robert Feroli, Pharm.D.
University of Maryland, School of Medicine: James I. Hudson, M.D.
University of Maryland, School of Pharmacy: Larry L. Augsburger, Ph.D.
Maryland Pharmaceutical Association: Paul Freiman

MASSACHUSETTS

Boston University, School of Medicine: Edward W. Pelikan, M.D.
Massachusetts College of Pharmacy & Allied Health Sciences: William O. Foye, Ph.D.
Northeastern University, College of Pharmacy and Allied Health Professions: Larry N. Swanson, Pharm.D.
University of Massachusetts Medical School: Brian Johnson, M.D.
Massachusetts Medical Society: Edward J. Khantzian, M.D.
Massachusetts State Pharmaceutical Association: Bertram A. Nicholas, M.Sc.

MICHIGAN

Ferris State College, School of Pharmacy: Gerald W. A. Slywka, Ph.D.
University of Michigan, College of Pharmacy: Ara G. Paul, Ph.D.
Wayne State University, School of Medicine: Ralph E. Kauffman, M.D.
Michigan Pharmacists Association: Salvador Pancorbo, Ph.D., Pharm.D.

MINNESOTA

University of Minnesota, College of Pharmacy: Edward G. Rippie, Ph.D.
University of Minnesota Medical School, Minneapolis: Jack W. Miller, Ph.D.
Minnesota State Pharmaceutical Association: Arnold D. Delger

MISSISSIPPI

University of Mississippi, School of Medicine: Richard L. Klein, Ph.D.
University of Mississippi, School of Pharmacy: Robert W. Cleary, Ph.D.
Mississippi Pharmacists Association: Phylliss M. Moret

MISSOURI

St. Louis College of Pharmacy: John W. Zuzack, Ph.D.
St. Louis University, School of Medicine: Alvin H. Gold, Ph.D.
University of Missouri, Columbia, School of Medicine: John W. Yarbro, M.D., Ph.D.
University of Missouri, Kansas City, School of Medicine: David Rush, Ph.D.
University of Missouri, Kansas City, School of Pharmacy: Wayne M. Brown, Ph.D.
Washington University, School of Medicine: H. Mitchell Perry, Jr., M.D.
Missouri Pharmaceutical Association: James R. Boyd

MONTANA

Montana State Pharmaceutical Association: Robert H. Likewise

NEBRASKA

Creighton University, School of Medicine: Michael C. Makoid, Ph.D.

University of Nebraska, College of Medicine: Manuchair Ebadi, Ph.D.

University of Nebraska, College of Pharmacy: David Newton, Ph.D.

Nebraska Pharmacists Association: Rex C. Higley, R.P.

NEVADA

University of Nevada, Reno, School of Medicine: Iain L.O. Buxton, D.Ph.

NEW HAMPSHIRE

Dartmouth Medical School: James J. Kresel, Ph.D.

New Hampshire Pharmaceutical Association: William J. Lancaster

NEW JERSEY

University of Medicine and Dentistry of New Jersey, New Jersey Medical School: Sheldon B. Gertner, Ph.D.

Rutgers University, College of Pharmacy: Thomas Medwick, Ph.D.

New Jersey Pharmaceutical Association: Stephen J. Csubak, Ph.D.

NEW MEXICO

University of New Mexico, College of Pharmacy: Carman A. Bliss, Ph.D.

New Mexico Pharmaceutical Association: Hugh Kabat, Ph.D.

NEW YORK

Albert Einstein College of Medicine of Yeshiva University: Dr. Walter G. Levine

City University of New York, Mt. Sinai School of Medicine: Joel S. Mindel, M.D., Ph.D.

Columbia University College of Physicians and Surgeons: Norman Kahn, M.D.

Cornell University Medical College: W. Y. Chan, Ph.D.

Long Island University, Arnold and Marie Schwartz College of Pharmacy and Health Sciences: John J. Sciarra, Ph.D.

New York Medical College: Mario A. Inchiosa, Jr., Ph.D.

State University of New York, Buffalo, School of Medicine: Robert J. McIsaac, Ph.D.

St. John's University, College of Pharmacy and Allied Health Professions: Andrew J. Bartilucci, Ph.D.

Union University, Albany College of Pharmacy: Barry S. Reiss, Ph.D.

University of Rochester, School of Medicine and Dentistry: Michael Weintraub, M.D.

Medical Society of the State of New York: Arthur Hull Hayes, Jr., M.D.

NORTH CAROLINA

Bowman Gray School of Medicine, Wake Forest University: Jack W. Strandhoy, Ph.D.

Duke University, School of Medicine: William J. Murray, M.D.

University of North Carolina, Chapel Hill, School of Medicine: Tai-Chan Peng, M.D.

University of North Carolina, Chapel Hill, School of Pharmacy: Richard J. Kowalsky, Pharm.D.

North Carolina Pharmaceutical Association: George H. Cocolas, Ph.D.

NORTH DAKOTA

North Dakota State University, College of Pharmacy: William M. Henderson, Ph.D.

North Dakota Pharmaceutical Association: William H. Shelver, Ph.D.

OHIO

Case Western Reserve University, School of Medicine: Kenneth A. Scott, Ph.D.

Medical College of Ohio: Robert D. Wilkerson, Ph.D.

Ohio Northern University, College of Pharmacy and Allied Health Sciences: LeRoy D. Beltz, Ph.D.

Ohio State University, College of Pharmacy: Michael C. Gerald, Ph.D.

University of Cincinnati, College of Medicine: Leonard T. Sigell, Ph.D.

University of Cincinnati, College of Pharmacy: Henry S. I. Tan, Ph.D.

University of Toledo, College of Pharmacy: Norman F. Billups, Ph.D.

Wright State University, School of Medicine: John O. Lindower, M.D., Ph.D.

Ohio State Medical Association: Ray W. Gifford, Jr., M.D.

Ohio State Pharmaceutical Association: J. Richard Wuest, Pharm.D.

OKLAHOMA

Oral Roberts University, School of Medicine: Jimmie L. Valentine, Ph.D.

Southwestern Oklahoma State University, School of Pharmacy: William G. Waggoner, Ph.D.

University of Oklahoma, College of Pharmacy: Loyd V. Allen, Jr., Ph.D.

Oklahoma Pharmaceutical Association: Carl D. Lyons

Oklahoma State Medical Association: Clinton Nicholas Corder, M.D., Ph.D.

OREGON

Oregon Health Sciences University, School of Medicine: Hall Downes, M.D., Ph.D.

Oregon Medical Association: Richard E. Lahti, M.D.

Oregon State Pharmaceutical Association: Mrs. Hallie L. Lahti

PENNSYLVANIA

Duquesne University, School of Pharmacy: Lawrence H. Block, Ph.D.

Medical College of Pennsylvania: Athole G. McNeil Jacobi, M.D.

Pennsylvania State University, College of Medicine: John D. Connor, Ph.D.

Philadelphia College of Pharmacy and Science: Alfonso R. Gennaro, Ph.D.

Temple University, School of Medicine: Charles A. Papacostas, Ph.D.

Temple University, School of Pharmacy: Murray Tuckerman, Ph.D.

Thomas Jefferson University, Jefferson Medical College: C. Paul Bianchi, Ph.D.

University of Pittsburgh, School of Medicine: Robert H. McDonald, Jr., M.D.

Pennsylvania Medical Society: Benjamin Calesnick, M.D.

Pennsylvania Pharmaceutical Association: Joseph A. Mosso

RHODE ISLAND

Brown University Program in Medicine: Michael C. Wiemann, M.D.

University of Rhode Island, College of Pharmacy: Christopher Rhodes, Ph.D.

SOUTH CAROLINA

Medical University of South Carolina, College of Pharmacy: Paul J. Niebergall, Ph.D.

University of South Carolina, College of Pharmacy: Robert L. Beamer, Ph.D.

Index

Brand names are in italics. There are many brands and different manufacturers of drugs and the listing of selected American and Canadian brand names and manufacturers is intended only for ease of reference. There are additional brands and manufacturers that have not been included. Asterisks indicate brands or drugs that are not available in the United States. The inclusion of a brand name does not mean the USPC has any particular knowledge that the brand listed has properties different from other brands of the same drug, nor should it be interpreted as an endorsement by the USPC. Similarly, the fact that a particular brand has not been included does not indicate that the product has been judged to be unsatisfactory or unacceptable.

Keep up to date on your medicines and health with USPC publications!

Just complete this coupon and return with payment to:
USPC, Inc., Order Processing Dept. 449
12601 Twinbrook Parkway, Rockville, MD 20852
Telephone: (301) 881-0666

FULL MONEY BACK GUARANTEE: If For Any Reason You Are Not Satisfied After Receipt Of Publication (s) Below, You May Return Purchase Within 30 Days For Full Refund.

☐ Subscription to *Advice for the Patient*® (*1986 USP DI*, Volume II), along with its *Updates*: $23.95.

☐ *About Your High Blood Pressure Medicines:* $6.95.

☐ Please send me literature on USPC's publications.

All orders must be paid in advance in U.S. dollars. Shipping costs for U.S. and Canadian orders are included in the price. Inquire for foreign order shipping charges.

☐ Enclosed is my check payable to USPC for $_____ .
   (Maryland residents add 5% sales tax.)

☐ Charge my: ☐ MasterCard ☐ Visa (Credit card orders must total $20.00 or more.)

Acct. No. _____ Exp. Date _____

Signature _____

Name _____ Title _____

Organization _____

Address _____

City, State, Zip _____

Telephone (   ) _____

Please allow 4-6 weeks for delivery. Prices subject to change without notice.